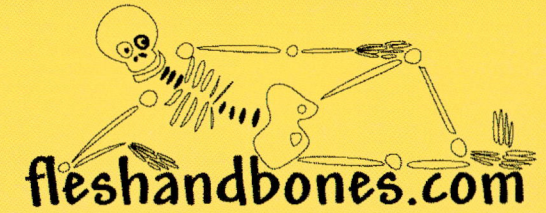

Paediatrics

Includes section on
Paediatrics in the Developing World

INTERNATIONAL EDITION · INTERNATIONAL EDITION

Commissioning Editor: Ellen Green
Project Development Manager: Jim Killgore
Designer: Sarah Russell
Project Manager: Frances Affleck

Paediatrics

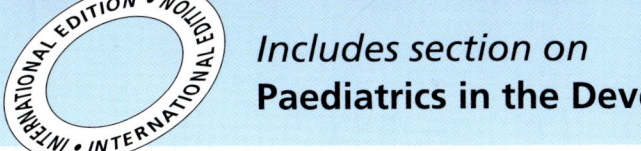

Includes section on
Paediatrics in the Developing World

Edited by

D.J. Field
MBBS(Hons) DCH FRCP FRCP(Ed) FRCPCH DM

Professor of Neonatal Medicine, University of Leicester,
Honorary Consultant Neonatologist,
Leicester Royal Infirmary, Leicester

J. Stroobant
MBBS FRCP FRCPCH MRCGP DCH DRCOG

Consultant Paediatrician,
The Children's Hospital, Lewisham,
London

Contributors

Sissay Amberber MD
Consultant Paediatrician, Gondar College of Medical Science,
Gondar, Ethiopia

C. Daman Willems BM FRCP FRCPCH
Consultant Paediatrician,
The Children's Hospital, Lewisham, London

E. Carter MA(CANTAB) FRCP(UK) FRCPCH
Consultant Paediatrician,
Leicester Royal Infirmary, Leicester

F. Craig MB BS MRCP(UK) FRCPCH
Specialist Paediatric Registrar, North Middlesex Hospital,
London

Sirak Hailu MD
Consultant Paediatrician,
Gondar College of Medical Science,
Gondar, Ethiopia

E. Wren Hoskyns
BMed Sci BM BS MRCP FRCPCH

Consultant Paediatrician,
Leicester General Hospital, Leicester

P.N. Houtman MBBS MRCP FRCPCH BSc(Hons)
Consultant Paediatrician,
Children's Hospital, Leicester Royal Infirmary, Leicester

T. O'Sullivan MRCP DCH FRCPCH
Consultant Community Paediatrician,
Lewisham Primary Care Trust, London

Tesfaye Tessema MD
Consultant Paediatrician and Dean,
Gondar College of Medical Science, Gondar, Ethiopia

K. Wheeler MB BS MRCP FRCPCH
Consultant Paediatrician,
John Radcliffe Hospital, Headington, Oxford

Illustrated by Ethan Danielson

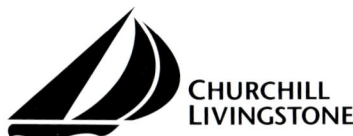

CHURCHILL LIVINGSTONE

EDINBURGH   LONDON   NEW YORK   PHILADELPHIA   ST LOUIS   SYDNEY   TORONTO   2002

CHURCHILL LIVINGSTONE
An imprint of Elsevier Science Limited

First published 1997
International edition first published 2002

ISBN 0443 05254 9
International edition ISBN 0443 071187

British Library Cataloguing in Publication Data
A catalogue record for this book is available from the British Library

Library of Congress Cataloging in Publication Data
A catalog record for this book is available from the Library of Congress

Note
Medical knowledge is constantly changing. As new information becomes
available, changes in treatment, procedures, equipment and the use of
drugs become necessary. The editors, contributors and the publishers have
taken care to ensure that the information given in this text is accurate and
up to date. However, readers are strongly advised to confirm that the
information, especially with regard to drug usage, complies with the
latest legislation and standards of practice.

The
publisher's
policy is to use
**paper manufactured
from sustainable forests**

Printed in China

PREFACE

We have tried in this book to give those that are new to paediatrics an insight into the subject. Each short chapter or 'learning unit' addresses a common problem in paediatric practice and discusses the conditions that may underlie that particular presentation. Emphasis has been placed on the underlying pathophysiology of symptoms and conditions so that the cause of a clinical problem is clear. This encourages a problem-solving approach to illness, based on a logical understanding of causation. The symptom-based approach has been used for the majority of the topics covered. However, one or two descriptive sections are included in order to 'set the scene'.

Similarly, some broad strategies of management are included and, where appropriate, the nature of health services for children has been discussed in general terms.

We hope that the book will be useful to all professional groups working with children; however, it has been written particularly with undergraduate medical students in mind.

The book is not intended to act as a comprehensive paediatric text. Our hope is to provide an easily understood and clinically related basis to the subject that will help direct students when they turn to more conventional (systems-based) texts.

1997   The Editors

PREFACE TO THE INTERNATIONAL EDITION

This edition of *Paediatrics: An illustrated colour text* has been developed with undergraduates training outside the developed world in mind. Additional sections have been added which are intended to widen the perspective of the book and provide greater emphasis to infectious disease and nutritional problems. Our international collaborators from Ethiopia and Dr Elaine Carter are largely responsible for these contributions.

2002   The Editors

ACKNOWLEDGEMENTS

The authors would like to acknowledge the following individuals who kindly provided illustrations for the book:

- Mr W Acclimandos, Consultant Ophthalmologist, Lewisham Hospital
- Dr Chen Chan, Consultant Paediatric Cardiologist, Glenfield Hospital
- Dr D Duckett, Department of Cytogenetics, Leicester Royal Infirmary
- Professor D Harvey, Professor of Paediatrics and Neonatal Medicine, Queen Charoltte's and Chelsea Hospital
- Dr D Lindsell, Consultant Radiologist, Churchill John Radcliffe Hospital
- Dr D McIver, Consultant Radiologist, Lewisham Hospital
- Mr A Monk, Cytogenetics Unit, City Hospital, Nottingham
- Dr A Rickett, Consultant Paediatric Radiologist, Leicester Royal Infirmary
- Dr G Stores, Senior Lecturer in Sleep Disorders, Park Hospital for Children, Oxford
- Dr R M Thomas, Consultant Paediatrician, Northwick Park Hospital
- Mr G Woodruff, Consultant Paediatric Ophthalmologist Leicester Royal Infirmary
- Dr J Vyas, Research Fellow, Department of Child Health, University of Leicester
- The Department of Medical Illustration, Leicester Royal Infirmary.
- Dr E Wraige, Dr A Lall and Mr W Thompson for the photograph used in the cover illustration.

CONTENTS

BASICS

CLINICAL EXAMINATION OF THE CHILD

Assessment of a medical or developmental problem in a child follows the same principles as for an adult: history, physical examination, and differential diagnosis based on an understanding of pathophysiology and clinical experience. The history is the most informative part of the assessment and much important information can be obtained from the parent or carer: it pays to listen carefully and allow the parents to explain their concerns and reasons for bringing the child for an assessment. Parents will accept an opinion from a clinician more readily if they feel that their own observations and concerns have been fully listened to. In most situations the child will not have a complex 'past medical history' and direct questioning in the history should concentrate on the likely abnormal areas rather than comprehensively covering all systems, unless the history suggests the need for detail. However, more information is essential to place the child in a family and social context as the appropriate management of any clinical problem must take account of the make-up of the family, who are the carers of the child (they may not be the child's parents), attitudes to illness within the family, and social circumstances which may influence the care of the child. See Table 1 for a check-list of essential points to be covered in history taking.

The process of taking the history, i.e. establishing a relationship with the parent, is not only important in itself but is an opportunity for the clinician to observe the child generally, and the relationship with the parent. Most importantly, it allows the

child to develop a trust of the stranger, reassured by the parent's own relaxed attitude.

PRINCIPLES OF THE INTERVIEW AND EXAMINATION

The most important points to bear in mind when examining children are listed below:

- Know the name and sex of the child.
- A relaxed, informal atmosphere with toys and a child-orientated setting are essential (Fig. 1).
- The age of the child determines the style of approach; the younger the child is the more cautious and gentle the process of examination.
- Examine children where they are most comfortable; young children will prefer to sit on their parent's knee or stand next to them. Older children will not mind lying on a couch.
- Talk to the child too, both to ask questions and to give explanations.
- Play with the child or say something amusing.
- Don't handle children roughly; leave the least pleasant part of the examination (e.g. ears or throat) until the end; tell them what you are going to do and be honest about any probable discomfort.
- Distraction is important either with a toy or by talking (Fig. 2).
- Examine opportunistically, respecting the child's modesty, undressing him/her in stages. It may not be possible to examine everything at the first attempt; know when to stop!

Table 1 **History check-list**

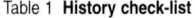

Main problem or complaint
Parents' specific anxieties
Other physical symptoms
Previous medical problems
Birth details
Growth
Developmental details and education
Feeding
Immunisations
Medication
Family composition and illnesses
Housing
Unusual stresses in family
Involvement of other health professionals, social
   services, etc.

- It is very useful to examine normal, healthy children, not only to gain familiarity with the process but to become confident in identifying the abnormal.

THE EXAMINATION

General impression
Before attempting to examine the relevant areas of the body, important information can be gathered by looking at the child generally first:

- shape of head
- unusual or characteristic facial features
- colour of skin: pink, blue, pale, yellow, mottled
- body proportions
- nutritional status
- similarity to parents
- obvious rashes
- body posture
- attitude and social interaction
- language
- play.

Hands
This is often a useful, non-threatening place to start the examination. Look for:

- shape
- extra digits
- abnormal digits
- colour
- clubbing
- nail abnormalities
- pallor
- rashes
- pulses.

Chest (to include the respiratory and cardiovascular systems)
Respiratory problems are the most common reason for children presenting to the clinician. It is also useful to examine this area early on as it does not require complete removal of clothing and the child may be cooperative before being disturbed by the continuing examination (Fig. 2).

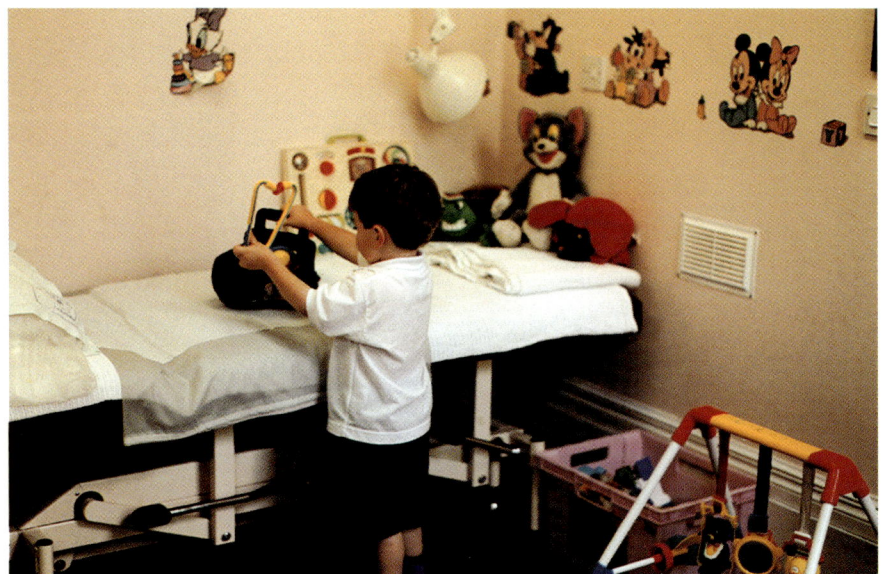

Fig. 1 **The interview setting.**

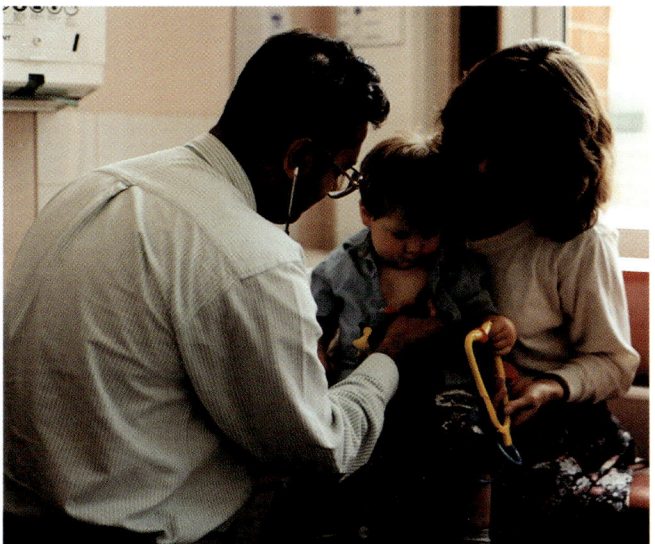

Fig. 2 **Chest examination.** Note how the child is being distracted by a toy stethoscope.

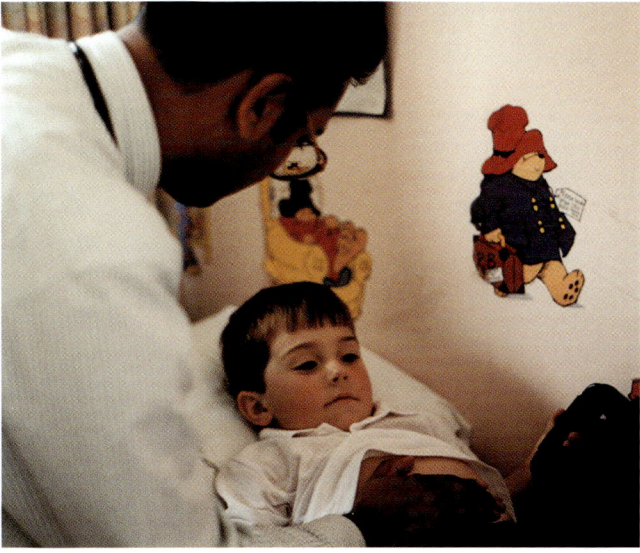

Fig. 3 **Examination of the abdomen.**

The main elements of chest examination are:

- Inspection:
  — shape
  — pattern and work of breathing
  — audible noises (cough, wheeze, stridor, grunting)
  — respiratory rate
  — chest movement — is it symmetrical?
- Palpation:
  — symmetry and expansion
  — trachea
  — transmitted sounds
  — thrills
  — apex beat.
- Percussion (rarely useful in infants and young children):
  — consolidation
  — pleural fluid.
- Auscultation:
  — breath sounds: crepitations (crackles), wheeze; ronchi (rattles), stridor
  — heart sounds
  — murmurs including site, loudness, character and length.

Abdomen

To be successful, examination of the abdomen (Fig. 3) must have the child quiet and relaxed; to persist with a crying, struggling child will aggravate the child, irritate the parents and will not reveal any abnormality. A young child or infant will be happier sitting or lying on the parent's knee; an older child will stand on the floor or lie on the examination couch. Clothing can be pushed out of the way without undressing the child or exposing all the areas of the abdomen completely. Look first; ask the child to point to any painful areas. The main elements are:

- Inspection:
  — swelling or localised lumps
  — distension
  — movement (abdominal wall and abdominal contents).
- Palpation: gently palpate the four quadrants first, determining areas of discomfort and obvious masses. Once the child is fully relaxed and cooperative, deeper palpation is possible, feeling specifically for the liver, spleen, kidneys, faeces, bladder or abnormal masses. It is unnecessary to examine the anus and rectum unless there is a specific indication. Most children will tolerate a rectal examination provided a full explanation is given beforehand.
- Percussion: may be useful to confirm the characteristics of palpated masses.
- Auscultation.

The genitalia can be examined at the end of the abdominal assessment if necessary but not routinely, particularly in girls. However, pubertal staging, testicular descent, hernias and vaginal discharge and discomfort, if present, will require assessment. Examination for sexual abuse is a specialised area and should be left to senior paediatricians.

CONCLUDING AN ASSESSMENT

The process of the clinical assessment as well as the direction of the questions asked should suggest a differential diagnosis. A management plan should then evolve. It is essential to allow parents the opportunity to ask questions about the assessment and to comment on and influence the management plan. They are usually excellent observers of their child's progress and of course will be responsible for carrying out any recommended treatment or advice. The success of any suggested management will depend on agreement and cooperation between them and a medical adviser; they must leave an assessment feeling that they have been fully involved in the process and that their concerns and questions have been satisfactorily and sensitively handled. It is useful to summarise the conclusions from the assessment and planned future management and to check with them that they have understood. It should be clear what future follow-up plans have been decided and from whom they should seek further advice.

Clinical examination of the child

- A comprehensive history will lead to likely diagnoses in most clinical situations; the examination serves to clarify the history's clues.
- Children should be examined opportunistically; a formal approach is unnecessary and often unsuccessful.
- Becoming familiar and comfortable with children is an important part of the experience of paediatric training.
- The parents or carers must be involved in discussing and planning the management of a child's health problem.

NEWBORN EXAMINATION I

When a baby is born, one of the parents' first concerns is that their baby is normal. In developed countries most deliveries occur in hospital. This provides an ideal opportunity to screen for a variety of diseases with good coverage of the population. This can be done by clinical examination or special tests. However, it is not necessarily the most appropriate time to identify disease. For instance, many neonates have transient murmurs as the ductus arteriosus is closing. This makes it difficult to screen for heart disease by auscultation alone. The other major objective of the newborn examination is to help parents with questions or problems they may perceive with their baby.

Babies with low birthweight or prematurity (Figs 1 & 2) are more likely to have difficulty coping with extrauterine life and these babies need special attention with early feeding, regular monitoring of the blood glucose and careful environmental control to keep the baby warm. Ideally, the baby should be kept in a thermo-neutral environment, defined as the ambient temperature at which energy expenditure is at a minimum. If the surroundings are too hot or too cold, the baby has to expend energy to maintain temperature.

HISTORY

Before examining a neonate, relevant information regarding the pregnancy and delivery should be obtained from the mother, midwives and nursery nurses. Other important facts should be available in the maternal notes and the charts of the care given to the baby since birth. A check-list for the

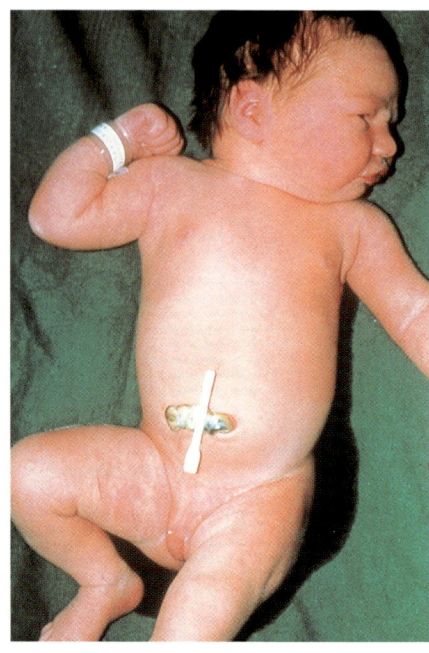

Fig.1 **Term baby.** The baby is 'chubby' (good sub-cutaneous fat), has good tone and is demonstrating the asymmetric tonic neck reflex (the fencer's position). There are prominent breast buds, the ears are normally formed and the skin colour is paler than a preterm baby.

areas to be covered is given in Table 1 and the relevance of major obstetric factors in Table 2.

EXAMINATION

There is considerable normal variation and there is no substitute for examining a number of newborn babies to gain an appreciation of the range of normality. Some normal parameters are given in Table 3. Always

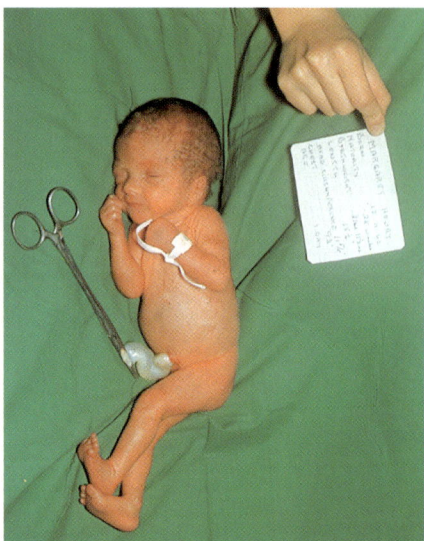

Fig. 2 **Preterm baby.** There is little subcutaneous fat and the legs are extended rather than flexed (an indication of reduced tone). The ears tend to be floppy because of reduced cartilage and the skin is thin and therefore looks red.

wash your hands before each neonatal examination. It is easiest when doing a neonatal examination to start at the top and work down (Table 4). However, it is worth listening to the chest and looking in the eyes with an ophthalmoscope at the beginning of the examination if the child is quiet. Pacifying a crying neonate is usually possible by putting a finger in his mouth and stimulating the sucking reflex or sitting the baby upright. Babies will also often open their eyes in this position.

Some of the more common abnormalities are shown on pages 6–7. It is unusual to pick up problems that the parents and nurs-

Table 1 **Check-list for neonatal 'history'**

Review maternal notes
- Previous children (gestation, birthweight, outcome)
- Family context (stable partner, employment, single parent)
- Family history of disease
- Consanguinity
- This pregnancy and labour (identified abnormalities or risk factors)

Ask mother and carers
- Identified problems or worries

Review baby's record chart
- Weight
- Feeding
- Urine
- Bowels
- Respiratory rate
- Temperature
- Blood glucose
- Bilirubin

Table 2 **Relevance of obstetric history**

Problem	Possible implication
Family	
Family history of inherited disease	Depends on mode of inheritance and which family member affected. Genetic advice may be necessary to assess risk. Screening tests may be possible on the baby
Consanguineous marriage	Increased risk of autosomal recessive disorders (particularly metabolic disease and mental retardation)
Pregnancy	
Twins/triplets	Risk of low birthweight, prematurity, birth asphyxia (particularly to last delivered)
Maternal diabetes	Risk of macrosomia, neonatal hypoglycaemia, respiratory distress and congenital malformation if control is poor
Infection	A number of infections in the mother may cause congenital infection in the baby (rubella, cytomegalovirus, chickenpox, etc.)
Abnormal investigations	Serious abnormalities can be identified on ultrasound (e.g. diaphragmatic hernia, heart disease, renal disease, spina bifida) or amniocentesis (chromosomal anomalies). Investigation and treatment can be prepared in advance of the delivery but at the cost of significant parental distress and ethical dilemmas
Delivery	
Shoulder dystocia	Fractured clavicle, Erb's palsy
Fetal scalp electrode	Scalp laceration
Long second stage of labour	Caput succedaneum formation
Difficult delivery	Cephalhaematoma, bruising
Breech delivery	Congenital dislocation of hip, bruising of buttocks, limb trauma

Table 3 **Normal newborn parameters**

Weight (kg)	2.5 – 4.0
Head circumference (cm)	33 – 37
Term pregnancy (weeks)	37 – 41
Haemoglobin (g/dl)	15 – 20
Time to first passing faeces and urine (h)	24
Usual amount of feed (ml/kg/day)	
Day 1	50
Day 2	75
Day 3	90
Day 4	120
Day 5	150

Table 4 **Check-list for neonatal examination**

Examine	Signs to look for	Comment
Colour	Cyanosis, plethora	Examine in good light — cyanosis is easy to miss
Cranium	Large/small head circumference	Hydrocephalus/ microcephaly
Face	Dysmorphism	Try to identify the specific abnormal features
Eyes	Red reflex	Use ophthalmoscope — red reflex is absent if cataract or retinal disease is present
Mouth	Cleft palate	Use little finger to feel the hard and soft palate
Neck	Sternomastoid 'tumour'	Head movement may be restricted
Pulses	Brachials and femorals	Absent femorals represent possibility of coarctation
Hands	Shape, creases, nails, accessory digits	
Chest	Shape, resp. rate, recession, auscultation	Heart murmurs (pp. 54–55)
Abdomen	Palpable masses	Liver is always palpable and kidneys usually
Umbilicus	Discharge, flare around	Suspect cord sepsis
Genitalia	Boys: testes	Cremasteric reflex may be very brisk
	Girls: labia and vaginal orifice.	
Anus	Check that it is present	Recto-vaginal fistula may allow the passage of meconium without an anus
Hips	Subluxation/dislocation	See page 98
Feet	Mobility	
Reflexes	Moro, grasp, sucking	
Tone	Posture during sleep	
	Posture on ventral suspension	

ing staff have not already noticed, except for hip abnormalities, murmurs and sometimes respiratory distress.

Congenital dislocation of the hip

Congenital dislocation of the hip (CDH), if detected early, can be treated by splinting alone. Those presenting in later childhood require major surgery (see p. 98).

Murmurs

Murmurs on their own are unlikely to be important but need follow-up until the murmur has gone or a diagnosis is made. Other cardiac signs (i.e. cyanosis, absent femoral pulses, respiratory distress or enlarged liver) require urgent investigation (see pp. 50–55).

Respiratory distress

Most babies known to be at risk of developing breathing problems (e.g. because of prematurity or meconium aspiration) are monitored on a neonatal unit, but there are occasional babies who are discovered at the neonatal examination to have respiratory distress. These infants need investigation for congenital lung problems (e.g. diaphragmatic hernia) and heart disease. They often receive antibiotics as respiratory difficulty may be the first sign of infection. This can be particularly serious when caused by a Lancefield group B, β-haemolytic streptococcus ('Group B strep').

SCREENING AND TREATMENT

Apart from the physical examination, blood testing for phenylketonuria and primary hypothyroidism is standard in the UK. In some districts, screening for cystic fibrosis (by measuring immunoreactive trypsin or identification of the CF gene) is also carried out, although the justification for this practice is controversial. Screening tests are dealt with in more detail on pages 14–15.

Vitamin K treatment is recommended for all neonates to protect against *haemorrhagic disease of the newborn*, which normally presents in the second week of life with generalised bleeding. It has a high

mortality and morbidity, particularly if there is intracranial bleeding. It is particularly common in breast-fed babies because breast milk delays the acquisition of gut bacteria which are the major source of 'dietary' vitamin K. Prophylactic treatment can be given orally or by i.m. injection. Although the i.m. route is more effective, it can be and has been fatally confused with syntometrine given to the mother at delivery.

SOCIAL PROBLEMS

The neonatal examination gives a chance for the paediatrician to assess the wider social situation in which the child will be brought up. In most developed countries, family size is small and many mothers have little experience of coping with their own or other babies. Whilst there may be a network of friends and relatives able to help and give advice, this role may be left to the health professionals. Some assessment of social circumstances is usually undertaken by midwives in the community prior to the delivery. However, new concerns regarding parenting skills may come to light after delivery but whilst the child is still in hospital. Occasionally, if the baby is felt to be at significant risk of neglect or harm, a case conference is called by social services to decide if any statutory action is necessary to protect the child.

ADVICE

It is best not to give much advice unless it is asked for by the parents or it comes up in the conversation. Gratuitous advice tends to be ignored and can undermine confidence.

There are numerous professionals who give advice (community and hospital midwives, breast feeding advisors, family doctors, health visitors, obstetricians, etc.) and it is often didactic and contradictory. At a time when parents often feel insecure anyway, such contradictory advice may make them very anxious. It is, therefore, important to support and encourage the parents to make their own minds up about how to look after their child. Most children do well whatever style of care they are given and there are very few instances in normal babies where the care is detrimental to health.

Breast feeding is dealt with on pages 36–37 and, although it has advantages over bottle feeding, it is usually too late to influence choice at the time of the neonatal examination.

Most parents of first babies will have a number of questions about child care that can be usefully answered. Parents with second children are likely to ask how the new baby will affect older children. In respect of siblings under 3 years old they can be told to expect a combination of affection for the new baby, jealousy and behaviour regression.

Newborn examination I

- Most abnormalities (except dislocation of the hips and murmurs) will have already been noticed.
- Listen and respond to the parents' worries.

NEWBORN EXAMINATION II

COMMON ABNORMALITIES

Some of the more common abnormalities found during neonatal examination are shown in Figures 1 and 2. Some need no treatment, just reassurance (e.g. cephal-haematoma, erythema neonatorum); others can be treated by the paediatrician (e.g. cord sepsis). But one of the main functions of the neonatal examination is to refer significant abnormalities on to the appropriate specialist (physiotherapist, orthopaedic, paediatric, ophthalmological surgeon, etc.).

Bilateral cephalhaematoma.

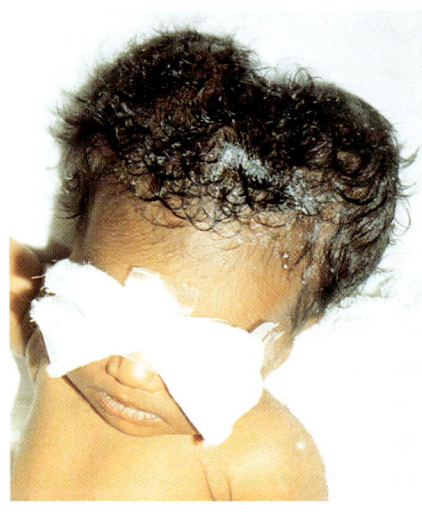

Congenital cataract.

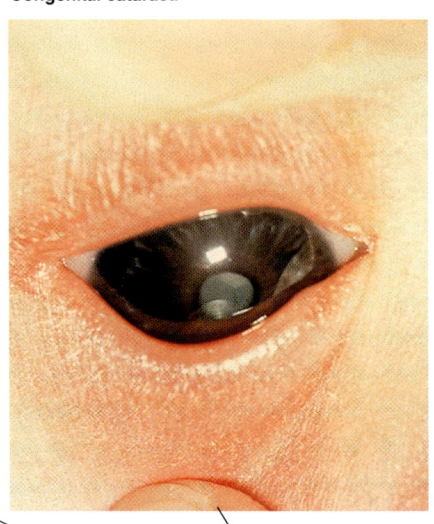

Milia. Normal crusting of pores, typically seen on the nose.

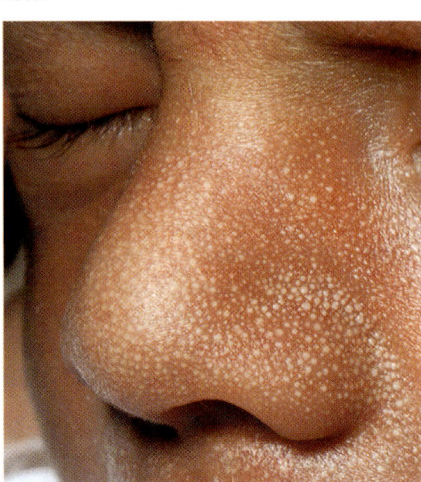

Accessory auricle.

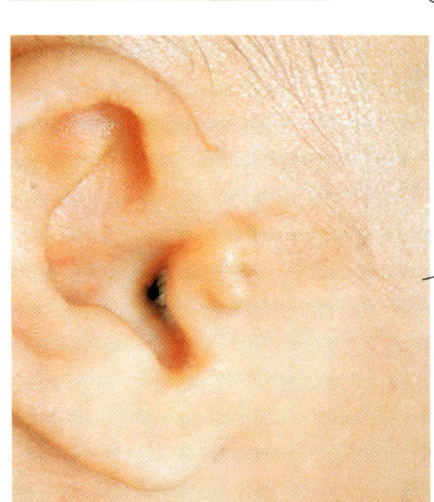

Fig.1

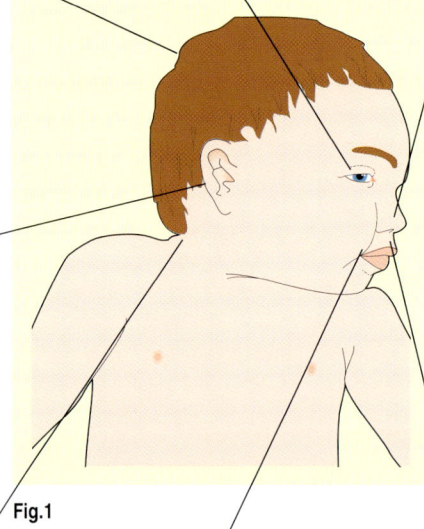

Down's syndrome facies.

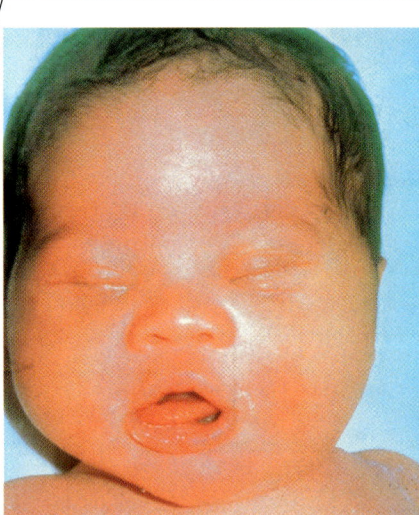

Neck webbing in Turner's syndrome.

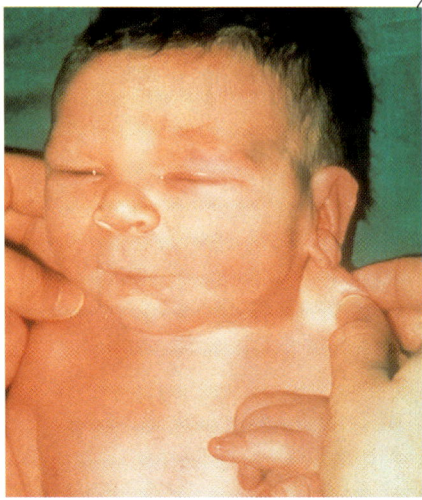

Cleft palate.

Bilateral cleft lip.

Simian crease typically seen in Down's syndrome.

Head lag. The baby is floppy and there is poor feeding secondary to birth asphyxia.

Distorted body proportions. The limbs are short compared to the trunk, particularly the femur and the humerus. The face is flat. The child has achondroplasia.

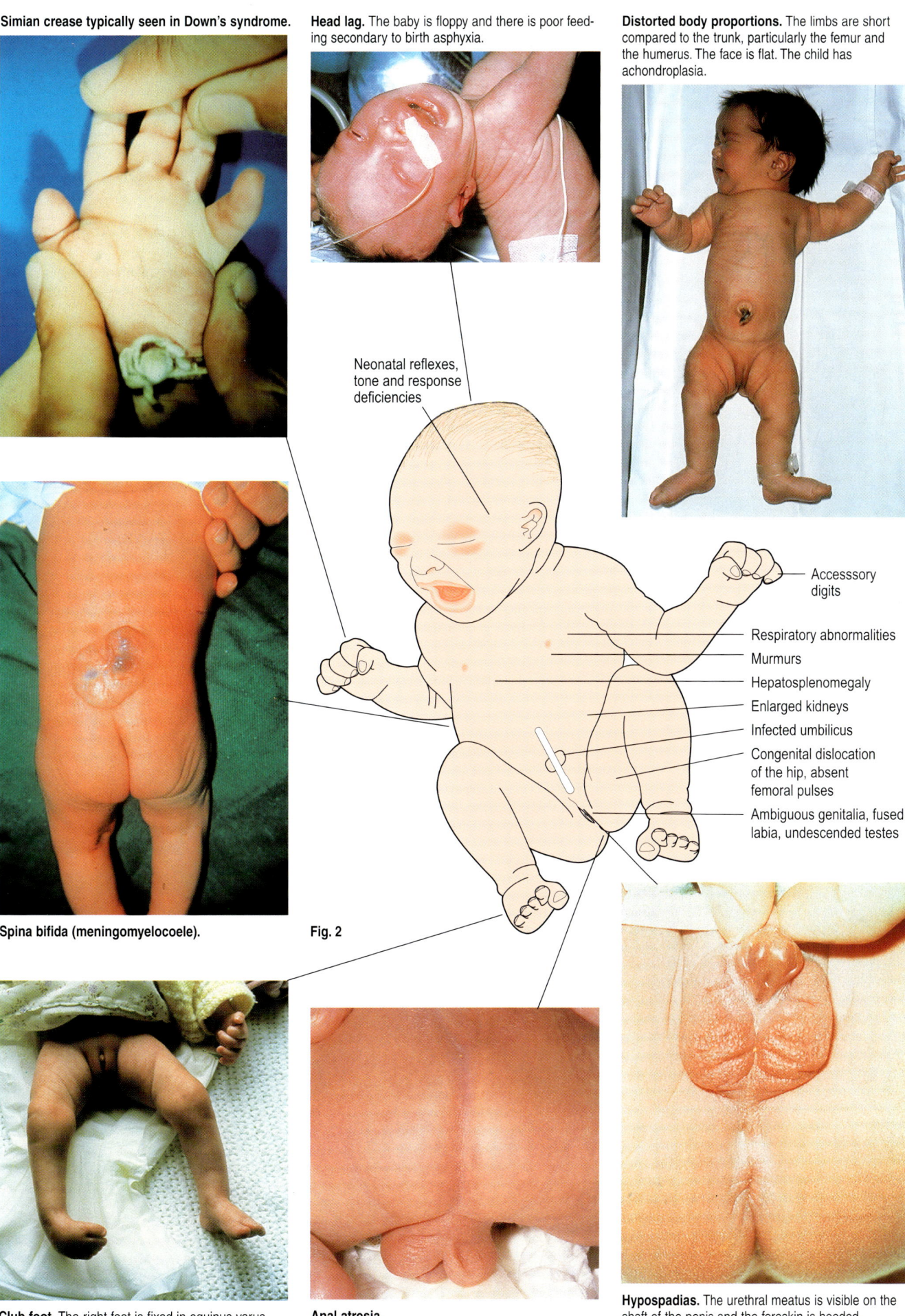

Neonatal reflexes, tone and response deficiencies

Accesssory digits

Respiratory abnormalities

Murmurs

Hepatosplenomegaly

Enlarged kidneys

Infected umbilicus

Congenital dislocation of the hip, absent femoral pulses

Ambiguous genitalia, fused labia, undescended testes

Spina bifida (meningomyelocoele).

Fig. 2

Club foot. The right foot is fixed in equinus varus.

Anal atresia.

Hypospadias. The urethral meatus is visible on the shaft of the penis and the foreskin is hooded.

RECOGNISING NORMAL DEVELOPMENT

Many parents become concerned that their child is not following a normal pattern of development, i.e. the child is late in acquiring a skill or is showing abnormal behaviour. In order to deal with such concerns it is essential to have an appreciation of natural variation.

The development of a child is dynamic. It is a continuous process from conception to adult maturity. The fetus develops over 9 months from undifferentiated cells in an embryonic sac into a newborn baby, with all the senses and basic life functions. The infant is wholly dependent. From birth to 5 years, the baby is transformed into a relatively independent child at school entry: mobile, dexterous, communicative, sociable and able to look after her/his basic living needs directly and to seek assistance where necessary. Throughout school years, the child develops — through family life, education, friendships, experimentation and risk taking — into the educated young adult, with career ambitions, able to have mature relationships, to make decisions and to take part in wider aspects of society beyond the family.

Normal development varies enormously. It is determined by a complex interplay between environmental factors (maternal health antenatally, in utero conditions, the birth process, economic and social conditions facing the family) and genetic factors. These factors may affect:

- rate of maturation (e.g. myelination of the nervous system)
- quality of a developing skill
- whether the child has the full potential to develop along normal lines.

The potential to develop and learn is inherited. Medical conditions may place limits on this. Environmental conditions and social opportunity will help minimise or maximise the realisation of that potential. For example, children are not born with language: they have to learn to listen, learn understanding, and learn how to express themselves. If a child is to realise his or her potential, there must be the opportunity to learn these skills from parents and teachers, from other children and from exploring a stimulating environment. The complex interplay of factors is summarised in Table 1.

The development of a child is assessed against a knowledge of the normal stages of development in children of various ages. These developmental 'milestones' are an average for a given population (Fig. 1). There is wide variation between different populations and within a given population, e.g. the age of independent walking can

vary from 7 to 17 months. However, if the infant is not walking by 18 months, the third centile for achieving walking, reasons need to be sought to explain the motor delay.

IMPORTANCE OF KNOWING ABOUT NORMAL DEVELOPMENT

Without a thorough knowledge of the normal stages of development, there are no criteria on which to decide whether a child needs further investigation or whether the parent(s) can be reassured and their anxiety removed: it is important to understand the processes which underlie development. False diagnoses of developmental delay cause great distress. However, to incorrectly reassure parents when they have noticed an area of real concern is worse

than to investigate or refer a child and then to find out all is well. A late diagnosis of developmental disorder, especially when the parents have long been worried, causes bitterness and resentment. Correct management is delayed.

Table 1 **Important points to remember in child development**

- Dynamic: early skills are the building blocks for later ones
- Sequence: development follows a sequence, with common variants
- Quality: quality of skill is more important than age 'milestone'
- Asymmetry: development of a hand preference before 1 year of age suggests a neurological abnormality
- Rate: depends on maturation (myelination) of the nervous system
- Maturation is from the head downwards (cephalocaudal)
- Newborn 'primitive' reflexes give way to voluntary control
- Generalised 'mass' reactions give way to specific individual responses
- Individual skills are gradually combined to give integrated function

Table 2 **Developmental examination**

Area of development*	Skills to assess or observe
Gross motor	Head and truncal control, balance, ability to use limbs for independent mobility, reaching and personal care
Hand–eye	Vision, visual awareness, scanning of shapes and puzzles, fine motor coordination, manipulation, drawing skills
Language and attention	Hearing, attention level, understanding of speech (receptive language), speech content (expressive language), speech quality (articulation, phonology)
Play and learning	Exploration of the environment, symbolic play, imaginative play, quality of play, problem solving, development of early concepts: prepositions, (in/on/under), size, shape, colour, number
Social and emotional	Relationships with others, quality of communication, social integration, behavioural development
Activities of daily living	Feeding, sleeping, dressing, toileting

* These areas overlap more and more with higher, integrated functioning, e.g. writing involves complex hand–eye coordination, good vision and language skills

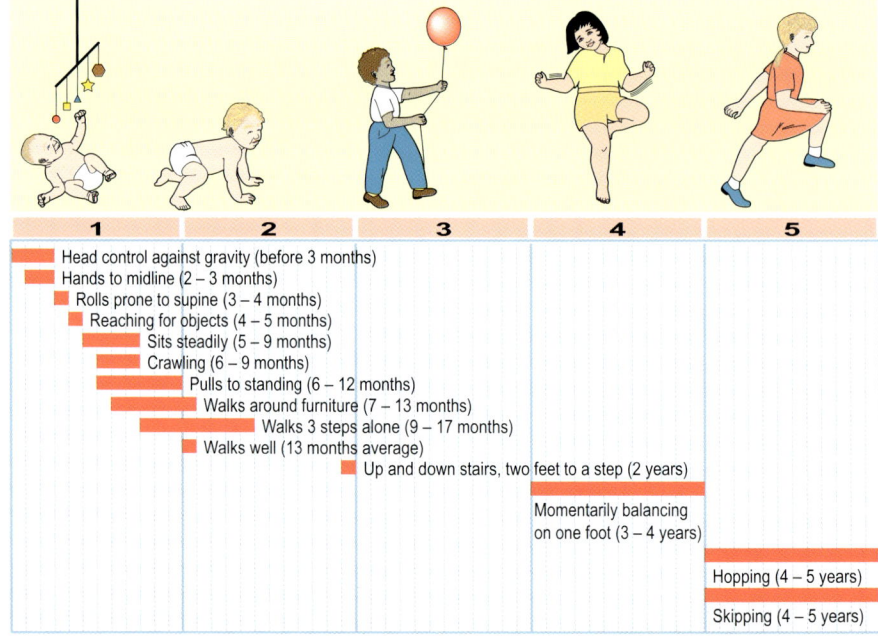

Fig. 1 **Motor development milestones.**

Head control against gravity (before 3 months)
Hands to midline (2 – 3 months)
Rolls prone to supine (3 – 4 months)
Reaching for objects (4 – 5 months)
Sits steadily (5 – 9 months)
Crawling (6 – 9 months)
Pulls to standing (6 – 12 months)
Walks around furniture (7 – 13 months)
Walks 3 steps alone (9 – 17 months)
Walks well (13 months average)
Up and down stairs, two feet to a step (2 years)
Momentarily balancing on one foot (3 – 4 years)
Hopping (4 – 5 years)
Skipping (4 – 5 years)

NORMAL VARIANT PATTERNS OF DEVELOPMENT

There are normal variations from the usual sequence of development. Family history is important: it is reassuring (but no more than that) if other members of the family have followed a similar course of development and turned out well, e.g. late in talking or walking. A number of different areas of development must be considered (Table 2). There are well-established variants in motor development (Table 3). The most common sequence is the child who sits/crawls/ stands/cruises-around-furniture/walks. Mean age of walking is 13 months. However, a large number do not follow this pattern. 'Bottom shufflers' are the most common variant. They fail to crawl but shuffle around on their bottoms or sides: a sit/shuffle/stand/walk sequence. They walk late and tend to be mildly hypotonic early on. Language development (Table 4) also varies and may follow a familial pattern. Isolated language delay, like motor development, may be benign. However, its significance should not be underestimated, and should lead to a test of hearing and a questioning about other areas of development. Seek advice before dismissing developmental concerns simply because family history suggests the reason for the child's delay. Follow up development for a few months if in doubt.

WARNING SIGNS

Parents are very good at picking up on developmental difficulties early. They must be listened to very carefully with appropriate examination and investigation. Be careful not to dismiss their concerns. Persistent moderate delay (developmental age only half to two-thirds of actual age followed over a 3–6 months' period) and severe delay when first recognised (development less than half the actual age) need further investigation. A history of loss of previously established skills or developmental arrest, with failure to gain new skills after a period of normal development, needs urgent investigation.

WHERE DO PARENTS DISCUSS THEIR CHILD'S DEVELOPMENT?

Throughout Britain there is a child health surveillance programme (Table 5). Through this, parents are offered the opportunity to discuss their child's development. Every child under 5 years has a named health visitor. Each geographical area has an agreed schedule of check-ups, often timed to coincide with the immunisation programme. The child health surveillance programme is delivered by the primary health care team or the community child health service and involves the health visitor in partnership either with the family doctor in the surgery or the community child health doctor in the health clinic.

THE OLDER CHILD

Development in the school-age child is by and large the domain of the educationalists. Parents will usually discuss any concerns firstly with the teaching staff. Developmental progress is redefined as educational progress.

Social and emotional development continues throughout childhood. The child gradually seeks greater independence and responsibility for decision making. This will be associated with risk taking behaviour and experimentation: with different interests, philosophies and ways of life. This can be a turbulent time both for the child or young adult and the parents or teachers! It is, however, helpful to be mindful that it is a normal, albeit traumatic, period of development in most instances.

Table 3 **Normal motor variants** (Unpublished data courtesy of P. Robson, King's College)

Motor pattern	Incidence in population	Mean ages child achieves milestone (months)		
		unsupported sitting	standing	walking alone
Crawl/stand/walk	83%	7	9.5	13.5
Stand/walk	6%	6	9	11
Bottom shuffling	9%	8.5	13.5	17
Creeping-rolling	1%	12	15	18

Table 4 **Early normal language development.** Complex language development gradually increases in later childhood.

Skill	Age
Listens: startles or widens eyes to sound	0–6 weeks
Turns to voice	4–7 months
Shows recognition of objects by using, e.g. brush, cup, socks, etc.	9–12 months
First words with meaning: 'mama', 'dada' to parents	10–15 months
Follows one-step requests with gesture, e.g. 'give me the doll'	15–18 months
Says 20+ words, two words with separate meanings, e.g. 'drink, daddy', 'mummy gone'	2 years
Understands two component tasks: 'give dolly a drink'	
Understanding is always a few months ahead of expressive language	
Identifies objects by their use, e.g. chair ('which one do you sit on?')	3 years
Early concepts developing: big/small, colours, meaning of 2	
Knows name, age, sex	3–4 years
More complex understanding with many questions	4–5 years
Sustained concentration and listening skills	5 years

Table 5 **Typical child health surveillance programme: ages when recommended screening occurs in Britain**

Age	Where	Who	Examination
Neonatal	Within 48 hours	Paediatrician/GP	Full physical examination
6–8 week check	Child health clinic	GP or community doctor	Full physical examination, development, growth
8 month check	Child health clinic	Health visitor, GP or community doctor	Development, hearing, growth, heart, testes, hips
2 year check	Home	Health visitor	Development, language and behaviour
3+ year check	Child health clinic	Health visitor, GP or community doctor	Development, growth
5+ year school entry	Primary school	School nurse and community doctor	Development, growth, vision and hearing, selective school medical

Recognising normal development
- Wide variation in healthy children is normal not exceptional.
- Newborn reflexes disappear gradually and are replaced by voluntary control.
- Observation of the quality of a skill is more important than simply noting the age of achieving the milestone.
- Note asymmetry.
- Developmental skills are learnt, not automatic.
- Receptive language (understanding) develops ahead of expressive language (talking).
- Age appropriate language development and attention skills are necessary for coping socially in school and learning to read and write.

THE BABY WITH AN UNUSUAL APPEARANCE

Unusual physical characteristics are common and part of nature. Some features in particular that are noted in a baby can be easily identifiable in other family members, e.g. a large head. Labour and delivery may produce short-term changes in appearance which, nonetheless, can be very alarming to parents (see Fig. 4). However, where an individual displays features which represent more than this normal variation they are described as *dysmorphic*. The various mechanisms by which this can arise are summarised diagrammatically in Figure 1.

Genetic problems leading to dysmorphism are of particular importance since:

- There is often a characteristic pattern of abnormality.
- There may be a risk of recurrence.

The types of genetic lesion are shown in Table 1.

Table 1 **Mechanisms for genetic dysmorphism**

Chromosomal	Whole chromosome addition, e.g. Down's syndrome, trisomy 21
	Whole chromosome deletion, e.g. Turner's syndrome, XO
	Partial chromosome addition, e.g. trisomy 4p syndrome
	Partial chromosome deletion, e.g. cri du chat, 5p⁻
Gene defects	Direct effect on appearance, e.g. albinism osteogenesis imperfecta (brittle bone disease)
	Secondary effects on appearance, e.g. thalassaemia, mucopolysaccharidosis

CLINICAL ASSESSMENT

Although some dysmorphic features do not appear until later life, and others are simply not noticed initially, the vast majority are apparent at or soon after birth. Abnormalities of this type, either singly or in combination, can be the marker of a complex disorder. Therefore, an urgent evaluation is required in order to establish whether further action is required. The essential steps are discussed below.

Family and past medical history

Pay particular attention to evidence of other relatives with similar problems to that under investigation (trying to confirm a genetic mechanism). Check whether parents were related before marriage (increased risk of genetic disease). Ascertain maternal drug intake (risk of teratogenicity, e.g. anticonvulsants associated with cleft palate), diet (poor diet may impair fetal growth), cigarette consumption

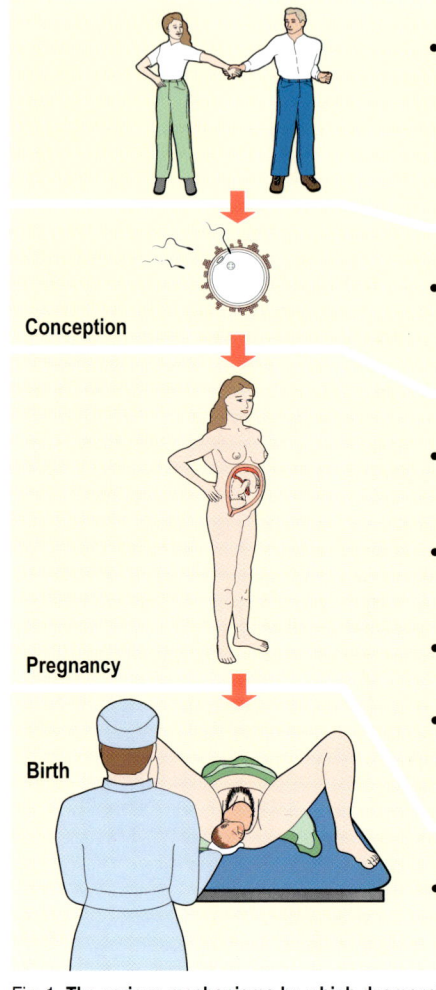

Conception

Pregnancy

Birth

- **Parental factors**
  - age (e.g. Down's syndrome in older mothers)
  - health
  - diet
  - pre-existing genetic abnormalities (e.g. achondroplasia)

- **Genetic factors** may arise de novo (e.g. trisomy 21) or allow recessive disorders to exhibit their effects (e.g. albinism)

- **Maternal exposure** to toxins may damage fetal development, e.g. fetal alcohol syndrome

- **Abnormal organ development** without specific cause identified, e.g. spina bifida or gastroschisis

- **Infections** may damage fetal development, e.g. rubella, toxoplasmosis, CMV

- **Hostile intrauterine environment**, e.g. amniotic bands causing compression injuries or even amputations

- **Traumatic abnormalities** during labour and at birth, e.g. caput succedaneum

Fig. 1 **The various mechanisms by which dysmorphic features may arise.**

(smoking may impair fetal growth) and alcohol intake (can produce fetal alcohol syndrome).

Ask in detail regarding previous pregnancies (some genetic disorders increase the risk of miscarriage) and health in the current pregnancy (seeking evidence of significant infection).

Physical examination

It is important to ascertain as thoroughly as possible the number and extent of abnormalities present. Some of the points of particular interest are shown in Table 2.

Investigations

Investigations should be conducted to either confirm the diagnosis (e.g. karyotyping in a child with suspected chromosomal defect) or to add further information about the nature of the child's problem (e.g. X-rays in a child with shortened limbs to assess the nature of the bony abnormality, or echocardiogram in a child with suspected congenital heart disease).

Table 2 **Key points of neonatal examination**

Head shape	Posterior flattening (bradycephaly) in Down's syndrome
Ear position	May be 'low set' (< 1/3 above lateral canthus) in chromosomal disorders
Eye shape	May be mongoloid slant in Down's syndrome
Red reflex	Absent with cataract, choroido-retinitis (part of congenital infection) or retinoblastoma
Palate	Always feel to ensure the palate is intact; cleft palate can be isolated but is part of many syndromes
Hands and feet	Variation (e.g. short incurving little finger, short big toe, prominent calcaneum) are features of a number of chromosomal lesions
Genitalia	Confirm normal anatomy — where this is not clear never assume genetic sex
Anus	Always confirm that the anus is present and patent; meconium may pass via a fistula without a normal anus (Fig. 2)
Back	Always turn the baby over to ensure that no spina bifida is missed

Consultation with a clinical geneticist

A consultation with a clinical geneticist should be sought regarding the significance of the observed lesion(s). Whilst geneticists are generally more familiar with patterns of abnormality, they will often employ a computer database to determine a differential diagnosis.

General points

It is essential to keep parents informed about progress at every stage. In practice, where the problem is complex, a firm diagnosis is often not reached for some time and parents should be warned of this possibility. However, many dysmorphic features are trivial (e.g. the presence of extra digits) and complete reassurance should be given at the earliest opportunity.

DOWN'S SYNDROME

Down's syndrome (trisomy 21) is the most important chromosomal defect producing a dysmorphic syndrome. This is not only because it is common (occurring in 1 in 660 births, the risk increasing with maternal age) but also because it is commonly associated with major abnormalities (see Table 3). These secondary phenomena place huge burdens both on the family and the health services.

It is usually the child's appearance which raises suspicion of the diagnosis (Fig. 3). The individual dysmorphic features associated with Down's syndrome all occur within the normal population. However, these features are rarely seen in combination. By contrast, in Down's syndrome a number (but not all) of these features are likely to be present.

The tendency for mothers carrying babies with Down's syndrome to have low levels of human chorionic gonadotrophin and high levels of alphafetoprotein (a fetal protein) in their blood, now forms the basis of a screening test. With time this may reduce the number of affected children delivered alive (pp. 14–15).

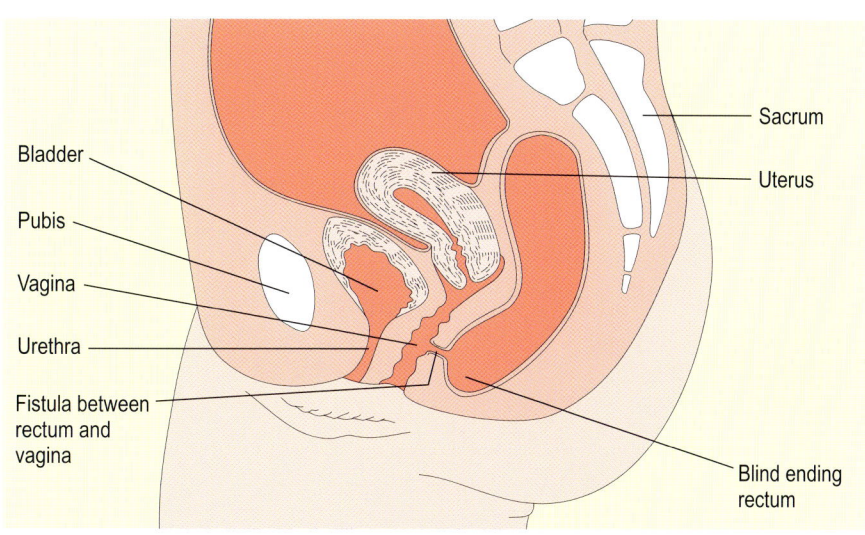

Fig. 2 **Imperforate anus in a female infant (sagittal section).** Fistulae are often present and may allow meconium to be passed in spite of ano-rectal atresia.

Bladder
Pubis
Vagina
Urethra
Fistula between rectum and vagina
Sacrum
Uterus
Blind ending rectum

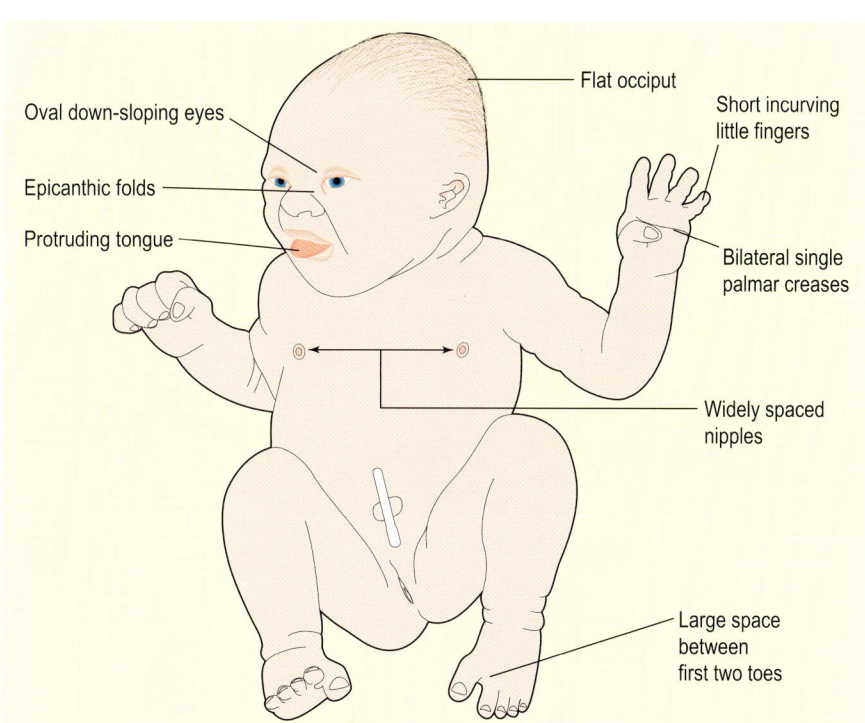

Fig. 3 **Some of the clinical features associated with Down's syndrome.**

Oval down-sloping eyes
Epicanthic folds
Protruding tongue
Flat occiput
Short incurving little fingers
Bilateral single palmar creases
Widely spaced nipples
Large space between first two toes

Table 3 **Major anomalies associated with Down's syndrome**

General	Hypotonia, poor feeding and relatively small stature in later childhood
Brain	Anomalies resulting in mental deficiency
Cardiovascular	Various major defects may occur particularly in structures derived from the endocardial cushions (e.g. VSD, arterioventricular canal defect, primum ASD)
Gastrointestinal	Duodenal atresia and Hirschsprung's disease
Eye	Strabismus or nystagmus

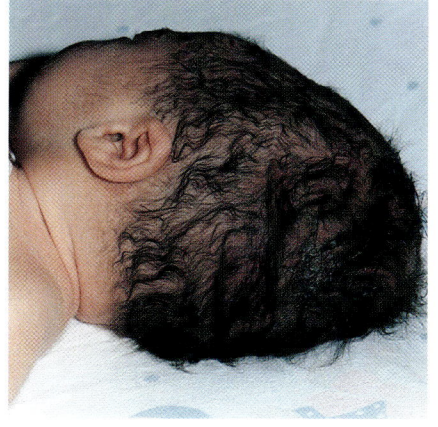

Fig. 4 **Child with caput succedaneum caused by birth trauma.**

The baby with an unusual appearance

- Attempt to ascertain whether there is a true abnormality or normal variation.
- Always look for recognised patterns of abnormality.
- Carry out appropriate investigations which add further information to the pattern of abnormality.

SOCIAL, PREVENTATIVE AND DEVELOPMENTAL PAEDIATRICS

PREVENTING ILLNESS

INTRODUCTION

Normal growth in a child depends not only on hormonal stimulation but also requires satisfactory nutrition, good general health and appropriate psychological stimulation. Normal development occurs through the complex interplay of both learning and neuronal maturation. Doctors have long recognised the need to intervene when either the child's environment or a previously undiagnosed medical problem threatens to reduce his or her long-term potential.

Priorities in this respect have varied not only with the individual but over time and between countries. For example, in many countries the provision of clean water (in order to reduce the incidence of gastroenteritis) and the abolition of malnutrition remain priorities, while in Western nations, increasing attention is being paid to the early detection of diseases such as cystic fibrosis and congenital hypothyroidism in order to ameliorate their long-term impact on the child. Despite this apparent contrast in the pattern of preventative care, many common themes can be identified within the schemes in place around the world.

SCREENING

In order to be of value, screening must be aimed at detecting a disease or condition that can be cured or for which the subsequent impact can be lessened by early intervention. The tests employed must be accurate in order to avoid undue anxieties over false positive results or missing cases following a false negative result. Costs must also be considered in relation to any programme of screening. In general, the incidence of the condition, the cost of early identification, potential savings in health costs later in life, and the reduction in suffering are all taken into account. Informed consent is an important part of any screening test and hence good counselling should ensure that parents fully understand what is being offered.

The tests described below are widely available in the Western world.

ANTENATAL SCREENING TESTS

The intention with antenatal screening is to identify major abnormalities with a view to offering counselling and, if appropriate, termination of pregnancy.

Maternal blood tests
Alphafetoprotein. This is raised in neural tube defect and some gastrointestinal abnormalities. It allows more specific tests (detailed ultrasound) to be focused on those most at risk.

Down's test. This test uses the fact that in women carrying an infant with Down's syndrome the alphafetoprotein is relatively high and the human chorionic gonadotrophin (HCG) is low — a risk is then calculated. This allows the more invasive specific tests (amniocentesis or cordocentesis and karyotyping) to be restricted to the high risk group.

Ultrasound
Whilst many women receive an ultrasound scan in order to check the growth of the baby against the estimated date of delivery, a smaller number also undergo scanning specifically to identify anomalies. Major problems (e.g. cardiac anomalies, diaphragmatic hernia) are reliably detected but the accuracy in diagnosing more minor defects (e.g. cleft palate) and the ethics of then offering termination are less clear cut.

POSTNATAL SCREENING TESTS
Blood tests in infants
Phenylketonuria (PKU). PKU has an incidence of 1 in 15 000 births. This test is the oldest of the infant screening tests. The aim is to prevent affected individuals from suffering the permanent brain damage which results from the accumulation of toxic phenyl ketones. This can be achieved by introducing a diet low in phenylalanine during very early life. The toxic products are measured in a spot of clotted blood collected from the baby, normally 7 days after starting feeds. Usually four samples are collected on to blotting paper and these 'spares' have enabled the introduction of the following two screens.

Thyroid stimulating hormone. Hypothyroidism occurs in 1 in 3000 births. Thyroid hormone is essential for normal neurone development and if a low level is not corrected by 4 months of age, permanent mental retardation results. The most common cause of hypothyroidism in infancy is a dysplastic or absent thyroid. As a result, affected infants have high levels of TSH which can be detected. The test will not detect hypothyroidism of pituitary origin but this is very uncommon. The test was initially thought to offer marginal benefit on financial grounds since the incidence of congenital hypothyroidism was felt to be only 1 in 15 000 to 1 in 20 000. However,

the test is sufficiently sensitive that it also picks up children with borderline thyroid function who would not have presented until later childhood.

Immunoreactive trypsin (IRT). This test used in screening for cystic fibrosis is less widely available. During the production of trypsin in the pancreas, a peptide (IRT) is cleaved from the molecule. Pancreatic damage or bowel disturbance in the period immediately after birth causes an increased amount of this marker to reach the blood, where it can be measured. Cystic fibrosis is the most likely cause of this situation arising but must be confirmed with a genotype and/or sweat test. Early treatment is felt to improve the outcome for many affected individuals. IRT is not reliable where other forms of gastrointestinal pathology are known to be present, e.g. intestinal obstruction.

NEWBORN PHYSICAL EXAMINATION

All babies are examined after birth by the midwife and again by a doctor within the first 48 hours of life. The primary aims are to ensure that the baby is well following birth and that the baby has no congenital abnormalities. It is vital to remember that at this time nothing can be assumed, e.g. the presence of eyes, an anus, an intact palate. These and other gross structural defects must be excluded as well as seeking more subtle problems such as a ventricular septal defect, a large kidney or congenitally dislocated hips. The time of the examination can also be used to answer any parental concerns and provide general advice regarding feeding, immunisation, etc.

SCREENING IN LATER CHILDHOOD

For many years children's health has been monitored throughout childhood by a series of informal contacts with health visitors, supplemented by occasional set medical reviews where growth, general well-being and development were all checked. With the increased availability of services and improved parental awareness, this unfocused approach is being replaced by population screening of a more limited kind (i.e. for those conditions where intervention is known to be of benefit, for example in hearing loss). However, greater priority is being placed on families where inadequate parenting skills and/or social problems and/or a chronic medical condition appear to jeopardise the child's future (Fig. 1).

IMMUNISATION

One of the great successes of modern medicine has been the role of immunisation in controlling infectious disease. The pattern in any one country reflects:

● Local priority (i.e. those conditions that have in the past caused major problems).
● Availability of a safe and effective vaccine (some vaccines are not sufficiently safe and/or effective to justify their routine use, e.g. cholera).

● The natural history of the disease (e.g. *Haemophilus influenzae* is a pathogen predominantly in children under 5 years of age, therefore boosters in older childhood are not necessary).
● The pattern of maternal antibody transfer. For some conditions babies receive high levels of immunity from their mothers, e.g. measles. Therefore, immunisation has to be postponed in order to ensure the baby makes a good response. For pertussis, little or no protection is acquired before delivery and therefore vaccination is needed at an early age.

Contraindications

There are very few absolute contraindications to the immunisations currently offered as standard within the UK. These are:

● The child must not be systemically ill at the time the vaccination is given.
● The child must not be immunosuppressed (congenital or acquired). HIV positive children are offered immunisation but BCG is excluded and killed polio vaccine is administered intramuscularly.
● There must be no history of reaction to a previous dose.

The current pattern in the UK is shown in Table 1.

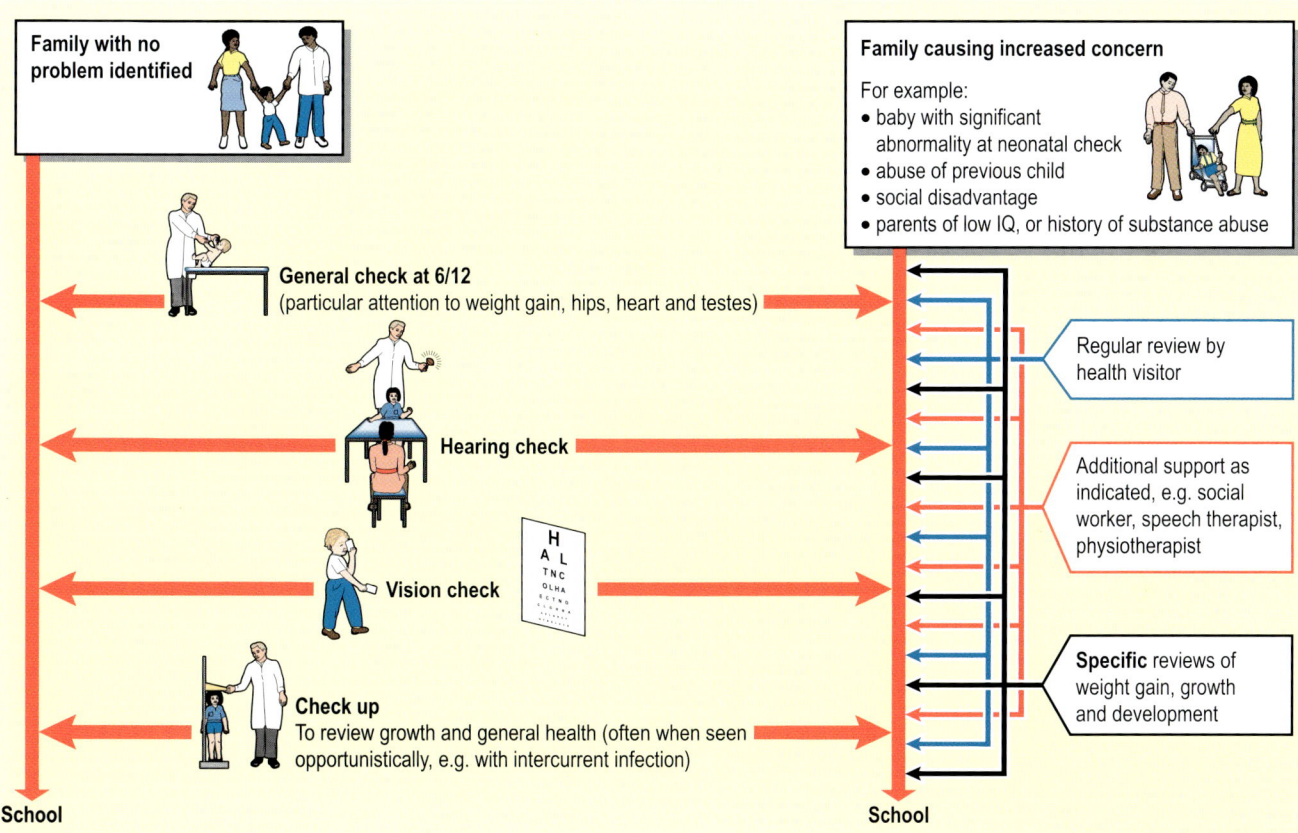

Fig. 1 **Screening in later childhood.**

Table 1 **Immunisation available in the UK**

Age	Disease/agent	Route
Birth	TB/BCG (live attenuated mycobacterium) in infants at risk because of ethnic origin or family history	Intradermal
2–4 months (3 doses)	Tetanus (toxoid) Diphtheria (toxoid) Pertussis (killed bacteria) *Haemophilius influenzae* (capsular antigen)	Intramuscular
	Polio (live attenuated virus)	Oral
2nd year of life	Measles (live attenuated virus) Mumps (live attenuated virus) Rubella (live attenuated virus)	Intramuscular
Pre-school	Tetanus, diphtheria, and polio boosters	As above
12 years	TB screening with BCG to at-risk children	As above

Preventing illness

● Preventative techniques are of particular value in children in order to maximise potential.
● Screening programmes must be carefully evaluated to ensure they are both effective and do not cause harm by creating unnecessary anxiety.
● There are very few contraindications to standard immunisations.

THE 'SLOW' CHILD (THE CHILD WITH DEVELOPMENTAL DELAY)

It can be difficult to identify the child with emerging developmental problems when the normal patterns and rates of development are so varied (see pp. 8–9). The clinical tools are:

- a good working knowledge of child development
- an ability to obtain information from parent(s), excellent observers of their child, who are accurate historians when asked the right questions
- a short developmental assessment, providing a profile of the child's development to support the history and on which to base an agreement with parents about appropriate further action
- depending on who is seeing the child (GP, hospital or community paediatrician), guidelines on: when and where to refer the child for full developmental examination, investigation and management and indeed when local review or no further action is required.

HOW DEVELOPMENTAL DELAY PRESENTS

Worried parents

Parents are frequently the first to notice their child's problem. In and of itself this may be sufficient to warrant further investigation, even if examination is non-contributory.

Child health surveillance

The purpose of screening programmes and surveillance is to detect developmental problems early (p. 14). The child with hearing loss, motor delay or language disorder should be identified early in order to provide for the special needs and, hence, to prevent avoidable secondary effects such as learning diffi-culty or behavioural problems (Table 1).

Professional concern

The child may give concern to professionals coming into contact with the family for incidental reasons, e.g. family doctor, nursery officer, school teacher or social worker.

PATTERNS OF ABNORMAL DEVELOPMENT

Developmental delay

In this situation, development continues along the normal route but the child persistently takes longer to arrive at each milestone compared with the normal range for the children of a given society or culture.

Table 1 **Warning signs of delayed development**

	General and social development	Fine and gross motor	Language and play
1st year: motor development dominant			
6–8 weeks	Not smiling back by 8 weeks, poor visual attention, poor eye contact	Significant head lag, floppy/increased tone	Silent baby, no coos or gurgles
8 months	Little social interest, not mouthing objects	Still fisting at 3 months	
	Poor interaction	Not rolling over, not weight bearing, not sitting even with support, no early palmar grasp of objects	No interest in objects, no pick-up of objects
	Poor feeding Unusually passive		Failure to develop babble by 10 months
Throughout first year	'Difficult', crying, irritable Persistent poor sleep pattern Posseting/vomiting Constipation	Not sitting alone by 10 months	
2nd year: language and social development more important			
12–18 months	Not recognising familiar adults Not recognising own name	Not getting into sitting position or pulling to stand by 12 months	Not recognising use of objects by 18 months, no first words by 15 months
		No mature fine pincer grasp by 14 months	Parental concern, vocabulary not expanding
18–24 months	Not giving or receiving affection, unaware of others' feelings	Unable to build Not walking 3 steps alone by 18 months	Not linking 2 words or following simple requests, no symbolic play with objects and toys
3rd and 4th year: language, play and learning dominant			
2½ years	Unable to tolerate social interaction, cannot play alongside other children, nor accept adult help with play Unaware of danger	Unsteady or wide-based gait 2–2½ years No circular scribble	Not using 50+ words meaningfully, cannot pay attention, lack of imaginative play
3–4 years	Unable to share play with other children Unable to develop play without adult help Persistent frequent tantrums	Immature walk/gait, immature pincer grasp, pick-up and release Cannot draw circle by 3½ years Cannot draw cross by 4 years	Not developing concepts, e.g. number, biggest/smallest, in/on/under; not understanding action words (eating, crying, etc.); nor identifying objects by use ('what do you sit on, cut with?' etc.), not joining 3 words, unintelligible speech

Moderate delay can be defined as a developmental age equivalent to or less than two-thirds of chronological age noted from history or clinical review over a 3–6 months period, e.g. a child of 36 months with development at 21–24 months. Severe delay is a developmental age one-half of chronological age or less (Table 2).

Developmental disorder

Here, the child's development is not following normal patterns but is aberrant or bizarre. Developmental progress may be made but it is disordered.

Indications of disorder include persistence of immature stages of development, e.g. the presence of primitive reflexes in the older child with cerebral palsy; patterns of development not seen in normal development at all, e.g. extensor body posturing in cerebral palsy; and atypical developmental profiles, e.g. the autistic child who is unable to use language for social interaction, but can recite TV adverts or jingles perfectly.

Developmental arrest or regression

In this case the child at first develops normally, followed by a period in which there is failure to gain new skills, a slowing in the rate of acquisition of new skills or the loss of previously established skills. Although uncommon, this presentation is highly indicative of a serious disorder.

Table 2 **Common or important reasons for delayed development**

- Primary acquired or inherited disorder affecting development
- Secondary effect on development of an existing chronic disorder, e.g. serious and/or chronic ill health, long-term hospitalisation, organic failure to thrive
- Sequelae of serious illness or injury, e.g. meningo-encephalitis, head injury
- Non-organic failure to thrive (i.e. non-stimulating environment) – social and child protection issues
- Emotional/psychological disorders

MANAGEMENT AIMS

Medical

An accurate assessment of a child's needs is necessary, together with a reasonable search for a diagnosis, following an investigation protocol for non-specific developmental delay or targeted investigations where specific disorders are clinically suspected. For the majority of children with non-specific learning difficulty there will not be a clear diagnosis (Table 3). Provision of physiotherapy, occupational therapy, speech and language therapy and psychology should be available, and the child will require ongoing specialist review as appropriate, e.g. orthopaedics for cerebral palsy, neurology for complex epilepsy.

Social

The medical specialists and care team should work with parents to share information, planning and decision making and ensure that financial benefits are made available (e.g. disability living allowance, invalid care allowance) and that housing needs are planned for.

The care team should also introduce families to relevant voluntary societies and self-help groups and endeavour to empower the child and family to manage the disability and to achieve as great a degree of independence as possible.

Finally, families should receive advice on health aspects relevant to decisions such as independent living, mobility, career and leisure in adult life.

Education and career

The care team can help by: providing advice to the family and local education authority to assist in correct school placement and educational provision; providing therapy, medical and nursing support throughout schooling; and assisting in the multidisciplinary planning of transition from school to adult life.

Community structure

This will involve the child development team and inter-agency liaison (see p. 20).

Table 3 **Common syndromes associated with delay**

Developmental disorder	Incidence, aetiology	Important features
Autism (including Asperger's syndrome)	2–3 per 1000 (much higher than previously thought) Boys:girls 3:1 (severe cases) 9:1 (more able) Definite genetic factor: increased familial recurrence Onset before 3–5 years	Triad of impairment: • impairment of social interaction and relationships • impairment of social communication, verbal and non-verbal • impairment of social understanding and imagination, with repetitive activity 70–80% have learning disability in addition
Attention deficit disorder (ADD)	Controversy over incidence: 5% of boys in USA less than 1% of boys in UK Boys far more than girls possible genetic factor Onset before 7 years	Physical restlessness Easily distractible, noisy Difficulty waiting for turn Interrupts in class or games Poor listening skills Inability to organise oneself for tasks or activities Dangerous activities, unaware of consequences Epilepsy more common
Fragile X syndrome (Fig. 1)	Most common chromosomal cause of severe learning disability in males X-linked 1 per 1200 boys; presents in girls also More severe expression in males: severity increases in successive generations	Learning disability Shy, social avoidance Hyperactivity Language disorder, echolalia Hypotonia, motor stereotypes Post-pubertal dysmorphism and enlarged testes Epilepsy more common
Williams' syndrome (Fig. 2)	1 in 5000 Single gene disorder probable Diagnostic genetic test: FISH Equal sex incidence	Typical facial dysmorphism: 'elfin' Coarse features, hypertelorism, long philtrum Typical language profile: unusually expression is in advance of understanding ('cocktail party chatter') Developmental delay usual Some achieve mainstream education Supravalvular aortic stenosis

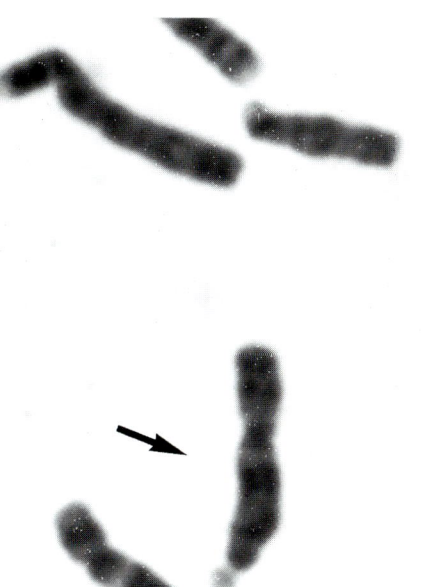

Fig.1 **Metaphase spread showing X chromosome with fragile site at abnormal section seen at the bottom of the figure.**

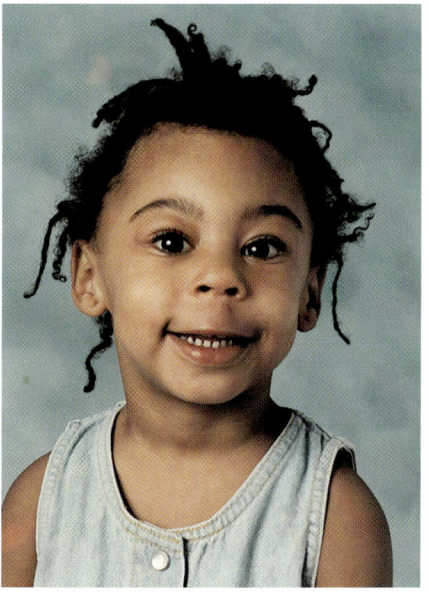

Fig. 2 **Facial dysmorphism in Williams' syndrome.**

The 'slow' child

- Assessment and/or investigations will provide an explanation of the child's problem in 30–40% of moderate and 60–70% of severe developmental delay.
- Family history is a vital part of the assessment and genetic counselling an essential part of management.
- Hearing must be adequately assessed in all cases of developmental delay.
- The community paediatrician plays a key role in coordinating management.
- Non-medical aspects are very important: liaison with education, working with voluntary groups, information on disability services and benefits.

THE DISABLED CHILD: CAUSATION

The able-bodied child develops integrated function in areas of sensory, motor, cognitive, language and communication, and social and emotional development. An impairment of one or more of these functions is caused by the absence or maldevelopment of, or damage to, normal physiological processes or anatomical structures. The child whose impairment restricts the ability to perform one or more activities at the age-appropriate level of development is disabled. The disability may prevent the child from reaching his or her full potential compared with other children in the comparable social and cultural environment. The result is, therefore, that the child is disadvantaged or handicapped. Not all impairment of function leads to a disability, for example a unilateral hearing loss may not affect a child's development. The disability only results in disadvantage or handicap if the child is prevented from taking part in everyday activities. This is in large part determined by society's attitude to people with disability and its determination, or otherwise, to pursue policies of integration and inclusion. Examples are shown in Figure 1.

Disability, from mild to profound, is present in 3% of all children; often there are multiple disabilities present. Incidences of some important forms of disability are given in Table 1. Thorough assessment and a careful investigation plan are always important in order that the child's problems are fully evaluated.

Although not possible in many cases, a positive diagnosis is very helpful for both parents and professionals and must be looked for:

- diagnosis helps parents to understand the disability and to manage it better
- parents get appropriate genetic counselling
- the prognosis may be clarified by the specific diagnosis
- known complications are managed better: secondary and tertiary prevention is planned
- a few rare but important conditions have specific treatments available.

Management

The aim of management is to provide comprehensive support for the family and to work with them to maximise the child's potential by minimising the handicapping effects of the disability, foreseeing and avoiding where possible, secondary complications of disability. The ideal is to allow a child every opportunity to participate in family, school and social life to the fullest extent possible and to assist the child and family in preparation for adult life (pp. 20–21).

HOW DOES DISABILITY PRESENT?

Disability may not declare itself, like other conditions, with a dramatic clinical presentation. Disability may be suspected before it is apparent. Known risk factors such as

Table 1 **Incidence of some forms of disability**

Disability	Incidence
Severe sensorineural hearing loss	1–2 per 1000
Severe visual impairment	1 per 2500
Significant motor impairment	3–4 per 1000
Cerebral palsy	2–3 per 1000
Duchenne muscular dystrophy	1 per 3000 boys
Autism (impairment of social understanding/interaction)	2–3 per 1000*
Learning disability (cognitive impairment)	25–30 per 1000
Severe learning difficulties	1 per 2500
Moderate learning difficulties	2–2.5 per 1000
Down's syndrome	1 per 700–1000**
* previously quoted as 3–4 per 10 000	
** incidence prior to antenatal screening was 1 in 600–700	

Definition	Example 1	Example 2
Impairment The absence, maldevelopment of, or damage to an anatomical or physiological structure	A unilateral congenital sensorineural hearing loss	Brain damage from bilateral large intraventricular haemorrhages in a preterm infant
Disability Where impairment causes a functional deficit. This is delayed or disordered development of one or more areas of ability significant enough to impair function	• Normal hearing in most daily circumstances • Normal language development • No special educational needs • **No disability**	• Impaired motor function caused by spastic cerebral palsy • Disabilities: impaired mobility and hand function • Other disabilities may coexist
Handicap or disadvantage The disability disadvantages the child and prevents the child from realising full potential	• Age appropriate development and independence skills • **No handicap** 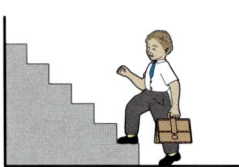	Restricted independence constitutes a disadvantage or handicap impeding full and equal access to social, educational and working opportunities 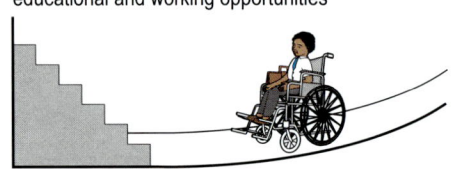

Fig. 1 **Impairment, disability and handicap — two examples.**

prematurity (Fig. 2) or the need for neonatal intensive care will alert health professionals and parents to the increased risk of disability occurring (Table 2). Child surveillance and health education programmes aim to identify disability early on, through screening and by helping parents to observe their child's development (pp. 16–17). Specific screening tests will target certain conditions, e.g. congenital hearing loss or visual impairment. The aim in identifying impairments early is to minimise disability and handicap. Where impairment is not detected early, it may present with secondary developmental delay, the effect of the unrecognised disability, e.g. hearing loss, presenting with language delay.

Parents are excellent observers of their child's development. Paediatricians learn to respond to parental concern, a common presentation of childhood disability. The parent may not know exactly what is wrong, but will provide accurate answers if a good history is taken.

DISABILITY IS NOT A DIAGNOSIS

Once concerns are confirmed and a disability recognised, an underlying diagnosis must be considered. After a full developmental assessment and physical examination, an investigation plan is made. This may be minimal if the cause of the disability is self-evident. Investigations are targeted to specific conditions where there are clinical

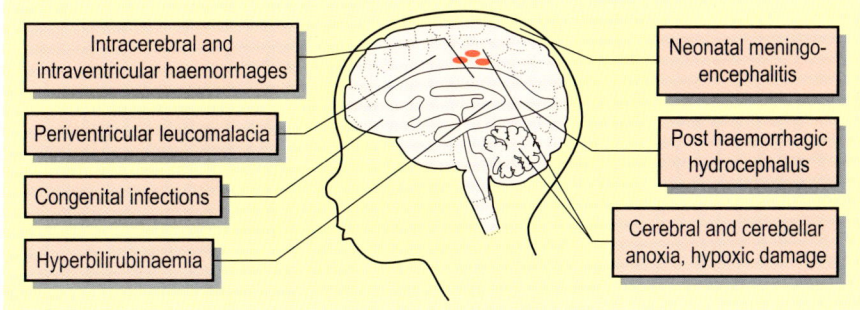

Fig. 2 **Mechanisms of brain injury in prematurity.**

Table 2 **Conditions associated with increased risk of disability**

Associations with pregnancy and delivery	Uncomplicated prematurity and low birth weight • 10% risk of disability below: — 32 weeks gestation or — 1500g birth weight Complications of prematurity and term delivery increasing risk of disability • intraventricular haemorrhage (Fig. 3) • periventricular leucomalacia • anoxia: birth asphyxia • birth injury • CMV, toxoplasmosis, other congenital infections • hyperbilirubinaemia • neonatal meningoencephalitis
Inherited disorders associated with disability	Known single gene disorders, e.g. Duchenne muscular dystrophy Chromosomal abnormalities, e.g. fragile X syndrome Many neurodegenerative disorders Hereditary spastic diplegia, athetoid cerebral palsy
Acquired conditions associated with disability	Post-meningoencephalitis Head injury Cerebrovascular accidents

pointers. In other situations, they should cover the commoner causes of disability, those with serious prognostic implications and treatable rare conditions (see pp. 11, 16, 17, 24–27 and 100–101).

EPIDEMIOLOGY

The pattern of disability has changed considerably over the last 50 years. In developed countries the effects of infectious diseases have diminished dramatically. On the other hand, children with congenital abnormality and those born prematurely have prolonged life spans due to much improved intensive and general health care. Extremely premature infants are now surviving but a relatively high proportion are disabled; some are profoundly and multiply disabled. In poorer countries the pattern of disability has changed alarmingly little.

The major causes remain malnutrition, infectious disease and war.

PREVENTION (Table 3)

Nutrition and clean water on a worldwide basis are key factors if much disability is to be tackled. Public health measures such as immunisation programmes have significantly affected child health and reduced disability in countries where the programmes operate. In developed countries, improved neonatal intensive care methods are allowing preterm babies to survive as normal infants where previously they would have died or survived with disability. However, as more extremely premature infants survive, some of these inevitably are disabled, some profoundly so.

Table 3 **Primary and secondary prevention of disability**

Primary prevention

• Preconceptual medicine, e.g. optimising daily folic acid intake may reduce the incidence of neural tube defects (NTD); withdrawing maternal sodium valproate prior to conception also reduces a known risk of NTD

• Good antenatal care of the mother

• Improved nutrition in pregnancy and early childhood

• Immunisation: the programme for *H. influenzae* B (HiB) has drastically reduced the incidence of meningitis. The MMR immunisation has reduced hearing loss from mumps and measles, and the rubella component means rubella syndrome is now rare (deafness, cataracts and congenital heart disease)

• Avoiding infection: listeriosis

• Improved neonatal care of the sick and preterm infant

• Health education, e.g. on accident prevention, raising awareness, e.g. symptoms of meningitis

Secondary prevention

• Genetic counselling: advising families of the known or estimated genetic risk
• Antenatal screening including fetal ultrasound screening for Down's syndrome; selective TOP/fetal medicine and neonatalogy; intervention where appropriate
• Neonatal population screening for selected conditions, e.g. PKU and hypothyroidism
• Targeted selective screening of at-risk groups, e.g. premature and sick neonates,
• Child health surveillance programmes responsive to parental concern for early identification of impairment

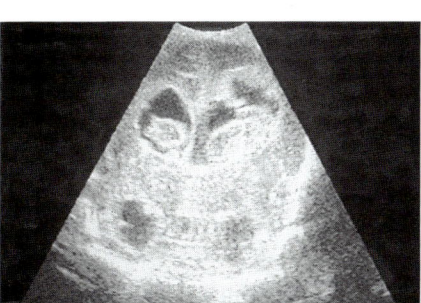

Fig. 3 **Grade IV intraventricular haemorrhage shown on ultrasound scan.**

The disabled child: causation

● Extreme prematurity holds a high risk of some degree of disability.
● Where one disability exists, it is essential to assess all other areas of health and development: this may require specialist skills.
● Parental involvement in decision making and sharing of information is essential.

THE DISABLED CHILD: MANAGEMENT

GENERAL AIMS

The general aims of disability management are:

- To work in partnership with the child and family in a manner which enables them to manage the disability effectively, through shared information, planning and decision making.
- To maximise the child's potential and minimise the consequences of disability through ongoing functional assessment of the child's needs, prevention of and screening for early signs of secondary disability.
- To provide services based on the child and family's needs, community-based where possible, to facilitate management of the child in the home, nursery or school environment.

MULTIDISCIPLINARY TEAM FOR CHILDREN WITH DISABILITY: NEEDS-LED ASSESSMENT AND PLANNING

To meet these management aims the disability team must be multidisciplinary; it must be good at interagency work (i.e. liaising with education authorities, social services, housing agencies, the voluntary sector, etc.); and it must be child- and family-centred. This means a form of working quite different from other areas of medicine: needs-led assessment and planning rather than diagnosis-oriented work, parental involvement in planning and sharing of detailed health information. It may be more important to identify a need and plan to meet it (e.g. how to achieve independence in personal hygiene through environmental aids) than to simply describe the medical findings (e.g. the angles of limb contractures in a child with muscular dystrophy).

Each district should have a child development team (Fig. 1) specialising in disability. Increasingly this is led by a community paediatrician. The team is responsible for helping the family care for their disabled child. The work of the team includes:

- assessment, diagnosis and management of the child with disability
- partnership with family doctor, local hospital services and tertiary paediatric resources
- partnership with Social Services, Education and voluntary sector agencies
- partnership with the child and family.

Assessment

A multidisciplinary diagnostic assessment will include a medical history and examination, an investigation plan and accurate assessment of a child's needs. A considered

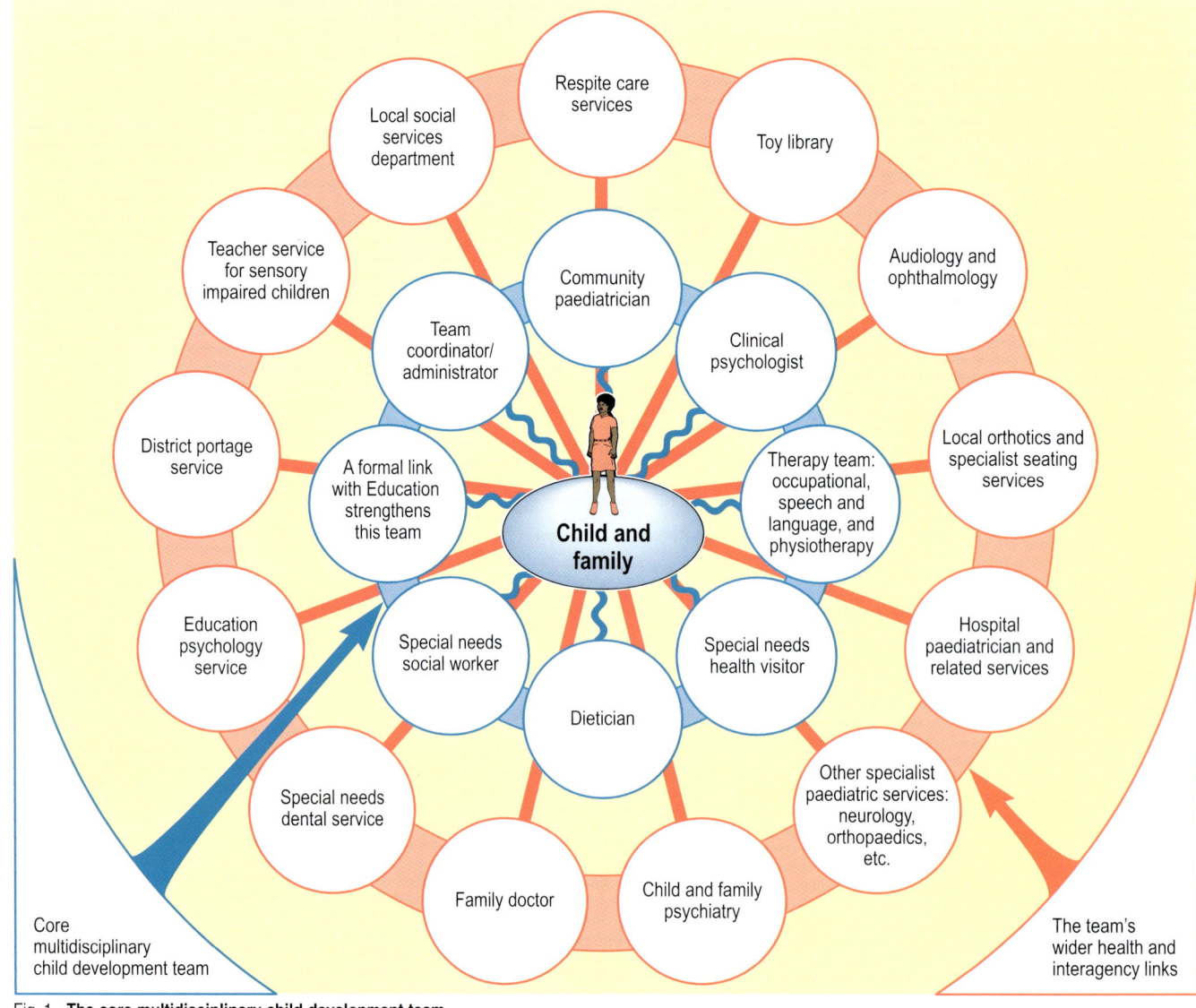

Fig. 1 **The core multidisciplinary child development team.**

search for a diagnosis will be made, following an investigation protocol for non-specific developmental delay and targeted investigations where specific disorders are suspected. Referral to hospital paediatric and tertiary specialist services for specific diagnostic or management issues will be made if necessary.

Development of a care plan and service provision

The care plan describes aims to meet the needs of the child highlighted by the assessment. It encompasses plans for medical treatment, the therapy programme, counselling and social support. It includes plans to liaise with other agencies. It is shared with the parents (and indeed the child when older), the family doctor and all professionals who need to know. Physiotherapy, occupational therapy, speech and language therapy and psychology input is planned. There may be joint programmes with a lead therapy. Further investigation or tertiary referral may be part of the care plan. Genetics advice is commonly required and may need sensitive timing. There may be a named key worker through whom the family can liaise with the team and with other agencies. The frequency of team or individual review is planned.

Aims of ongoing review

Follow-up reviews look at the child's development over time and at the care plan, adjusting it as necessary. Care is taken to prevent or detect early signs of secondary complications of the disability. *Secondary prevention* includes good seating and positioning management to reduce the risk of contractures or dislocated hips. Secondary effects include behavioural problems in autism or depression in a boy with muscular dystrophy. *Tertiary prevention* would include surgical correction of contractures or relocation of a dislocated hip, to restore mobility or seating position and to avoid longer-term joint pain. Review of growth and nutrition is always important: a feeding team is an essential subunit of the child development team and should draw on expertise from the community team, the dietician and the hospital paediatric medical and surgical services.

Use of specialist services

Specialist services fulfil key roles, e.g. the orthopaedic clinic for children with cerebral palsy, the neuropathic bladder clinic, child psychiatry, audiology, ophthalmology, etc. Close links with the hospital paediatric team are essential. The paediatric neurologist is an invaluable resource in diagnosis and management and may lead the management of

certain conditions, such as complex epilepsy. Genetic counselling should always be considered: the geneticist may help with the diagnosis and assessment of recurrence risk.

Aids and appliances

A responsive efficient service is vital for a child's orthotics needs (splints, braces, mobility aids). In addition, there are needs for specialist seating, lying and standing equipment, bathing aids, special utensils, etc. Environmental control aids may be needed to enable the older child to answer the phone, the front door, to use electric devices, etc. Augmentative communication aids, switch mechanisms and microcomputers, may turn an isolated non-communicating child into a participating, communicative one. Hearing aids and aids for the visually impaired are examples of specific equipment needs for certain disability groups. Housing adaptations are commonly required as the disabled child grows.

Education and careers advice

Notification to the Local Education Authority under section 332 of the 1996 Education Act ensures that educational needs are planned well in advance to assess whether mainstream schooling will be successful or special educational provision more appropriate. The team must notify the Local Education Authority (LEA) of children under 5 with disability known to them. A full assessment will be called for by the LEA where a child has or is likely to have special educational needs (SEN). Health professionals provide advice from their perspective on how the child's health needs impact on the educational needs, and advise on what requirements the child may have. A statement of SENs is a legal document committing the LEA to the provision of the resources outlined in the document. The team will be centrally involved in providing advice to family, the LEA and schools on an ongoing basis to assist in successful school placement and meaningful access to the educational provision.

The transition to adulthood is a vital time for the disabled young adult. The health team will join with the family, Education and Social Services to plan in areas of health needs, education and career plans, leisure and social needs and independent living, such as housing and mobility.

Social support and financial benefits

Support in this vital area may help families cope with the many practical and financial difficulties, including the loss of income incurred if a parent has to give up work to care for the disabled child. Services provided should include:

- *Advice on financial benefits:* Disability Living Allowance (DLA) and Invalid Care Allowance are two important benefits most frequently received. The Family Fund will often pay for equipment or expenses the family might otherwise be unable to afford.
- *The orange badge scheme* allows a disabled car user's badge for the carer of a disabled child.
- The team will also provide an *information resource* about local and national disability services.
- Introduction of families to relevant *voluntary societies and self-help groups.*
- An *underlying aim is to empower child and family* to manage the disability and to achieve as great a degree of independence as possible.

Respite care

Parents need their own time for rest, leisure or for personal appointments. Respite care is important for the health of the family and should be enjoyed by the child also. Social Service departments usually organise this service and find respite care families who will take children for regular breaks.

Voluntary societies and parent support groups

These are usually very helpful for families and an important source of information and support. They include the large national bodies such as SCOPE (cerebral palsy), National Autistic Society, Down's Syndrome Association, RNIB (visually impaired), NDCS (deaf children) and Contact a Family. Locally, there are often branches of the parent bodies and many independent self-help groups. The groups provide newsletters and keep the parents very well informed. They can also put parents in touch with other parents and this can be an invaluable avenue of support for the family.

The disabled child: management

- Management has to be multidisciplinary and interagency, with close cooperation between hospital, community and GP.
- Aims of management: to maximise potential and to minimise the handicap, to prevent or minimise secondary complications.
- A holistic approach is important to the child's health, including attention to nutrition and emotional well-being.

SQUINT

Squint is defined as the eyes not being aligned in the correct parallel manner. It is classified according to:

- *Direction of squint*, e.g. convergent (medial deviation of the eye) or divergent (lateral deviation of the eye).
- *Constancy of squint*, e.g. manifest (present all the time) or latent (present intermittently, e.g. when tired).
- *Function of extra-occular muscles*, e.g. paralytic (a muscle is paralysed) or concomitant (there is no paralysis).

CONCOMITANT SQUINT

This is the most common type of squint and is often familial. Treatment at an early age is essential before the vision in the squinting eye is suppressed by the occipital cortex to avoid the confusion of having double vision. This eventually leads to the eye not being able to see at all with permanent blindness (amblyopia). Therefore, children with suspected squints must be referred to an ophthalmologist before the age of 6 months since, if treatment is delayed beyond this time, permanent suppression of vision may already have occurred.

In this condition the muscles are not paralysed. Each eye can look in all directions individually, with a full range of extra-occular movements, but the eyes are malaligned, so that they do not look in parallel.

It is caused by anything which interferes with sensory or motor function of the eye, for example:

- poor vision secondary to obstruction of light entering the eye, such as a cataract or a corneal opacity

- blurred vision due to hypermetropia or myopia
- retinal abnormality, e.g. retinopathy of prematurity or retinoblastoma (Fig. 1)
- muscular imbalance of the extra-occular muscles, e.g. a muscle is too long or too short.

PARALYTIC SQUINT

Here, one or more of the extra-occular muscles is paralysed. The affected eye deviates in the opposite direction to the action of the paralysed muscle. The squint is present at all times, i.e. it is manifest. It is more noticeable when the eye looks in the direction of the action of the paralysed muscle. If it occurs in a young child, amblyopia may result. If it occurs in an older child, when the eye has already learned to 'see', double vision results because the extra image cannot be suppressed at that stage. The vision is therefore not lost in the squinting eye. The diplopia is maximal when looking in the direction of the paralysed muscle.

Such a squint can result from an abnormality of the eye muscle itself or the nerve supplying it. A cause must always be sought since a paralytic squint is often a sign of serious underlying pathology, e.g. a space-occupying lesion of the brain damaging the nerve supply in squint of sudden onset, or cerebral palsy when the squint is longstanding.

PSEUDOSQUINT

A number of infants appear to have a squint on initial inspection but formal testing does not confirm the diagnosis. This situation is called pseudosquint (Fig. 2). Hypertelorism (widely spaced eyes), epicanthic folds or mild facial asymmetry can all result in this optical illusion. No intervention is required.

EXAMINING AN EYE WITH A SQUINT

1. Establish the presence of a squint

Observe the eyes to see if the light reflection from the cornea is symmetrical. The light from a window can be used, or a torch shone in the eyes from 1 to 2 feet. Get the child to look in all directions to see if the squint becomes apparent or more obvious when looking in a particular direction. Ask the mother if she has noticed a squint at any time.

2. Establish if it is paralytic or concomitant

Examine the movement of each eye individually. If each eye moves fully in all directions when examined separately, the squint is concomitant; if one eye is unable to look in a particular direction, the squint is paralytic.

3. Further assessment of a concomitant squint

- *Check which is the squinting eye.* This can be difficult to establish. The 'cover' test is used. The child looks at a fixed object. One eye is covered up and then uncovered. This process is then repeated with the other eye. The squinting eye moves to take up fixation when the normal eye is covered. This is explained in more detail in Figures 3 and 4. Note that this process can make a latent squint more obvious and that both eyes may squint intermittently. In such a case both eyes are seen to move when tested. This is because the eyes take it in turns to fix on the object.

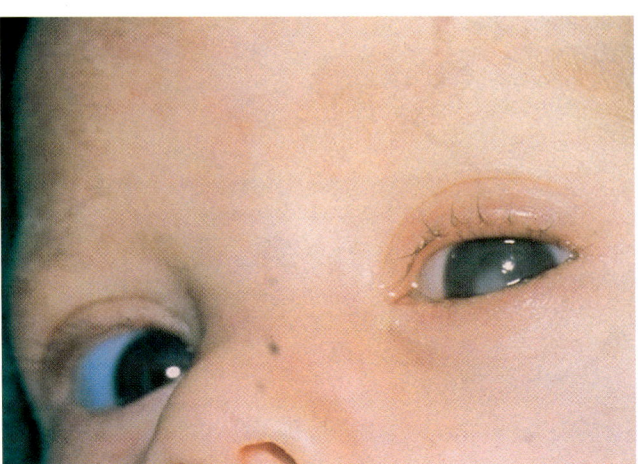

Fig. 1 **Retinoblastoma with squint.**

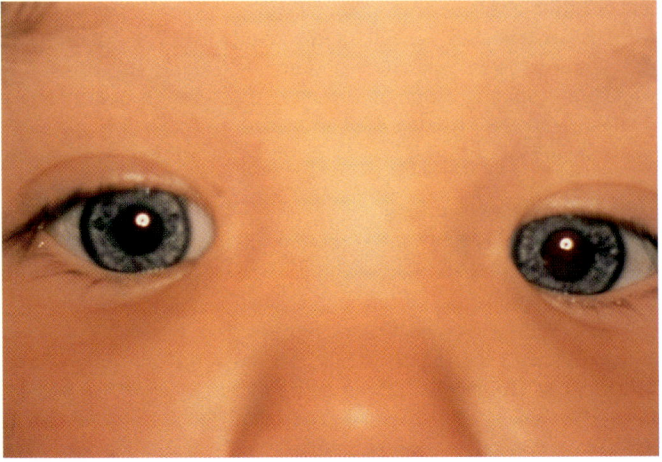

Fig. 2 **Pseudosquint.**

- *Check to see if there is a pathological cause.* Examine for cataracts, a corneal opacity and retinal disease.
- *Check the visual acuity of each eye.* The non-squinting eye would be expected to have normal acuity. The squinting eye usually has reduced acuity. Test to see if the child can see small objects with each eye separately: small sweets or beads can be used. If both eyes squint visual acuity is usually preserved in both eyes because they take it in turns to be the 'seeing' eye.
- *Examine for refractive defects.* This is usually performed by an orthoptist.

4. Further assessment of a paralytic squint

Determine the direction of greatest squint, indicating which muscle is paralysed, e.g. a medial squint with maximum diplopia on lateral gaze of that eye is caused by paralysis of the lateral rectus muscle, supplied by the sixth cranial nerve. Associated abnormalities of the eye may be present. For example, paralysis of the 3rd cranial nerve results in an associated ptosis and a dilated pupil. There may be signs of intracranial pathology, such as raised intracranial pressure (slow pulse, raised BP), other cranial nerve palsies or abnormal neurology in the limbs.

TREATMENT OF CONCOMITANT SQUINT

The aims of treatment are to: improve acuity in the squinting eye and improve alignment of the two eyes for cosmetic reasons and to provide depth of vision. Treatment consists of: glasses to correct refractive errors, patching of the good eye to improve the acuity of the squinting eye (Fig. 5) and surgery. Once glasses and patching have improved the acuity, the muscles can if necessary be shortened or lengthened by a simple operation to correct the alignment.

Part One

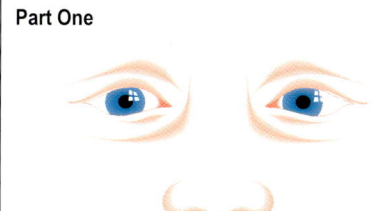

Step 1
Get the child to fix on an object. The good eye will look straight forward and this eye will be placed centrally: the right eye in this case. The squinting eye is turned inwards (medially).

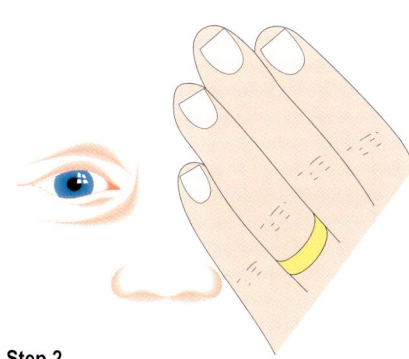

Step 2
Cover up one eye. If the squinting eye is covered, the good eye remains fixed on the object, so **no movement** will be observed.

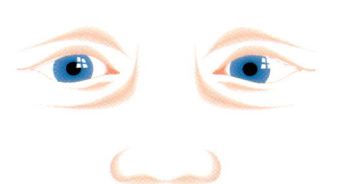

Step 3
When the hand is removed, there is still **no movement** as the good eye continues to watch the object.

Part Two

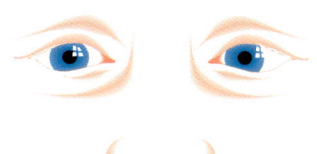

Step 1
The child fixes on an object again. The good eye is placed centrally and the squinting eye is turned inwards.

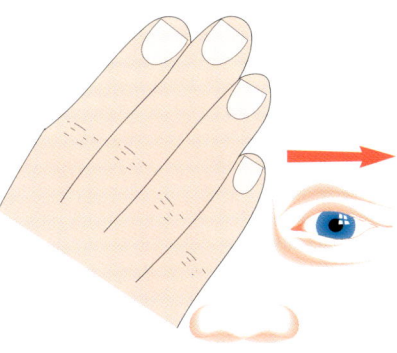

Step 2
The good eye is now covered, so the squinting eye must take over in order for the child to continue looking at the object. To do this, the squinting eye **moves** to take up a central position.

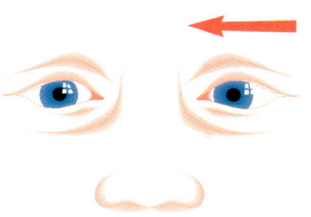

Step 3
When the hand is removed, the child prefers to view the object with the good eye. This eye therefore takes over fixation, so the squinting eye **moves again** back to an inwardly turned position.

Fig. 4 **The cover test.**

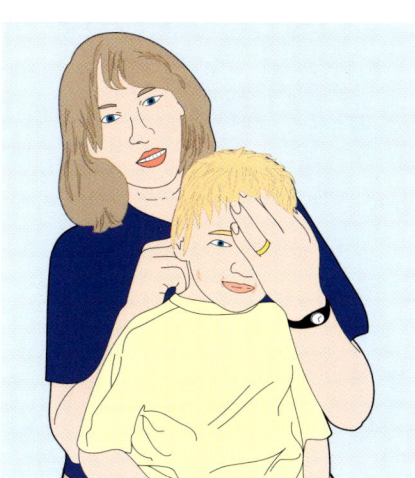

Fig. 3 **Position for performing cover test.** The child looks directly at the observer.

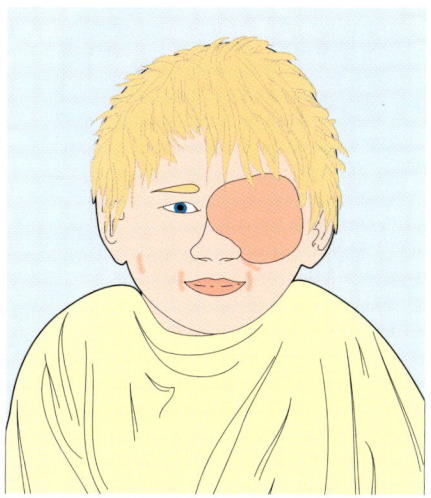

Fig. 5 **Eye patch used as treatment for squint.**

Squint

- Full CNS examination must be performed in all children with a paralytic squint.
- Acute paralytic squints must be investigated *urgently*.
- All concomitant squints should be refered to an ophthalmologist by the age of 6 months.
- Concomitant squints are often hereditary.
- NAI may present with a paralyic squint, secondary to a subdural haematoma.

VISION

Visual experiences are an integral part of a child's early development. We learn through observing, experimenting with copying what we see and refining our efforts. Significant congenital visual impairment, therefore, impacts on all aspects of early development and the child may present in infancy with global delay. In contrast, a deaf child may be thought to have normal development for many months. One child per 2500 is born with significant visual impairment requiring special educational provision. Less serious problems are relatively frequent. The most common are the correctable refractive errors: long sight (hypermetropia), short sight (myopia) and astigmatism. Strabismus, or squint, is also very common and has many alternative local terms: 'cast', 'turned eye', 'lazy eye', 'boss-eye'. Squint is covered separately on pages 22–23.

VISUAL PATHWAYS

Visual impairment can originate at any point along the visual pathway from the eyelids and cornea to the occipital cortex (Fig. 1). The sense of vision requires the combined function of the optical components of the eye and the neural pathways, including the integrative processing of visual information with the associated information of sound, touch, movement and memory of past experiences. The occipital cortex is responsible for the conscious perception of visual images and the interpretation of the messages received.

Myelination of the optic pathways is not mature at birth. Maturation and normal development of the optic pathway is dependent on exposure to light stimuli from birth. Where this is impeded, as with undetected or uncorrected congenital cataract or severe ptosis, visual loss may be permanent by 3 months, hence the importance of early recognition and surgical correction within the first few weeks of life.

Delayed maturation of the visual pathway causing abnormal visual responses for up to a few months of age may be part of the range of normal variation. However, it can also be an early sign of developmental problems which only declare themselves at a later age.

VISION TESTING

There is no widely applicable test of visual acuity in infancy and early childhood. Assessment of a child suspected of having impaired vision is, therefore, a specialist task.

Normal mature visual acuity for distance is 6/6 and is achieved by 7 years. A person with 6/6 vision can identify letters from 6 metres distance which an average adult could also see from 6 m. A visually impaired person with 6/60 vision identifies at 6 m what an average adult could see from 60 m distance. Letters of varying size are used to replace the need for testing over distance and the test is done in adults and childrem at 6 m. Reduced letter size allows testing of the young child at 3 m. If distance vision is normal, near vision is nearly always normal too in young children. Refractive errors can usually be corrected by spectacles.

VISUAL IMPAIRMENT

Visual impairment is described in terms of uncorrected and corrected visual acuity (Table 1). In Britain, people whose corrected vision remains significantly impaired are

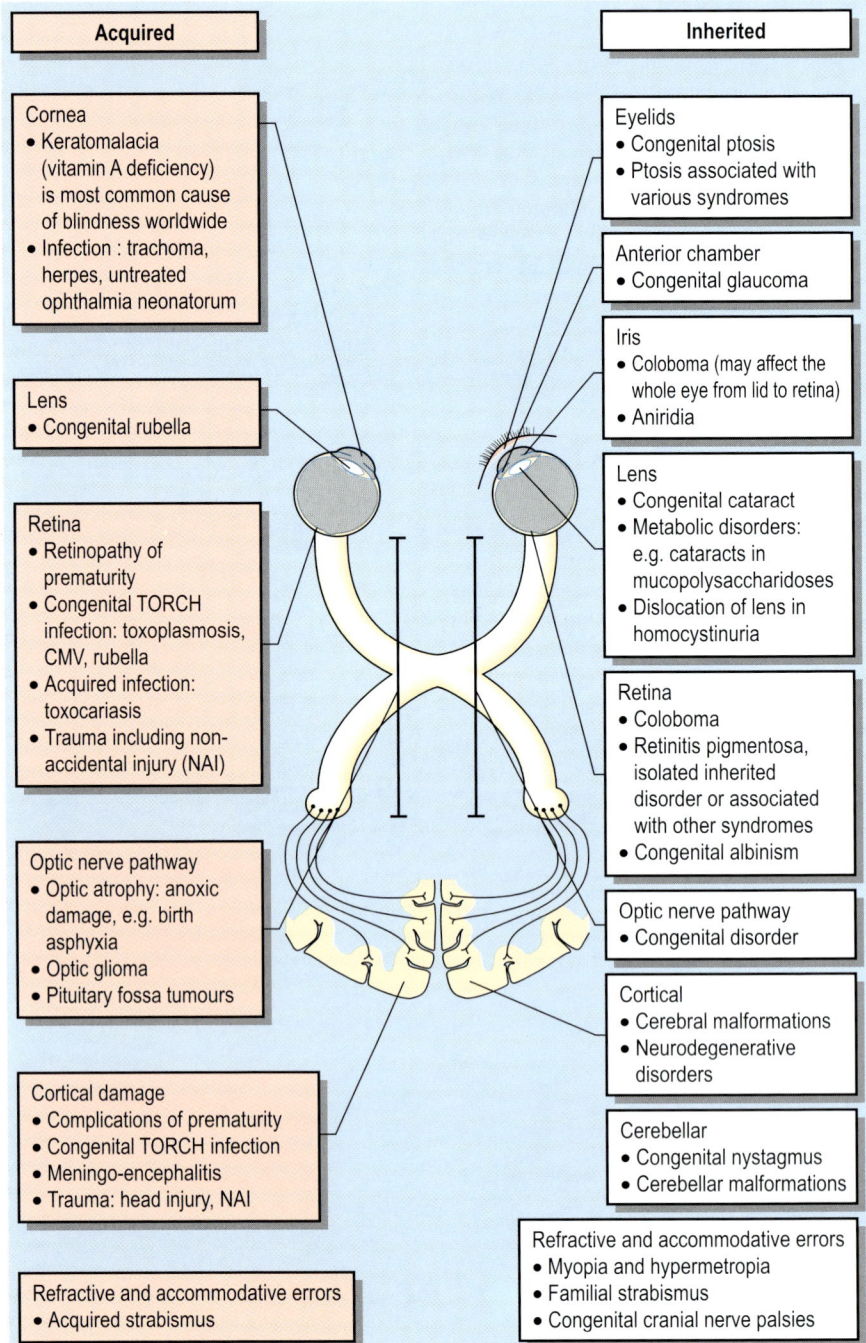

Fig. 1 **Causes of visual impairment.**

Acquired

Cornea
- Keratomalacia (vitamin A deficiency) is most common cause of blindness worldwide
- Infection : trachoma, herpes, untreated ophthalmia neonatorum

Lens
- Congenital rubella

Retina
- Retinopathy of prematurity
- Congenital TORCH infection: toxoplasmosis, CMV, rubella
- Acquired infection: toxocariasis
- Trauma including non-accidental injury (NAI)

Optic nerve pathway
- Optic atrophy: anoxic damage, e.g. birth asphyxia
- Optic glioma
- Pituitary fossa tumours

Cortical damage
- Complications of prematurity
- Congenital TORCH infection
- Meningo-encephalitis
- Trauma: head injury, NAI

Refractive and accommodative errors
- Acquired strabismus

Inherited

Eyelids
- Congenital ptosis
- Ptosis associated with various syndromes

Anterior chamber
- Congenital glaucoma

Iris
- Coloboma (may affect the whole eye from lid to retina)
- Aniridia

Lens
- Congenital cataract
- Metabolic disorders: e.g. cataracts in mucopolysaccharidoses
- Dislocation of lens in homocystinuria

Retina
- Coloboma
- Retinitis pigmentosa, isolated inherited disorder or associated with other syndromes
- Congenital albinism

Optic nerve pathway
- Congenital disorder

Cortical
- Cerebral malformations
- Neurodegenerative disorders

Cerebellar
- Congenital nystagmus
- Cerebellar malformations

Refractive and accommodative errors
- Myopia and hypermetropia
- Familial strabismus
- Congenital cranial nerve palsies

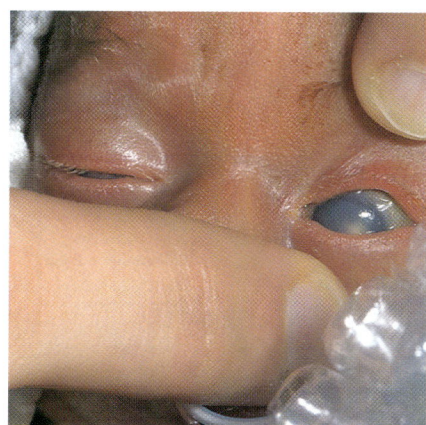

Fig. 2 **Eye of newborn with both corneal opacification and cataract.** Both abolish the red reflex.

registered partially sighted or blind. They are entitled to certain services and benefits through registration.

IDENTIFICATION

Parental observation and health education

Parents may notice altered visual alertness, responsiveness, following behaviour or squint.

Neonatal examination and 6 week check

These assessments look for congenital abnormalities and confirm the presence of a normal red reflex. The red reflex is produced using an ophthalmoscope at 12–18 inches on +3 setting. The posterior chamber is illuminated and light reflects back from the retina through the lens. Normal reflex excludes congenital cataract (Fig. 2). Fundoscopy of very premature infants is used to detect retinopathy of prematurity.

Infancy–2 years

There is no easily administered test for visual acuity but visual behaviour and development are important. Visual interest and ability to follow faces or objects are noted. The quality of developing hand–eye coordination gives good qualitative information about visual function.

3–5 years

The cover test can be performed to check for squints (pp. 22–23). Visual acuity can

Table 1 **Visual acuity and impairment**

Partially sighted	Corrected visual acuity between 4/60 and 6/24 in the better eye
Blind	Corrected visual acuity of 3/60 or less in the better eye (3/60 — equivalent to needing to be 3 m from letters which a normally-sighted person can read from 60 m)
Amblyopia	Permanent (non-correctable) reduction in acuity in one or both eyes

be tested using standardised charts in which the child matches letters identified by the tester at a distance.

School age

Most children manage the standard 6 m Snellen chart at school entry screening (5 years).

MANAGEMENT

General management

The work of the multidisciplinary team in supporting the parents and child with disability is described on pages 20–21.

Specific management

Medical. Early surgical treatment in the neonatal period is necessary for congenital cataracts. Very preterm infants need a careful ophthalmic follow-up to watch for retinopathy of prematurity, which can be managed with laser treatment if detected early. Refractive errors are often managed in children under 5 years by orthoptists and ophthalmic surgeons, later on by opticians.

Genetic. Genetic assessment is important because 50% of significant visual impairment is inherited and 50% is part of more complex disability where genetic advice may help in diagnosis and counselling of parents.

Developmental and educational. Full developmental and audiological assessment are critical and need to be carried out by a specialist team. It is vital to confirm if hearing and underlying developmental ability are normal. The teacher for visually impaired children is a vital part of the multidisciplinary team and is usually the key worker. Blind children and most who are registered as partially sighted will require special educational provision, often in a school for the blind.

Social. In addition to the usual disability benefits, registration of the child as partially sighted or blind has some attendant benefits. Some Social Services departments have specific social workers for the visually impaired.

PREVENTION

Primary

Awareness of the risks to the premature and sick neonate and improved intensive care have greatly reduced the incidence of retinopathy of prematurity. Rubella immunisation has led to the virtual disappearance of the congenital rubella syndrome of hearing loss, cataracts and heart disease. Hib vaccine has dramatically reduced the incidence of blindness secondary to

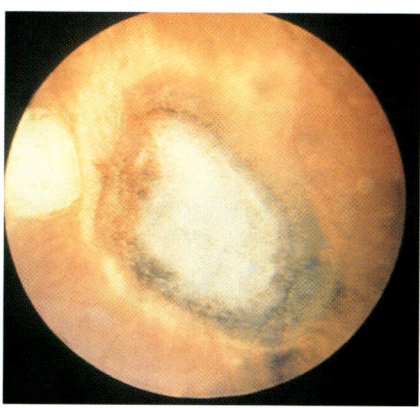

Fig. 3 **Chorioretinitis.**

Haemophilus influenzae meningitis. Public awareness of congenital toxoplasmosis has increased although the prevalence is higher in France and elsewhere than in the UK. Public health campaigns are probably the best way to reduce the incidence of acquired toxocariasis from dog and cat faecal material. Children with diabetes must be helped to understand the importance of good diabetic control to avoid longer-term complications, including diabetic retinopathy and cataracts.

Secondary

Early identification and treatment of correctable conditions such as cataract and squint are major reasons for the relevant parts of the child health surveillance programme. Management of amblyopia remains controversial. Effectiveness of early recognition and intervention has not been proven.

Tertiary

The multidisciplinary team and interagency cooperation have as their aim to minimise the effects of visual disability and to maximise potential through good health management, provision of aids, specialist teaching advice, social services and voluntary agency support.

Vision

- All children with developmental delay must have their vision assessed, and retinoscopy may be necessary.
- Up to 50% of blind children have coexisting and related disabilities.
- Genetic counselling is an important part of the investigation and management.
- Management of visual impairment requires a multidisciplinary team approach.

HEARING

HEARING LOSS

Hearing is necessary for a child to acquire normal language and good quality speech. Hearing impairment must be bilateral to significantly affect language development. Two children per 1000 have permanent sensorineural hearing loss (SNHL) requiring hearing aids and 1 per 1000 will need special educational provision. Far more children have conductive hearing loss (CHL) that is mild, fluctuating and usually temporary, caused by middle ear problems.

Hearing loss (HL) is defined as a hearing threshold worse than 20 decibels (dB) at a given frequency. The decibel is a measure of sound energy on an arbitrary scale where zero is the quietest sound heard by the average adult. Severity of hearing loss is described by the *average* hearing threshold across the frequency range for the better ear (Table 1).

Table 1 **Grades of hearing loss**

Normal hearing	20 dB or less
Mild HL	21–45 dB
Moderate HL	46–70 dB
Severe HL	71–90 dB
Profound HL	91 dB or worse

Types of hearing loss

In general, hearing problems of the external and middle ears — conductive hearing loss (CHL) — affect low frequency sounds most (particularly vowel sounds) whereas sensorineural hearing loss (SNHL) selects the higher frequencies (particularly consonants) and may affect the whole frequency range (Fig. 1). Middle ear problems are so prevalent that a mixed hearing loss with CHL and SNHL components present is not uncommon.

High frequency loss (always SNHL) is permanent and more disabling because consonants are more discriminatory for interpretation of speech. Hearing aids are usually beneficial here. Low frequency loss (usually CHL) can impede development but is usually amenable to treatment. Hearing aids are rarely necessary and are restricted to children who cannot be treated surgically.

Sound is received through the external auditory canal and vibrates the tympanic membrane, which augments sound energy and transmits it along the ossicular chain in the middle ear. The stapes bone passes on sound vibrations through the oval window of the cochlea and along the two-and-a-half spirals of sound-sensitive cochlear hair cells. These cells discriminate between the range of frequencies of sound and send impulses along the auditory nerve to the

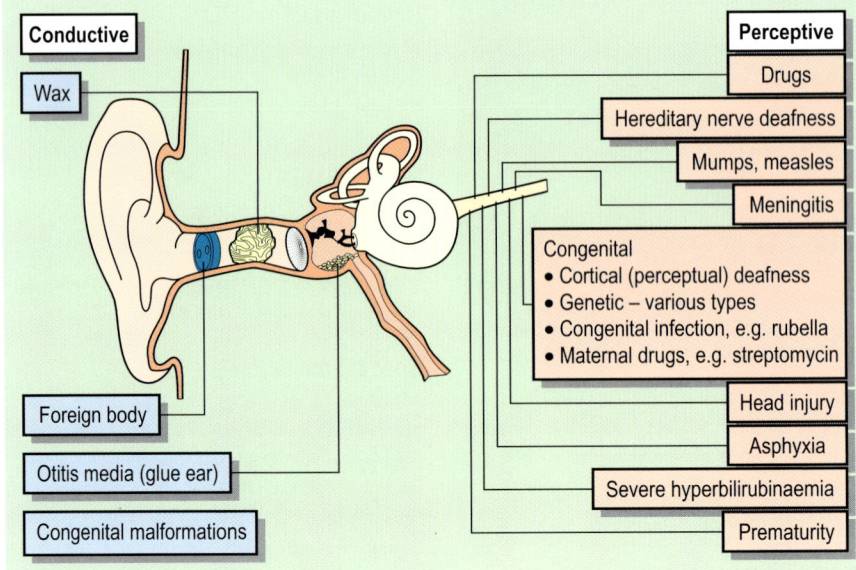

Fig. 1 **Causes of deafness in children.**

brain stem. Nerve pathways carrying the impulses from each ear cross over at brain-stem level. From there, information is transmitted to the cerebral cortex where it is interpreted. Problems with hearing can arise at any point along the auditory pathway.

External ear

Wax and foreign bodies only cause impairment if totally occluding the canal. Congenital atresia is rare, and is usually associated with middle and/or inner ear abnormalities.

Middle ear

Otitis media with effusion (OME or 'glue ear') is very common and is often associated with recurrent acute otitis media. Cleft palate and anomalies of the middle ear, e.g. Treacher–Collins syndrome, predispose to OME. Repeated episodes of acute suppurative otitis media may lead to perforation of the tympanic membrane.

Inner ear: the cochlear and VIII nerve

The majority of SNHL is explained by cochlear abnormalities.

Cortical deafness

Damage to the cerebral cortex may disrupt the ability to interpret sound impulses, despite normal hearing pathways up to brain-stem level.

IDENTIFICATION

The majority of hearing impaired children are identified either by recognising that

they are at high risk or by parents raising their concerns. Screening programmes are aimed at early identification of hearing impairment amongst otherwise normal children, since early intervention can significantly improve language and general development. Current approaches to early identification include:

- parental observations focused through health promotion advice in the parent-held records
- selective neonatal screening of high risk groups (Table 2)

Table 2 **Causes of childhood hearing loss**

Sensorineural hearing loss	Causes where CHL may coexist
Hereditary sensorineural deafness (50%)	
Congenital syndromes (numerous)	
Down's	*
Pendred's (hypothyroidism)	
Alport's (nephritis)	
Treacher–Collins	*
osteogenesis imperfecta	*
otosclerosis	*
Antenatal/perinatal factors (20%)	
prematurity	
maternal toxins, e.g. streptomycin	
congenital infection, rubella and CMV	
neonatal meningitis	
aminoglycoside-induced ototoxicity	
birth asphyxia: anoxic damage	
hyperbilirubinaemia (now a rare cause in the UK)	
Acquired (30%)	
trauma (head injury, fracture base of skull)	
meningitis	
viral infections: measles, mumps	

- population screening (see methods below)
- selective secondary screening of children known to be at risk (e.g. following head injury or meningitis)
- assessment of children presenting with problems associated with deafness (e.g. parental concern about hearing, language delay, recurrent ENT problems).

METHODS OF AUDIOLOGICAL TESTING

Evoked-response audiometry (ERA)
Brain-stem evoked response (BSER) tests electrical responses at brain-stem level to frequency-specific sounds. Oto-acoustic emissions test the sound 'echo' received back from the cochlea in response to sound presented to the ear. ERA can be used at any age, but may require sedation or a general anaesthetic in children over 3 months up to the age when cooperation can be guaranteed.

Developmental-based audiometry
Distraction hearing test
This is performed as part of the child health surveillance screening programme between 7–8 months. It is also used as part of the diagnostic assessment up to a developmental age of 18–24 months. It relies on the developmental ability of the baby to turn to localise the source of a range of sound frequencies offered at less than 35 dB sound level.

McCormick toy test
Between 3–3.5 years most screening programmes often use this freefield speech-based test. It is also used in the diagnostic clinic for children aged 2–4 years, i.e. until pure-tone audiometry is possible. There are seven pairs of common toys with matched sounds (e.g. tree/key, cup/duck). The test requires the child to identify toys named by the tester at less than 40 dB sound level.

Pure tone audiogram (PTA) with headphones
Frequency-specific sounds 0.5–8 kHz are presented to ascertain the quietest thresholds heard in each ear. This test is performed on all children aged 5–6 years in school. Children are referred on to hearing specialists if thresholds are worse than 25 dB. PTA is the gold standard audiological diagnostic test at all ages once cooperation is possible (variable success between 3–5 years).

Tympanogram (impedance measurement)
This is a measurement of compliance of the tympanic membrane and of middle ear pres-

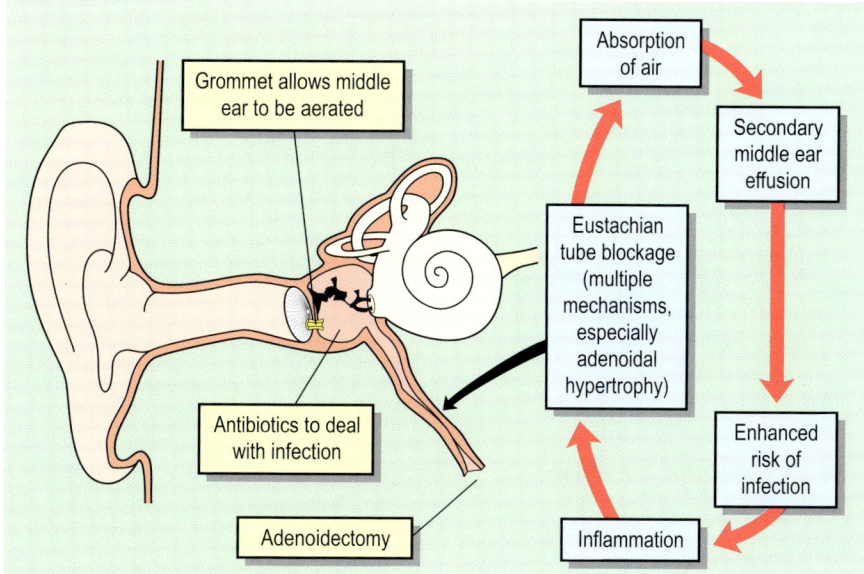

Fig. 2 **Glue ear mechanisms and treatment.**

sure. It is a diagnostic tool for middle ear disorders and can also aid assessment of nerve pathways through the stapedial reflexes. It requires minimal cooperation.

CONDUCTIVE HEARING LOSS

Otitis media with effusion (glue ear) (Fig. 2) is the most common cause of hearing loss in children (30–50% of infants and 10% of primary school children have middle ear fluid at any one time, 4% having persistent problems).

It results from occlusion of the eustachian tube, usually by large adenoids and repeated upper respiratory infection. Treatment is designed to aerate the middle ear either by 'unblocking' the eustachian tube (adenoidectomy) or placing a small tube across the ear drum (grommet). The natural history of the condition is spontaneous resolution, however this may take some years.

MANAGEMENT OF PERMANENT HEARING LOSS

General management
The work of the multidisciplinary team in supporting the parents and child with disability is described on pages 20–21.

Specific management
- **Medical.** Confirmation of hearing loss necessitates investigation.
- **Ophthalmic examination.** Hearing loss and chorioretinitis may coexist in congenital infections: rubella, toxoplasmosis or CMV.
- **Genetic counselling.** At least 50% of uncomplicated congenital sensorineural

HL is hereditary, and many more complex syndromes with genetic implications need to be considered in the differential diagnosis.
- **Hearing aid service.** The child must be assessed promptly for hearing aids. Babies grow quickly and need new fittings for fresh moulds for the hearing aids every 6–12 weeks.

Development and education
Full developmental examination is essential as part of the overall assessment. Educational needs must be planned well in advance to assess whether mainstream school will be successful or special educational provision is more appropriate.

Social support
In the UK there are two national societies, the National Deaf Children's Society (NDCS) and the Royal National Institute for the Deaf (RNID). Local parent support groups may exist.

Hearing
- Undiagnosed hearing loss may present as language delay, global developmental delay or behavioural difficulties.
- Selective neonatal screening will identify 50–60% of cases of sensorineural hearing loss.
- Audiological assessment is essential without delay following meningoencephalitis.
- Conductive hearing loss is very common.

BEHAVIOUR

Although the number of children attending the paediatric clinic with significant psychopathology is small, many children have psychological dysfunction which influences their physical health. Appreciating this component of any problem depends on a good understanding of the child's level of development and experience. All children are different and for some several interviews may be needed to assess important factors.

HOW TO COMMUNICATE WITH CHILDREN

Communicating effectively with children is often very difficult. With preschool children it is best to start with play. In school children, verbal language becomes increasingly relevant. In establishing *rapport*, younger children usually respond better to direct questions. Topics they will be able to talk about include the family, friends, favourite toys, food and daily activities. Older children prefer a more 'open' technique of interview, and will often have their own agenda for discussion, which may easily be stifled. Consider the child's developmental skills: a younger child will not usually respond to questions like 'Tell me about your family' but may be better at 'What does your brother like playing with?'. A child below 10 years will not usually be able to give significant information about the time of onset and the course of the illness.

BABIES

Sleep problems

These are common and usually take the form of difficulty in getting the child to sleep (see p. 34). In well babies this usually resolves quickly, so parents can be told of the good prognosis at the outset. Important areas to assess in terms of possible intervention include the baby's daily timetable, the parents' relationship with each other, and the parenting they themselves experienced. Many parents will have been offered lots of advice already and feel confused. Further advice may, therefore, be less helpful than listening to the parents, understanding their difficulty and showing interest in their baby. To get it to sleep, the parents must learn to put the baby down — often they find this very difficult — but the baby needs time on its own, and needs privacy. Babies who only sleep when 'rocked off' by a parent are being tranquillised rather than satisfied — the baby becomes dependent on this behaviour.

YOUNGER CHILDREN

Temper tantrums

These are common around the age of 2: at this age a child has a high level of speech and understanding, and is developing more complex (symbolic) thought, yet the child is still 'self-centred' and does not understand how his actions affect others. He discovers that he can influence his surroundings, e.g. sphincter control/control of his parents. There is a conflict between his newly-developing independence and a wish to return to babyhood. It is a normal phase of development, during which time the child needs to learn his limitations, but it is very stressful to parents. Often by the age of 2 there is a new sibling, aggravating the tension between child and parents.

Parents can be advised that all children have differing personalities, and the genetic component cannot be altered. However, there is much the family can do to improve matters. Tantrums should be ignored, however hard for the parent. When the tantrum is over, the child is then treated as normal. Any inconsistency will lead to failure, and the parent must show full commitment to obtain success.

Communication problems

Problems with speech are very common; the frustration engendered by being unable to communicate often leads to behavioural problems. The important causes include speech delay (either specific or part of generalised developmental delay), hearing loss (congenital or, more commonly, secondary to acquired middle ear disease) or sensory impairment (e.g. visual loss or lack of stimulation). It is important to understand that under these circumstances bad behaviour is not the primary problem.

A very small proportion of children with communication difficulty have *autism*, a rare and poorly understood condition affecting communication, restricting socialisation and often associated with a stereotyped repetitive social repertoire of interests and activities. This term is often overused: to be relevant to a child, symptoms should be present by 3 years, with both verbal and non-verbal communication difficulties and failure to develop social relationships. Many of these children also have major non-specific learning deficits.

Mutism is another rare condition (not to be confused with the speech problems of profound deafness or developmental delay). It often takes the form of *elective mutism*, whereby the child 'elects' to talk only in certain circumstances, for example at

home rather than at school, or to specific individuals only. Some of these children have suffered some specific psychological trauma.

Disorders of attention

Again, terms such as 'hyperactivity' are much overused, but can be reasonably applied if there is marked inattention and restlessness occurring in at least two places (e.g. not just at home) in a child whose problems started before the age of 6 years and have continued over at least 6 months. It can often be associated with developmental delay, but in other cases is the forerunner of more antisocial behaviour, as in conduct disorders. The prognosis is variable; some success has been achieved with formal psychotherapy and the use of the amphetamine, methylphenidate.

Conduct disorders

Social factors mainly determine whether behaviour is acceptable or not. 'Testing out' the environment is normal, particularly in young children. However, if boundaries are uncontrolled, serious problems can develop. The signs are different depending on age: the preschool child may have prolonged temper tantrums; in middle childhood there is deliberate aggression, teasing and swearing, and often cruelty to animals. Frank violence, truancy and drug abuse takes over as the child gets older, bringing the attention of the law. As in many behavioural disorders, there is hardly ever one single cause (Fig. 1).

Emotional problems presenting with physical symptoms

Recurrent non-specific abdominal pain is amongst the most common problems presenting to paediatricians. Although a careful clinical evaluation is required, in most cases no underlying disease process is found. A specific emotional or psychological cause is often not discernible, and management is concerned principally with reassuring the child, and especially the parents. Other common symptoms associated with anxiety include:

- headaches, dizziness and fainting
- recurrent sore throats
- palpitations and chest pain
- muscle pains.

Tics

These are repetitive, purposeless movements in the absence of a neurological cause. They usually involve the face (blinking or grimacing) or the neck (nodding) or both. They become worse at times of stress. In a mild form they are actually quite common. It is important to reassure the family that the problem will usually resolve with time, in order to minimise any further anxiety.

School refusal and truancy

It is important to distinguish these conditions. In *school refusal* or 'phobia', the child is afraid to depart from the home environment for that of school: anxiety or depression often play a major part. Symptoms of physical disease, as above, are common. Guidance and therapy are likely to be beneficial. *Truancy* is usually part of a conduct disorder, and parents often compound the problem, even expecting children to be at home.

Feeding problems

These are covered elsewhere (pp. 36–37).

ADOLESCENCE

Depression

Until recently, depression in children has been underestimated, but the incidence has been suggested to be as high as 4% in 14-year-olds. There may be any of the following: sleep disturbance, loss of appetite, school failure, social withdrawal, bad behaviour and fatigue. The causes are uncertain, but there may be an unhappy family or depressed parent; an adverse life event; loss of a parent or grandparent; or sexual abuse. Treatment is with individual and family therapy, where the possible causes are explored, and attempts are made to promote normal grieving, improved family and school functioning and environmental change as appropriate. Antidepressants require careful consideration but may be helpful in some cases.

Chronic fatigue syndrome

This condition causes severe physical and mental fatigue following modest physical or mental effort. Often there is depression or anxiety, and symptoms of physical disease (as above). It is more common in girls and can lead to extensive loss of schooling. Management is aimed at restoring a normal lifestyle over a period of months involving:

- paediatrician
- pychologist
- physiotherapist
- teachers.

The distress of the child must be acknowledged, while at the same time an organised and gradual return to normal activities is undertaken, e.g. starting back at school half days.

Eating disorders

These are covered elsewhere (pp. 36–37).

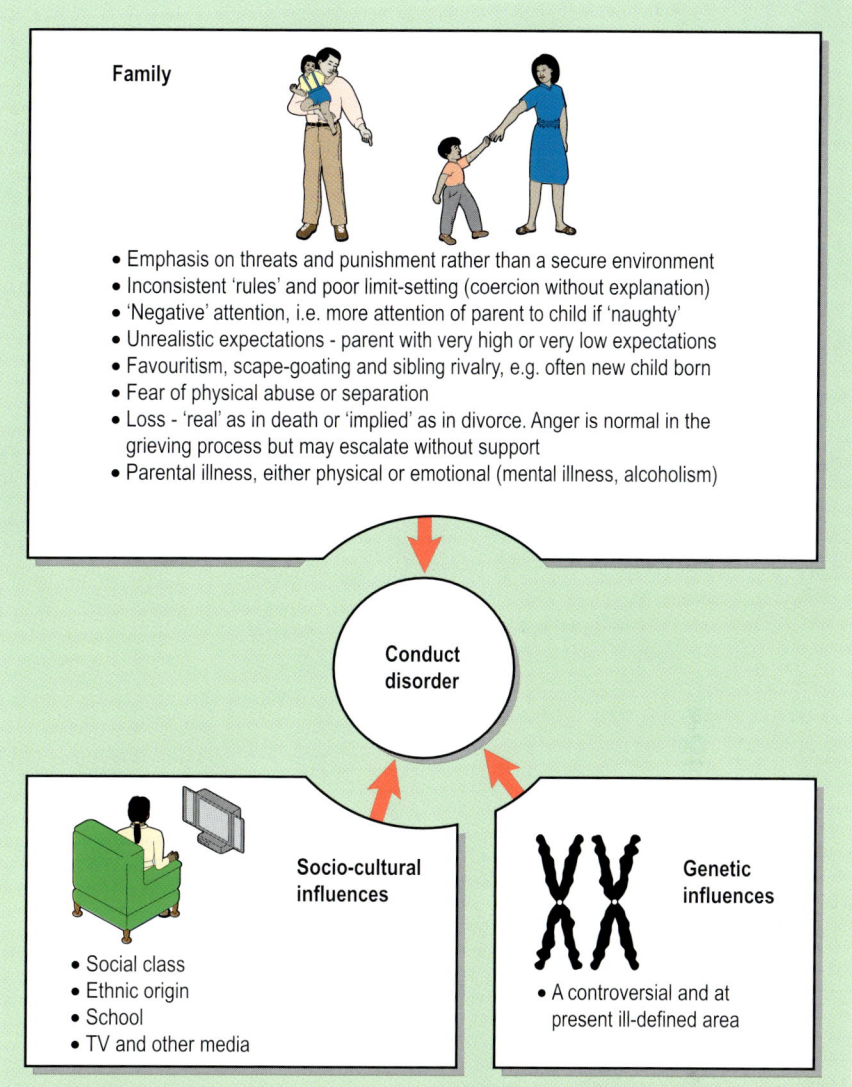

Fig. 1 **Factors thought to be associated with conduct disorders.**

Within figure:

Family

- Emphasis on threats and punishment rather than a secure environment
- Inconsistent 'rules' and poor limit-setting (coercion without explanation)
- 'Negative' attention, i.e. more attention of parent to child if 'naughty'
- Unrealistic expectations - parent with very high or very low expectations
- Favouritism, scape-goating and sibling rivalry, e.g. often new child born
- Fear of physical abuse or separation
- Loss - 'real' as in death or 'implied' as in divorce. Anger is normal in the grieving process but may escalate without support
- Parental illness, either physical or emotional (mental illness, alcoholism)

Conduct disorder

Socio-cultural influences

- Social class
- Ethnic origin
- School
- TV and other media

Genetic influences

- A controversial and at present ill-defined area

Drug dependency

Teenagers are vulnerable to drug dependency — they enjoy competing, 'having a good time' and experimenting. The most at risk include those with low self-esteem, or who are lonely and inadequate individuals. Typical drugs used include narcotics, tranquillisers, neuroleptics and antidepressants. Drug abuse is a progressive disorder, and can have devastating social, legal, physical and educational consequences. Management strategies include improving the child/parent relationship, self-help groups, psychotherapy and sometimes inpatient or foster care programmes.

AVAILABLE METHODS OF THERAPY

Usually simple guidance is all that is needed. When problems are more significant, the services of a child psychology team are important. Some conditions, such as sleeping and feeding problems in babies, and chronic fatigue, respond well to behav-ioural techniques, while others such as depression require mainly psychotherapy. Many conditions benefit from both. However, recently there has been a greater emphasis on family therapy, where the whole family attend sessions and the dynamics are observed and discussed.

Behaviour

- Always be alert to the possibility of an emotional cause for physical symptoms.
- Positively exclude organic disease before making a diagnosis of psychological disorder.
- Physical symptoms of emotional problems vary with age.

WETTING

NORMAL DEVELOPMENT OF BLADDER CONTROL

Patterns of urination in young children and babies are very variable. Babies commonly empty their bowels and pass urine immediately after feeding. After 6–8 months this pattern is less obvious, but it is rare to develop voluntary control of bladder function before 15–18 months of age. Usually the first indication of voluntary control is a self-interest in having just passed urine, children often pointing this out to the parent. Around this time they are able to communicate with increasing reliability if asked whether they feel they are likely to empty their bladder imminently. Urinary urgency is common at this stage and the child will often tell a parent just before micturition, without giving any chance for preparation. The urgency gradually lessens, and this is usually the time for potty training to start. At first the parent will do most of the work of preparing the child for the toilet, but the child soon takes over, often with considerable pride, and takes down clothes in preparation. This is usually the time to dispense with nappies during the day. In the next few months the child is still usually wet at night, but the retention span gradually increases so that by 30 months, two-thirds of children are dry at night.

DEFINITIONS

The term *enuresis* is usually defined as involuntary urination occurring in a child in whom bladder control would be expected. Primary enuresis refers to a child who has never been properly dry, and secondary enuresis when there has been at least a 6-month period of bladder control. Wetting only at night (nocturnal enuresis) is distinguished from daytime and diurnal enuresis. However, there are no specific age limits at which these terms can start to be applied, and in the individual child it is important to describe a wetting problem more directly.

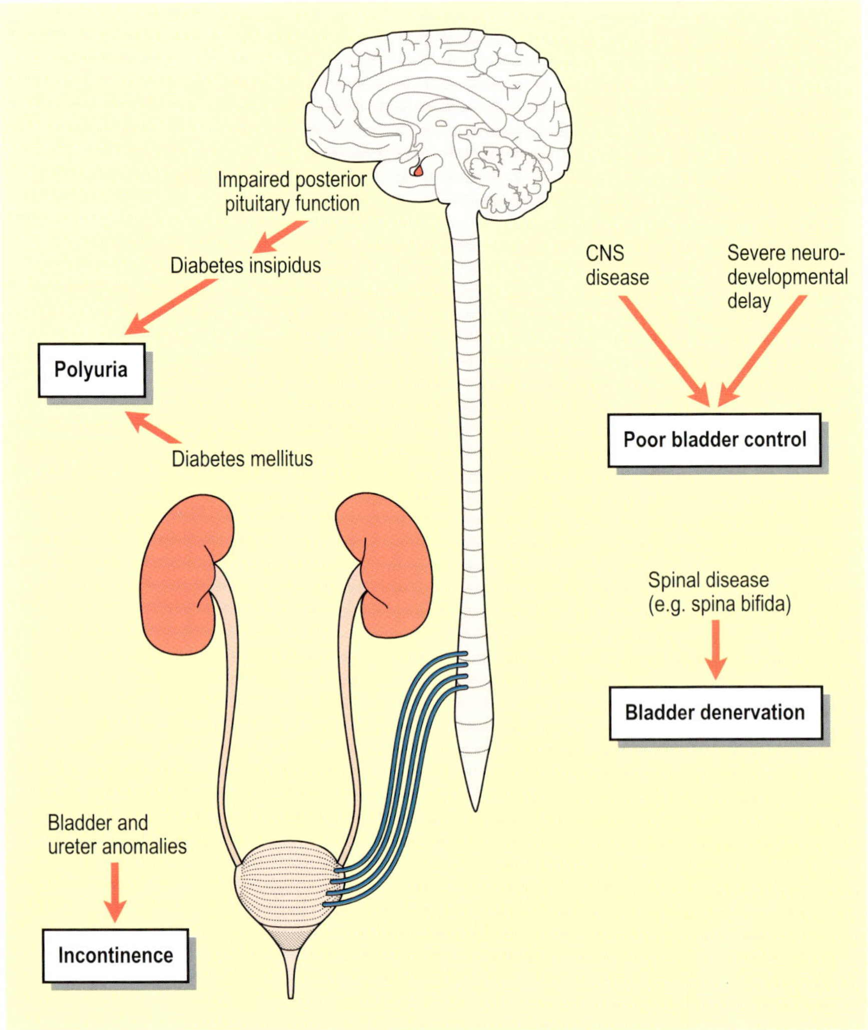

WHEN TO WORRY ABOUT WETTING

There are no strong divisions between normality and abnormality. In the majority of cases the picture is consistent with failure to change from the normal state in the first year of life, and management of these maturational aspects is dealt with below. However, there are certain features which, if present, point to concern for other causes of wetting, and make relevant investigations important (Fig. 1).

Secondary enuresis

Return of wetting in a child with previously consistent bladder control suggests either urinary tract infection or some specific psychological stress at home or at school. Sexual abuse should be considered. Nocturnal epilepsy is an unusual cause. Often though, a more detailed history will reveal a relapsing pattern of wetting without prolonged periods of dryness, and these children are not really different from those with primary enuresis.

Daytime enuresis

This is uncommon without nocturnal problems, and suggests an organic cause.

Incontinence

This is not always synonymous with enuresis. Continual dribbling, or dampness, suggests lower urinary abnormalities such as an ectopic ureter opening into the urethra, or a bladder diverticulum (Fig. 2). Neurological abnormalities as in spina bifida may result in a neuropathic bladder. Such children have complicated patterns of micturition with high pressures being produced in the upper urinary tract by uncoordinated bladder contractions. Further assessment involves urodynamic studies of

Impaired posterior pituitary function

Diabetes insipidus

Polyuria

Diabetes mellitus

CNS disease

Severe neuro-developmental delay

Poor bladder control

Spinal disease (e.g. spina bifida)

Bladder denervation

Bladder and ureter anomalies

Incontinence

Fig. 1 **Pathological causes of problems with micturition.**

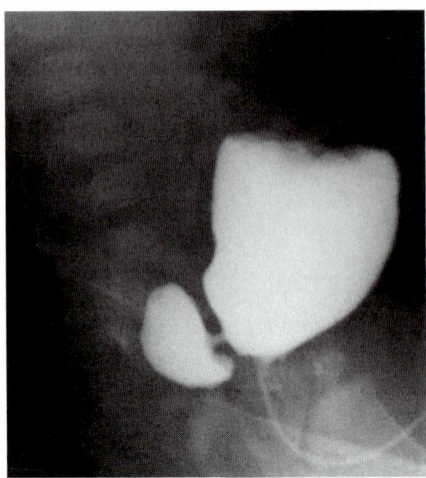

Fig. 2 **Cystogram showing a bladder diverticulum posteriorly.**

bladder function, and often treatment with intermittent self-catheterisation in cooperative children.

Polyuria

Parents may notice this as urinary frequency, but in polyuria large amounts are passed at each urination. More often it presents as polydipsia. Causes of polyuria include the following.

Habitual excessive drinking. This is the most common cause and is often started by inappropriate fluid feeds, e.g. as a comforter, in late infancy. Unfortunately, if this problem becomes chronic, it can result in a relative inability to concentrate the urine making distinction from organic causes more difficult.

Osmotic diuresis. Always check for glycosuria (diabetes mellitus) if there is acute onset of thirst and polyuria.

Failure to concentrate the urine. Babies have somewhat limited concentrating ability but after the first year of life it is normal to achieve urinary concentrations above 800–1000 mosm/kg. This may help the development of bladder control. Diabetes insipidus in childhood is either central (usually idiopathic), or nephrogenic (X-linked) with failure of the renal tubules to respond to normal levels of antidiuretic hormone. In these children urine osmolality is rarely over 200–300 mosm/kg even in dehydration. In chronic renal failure the kidneys respond poorly to changes in fluid intake, particularly because of the renal tubular damage. More specific causes of renal tubular damage may result in more complex problems such as the Fanconi syndrome, which, as well as polyuria, also causes (renal tubular) acidosis, hypokalaemia, hypophosphataemia, glycosuria and amino-aciduria. The pattern of loss from the renal tubules varies depending on the underlying diagnosis. Some syndromes are progressive and eventually lead to chronic renal failure.

APPROACH TO WETTING

Wetting becomes a problem when it interferes with the normal lifestyle within a family. Prevention is better than cure, and consistency is probably more important than any specific method of toilet training. The avoidance of prolonged conflict with the child means not forcing the use of a potty. There should be no fuss when the inevitable accidents occur. This all depends on parental personality and education, and professionals such as health visitors can be very useful in allaying anxiety at an early stage.

When a problem is established, further facts are useful to tell the parents:

- children vary greatly in the age at which they acquire control: about 10% of 5-year-olds are wet at night, but the number reduces considerably every year such that only about 2% of 12-year-olds are regularly wet
- enuresis is more common in boys
- a family history of wetting is common
- fluid restriction is not effective (except when previously excessive)
- constipation exacerbates problems of wetting.

Such discussions by themselves often make the problem less pronounced. Social conditions at home are also important: a washing machine will make changes of clothes and bedclothes much easier. Plastic undersheets are invaluable. Treatment and intervention are not usually considered until the child is about 7 years old; this is because of the natural resolution of enuresis in children around this time and the relatively poor rate of success in younger children. School nurses and social services may play a major role in family support.

Specific strategies for treatment of nocturnal enuresis include:

- **Star charts.** The child is encouraged to attach a star to a chart or calendar when he has not been wet and a reward is given for several dry nights in a row (Fig. 3). This encourages a positive approach to toilet training.
- **Alarm clock systems.** Children are taught to set an alarm clock for a time during the night before they are wet (say 2 a.m.), and the time set can be gradually put forward until the child is eventually dry all night.

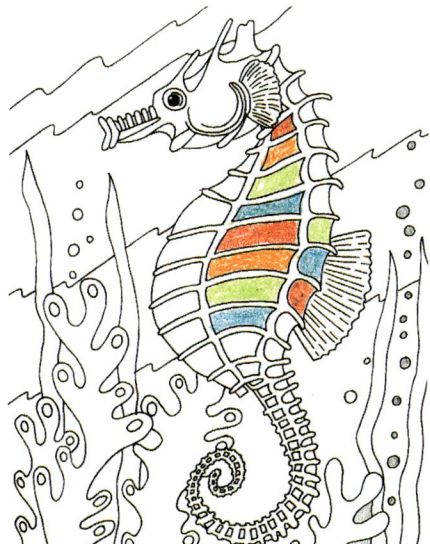

Fig. 3 **'Starcharts' can be individually tailored to the child's interests.** In this case the child colours in more of the picture after each dry night.

- **Buzzer and pad systems.** This is a similar pattern of therapy to that above, except that voiding triggers off an electric bell, and the child is wakened (Fig. 4). Both these methods are thought to work by 'conditioning' the child to respond appropriately around the time of micturition and, if successful, not only stop the child urinating in the bed, but also inhibit micturition at night altogether, presumably by improving bladder function.
- **Drug treatment.** DDAVP (synthetic antidiuretic hormone) is used successfully to inhibit urine production at night. In the past, other drugs such as tricyclic antidepressants have been used but these are rarely indicated now. Any drugs used for this condition should be given a limited trial period. Even if successful, relapse is common on stopping. However, they can be very useful for special occasions in order to relieve embarrassment, e.g. staying with friends, or on holiday.
- **Contact with special groups** such as the Enuresis Resource and Information Centre (ERIC). Such groups provide resources and advice to help parents and health professionals.

Daytime enuresis without a specific cause also often responds to psychosocial support and toileting guidance programmes.

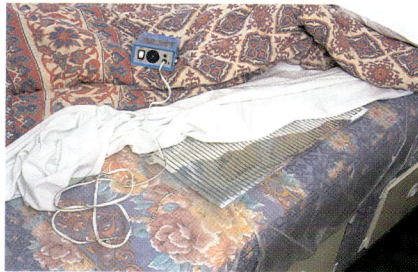

Fig. 4 **Pad-alarm system.** A low-current electrical circuit is completed by urine contact with a pad, setting off a buzzer alarm.

Wetting

- A return to daytime wetting in a previously dry child always requires investigation.
- Investigation and treatment of nocturnal enuresis should be delayed until 6–7 years of age.
- Punishment for enuresis is not helpful.

CONSTIPATION AND SOILING

NORMAL DEVELOPMENT

By the fourth week of gestation the intestines have formed a defined tube. From the fifth week, excess growth of the endoderm relative to the mesoderm results in partial blockage of the lumen. Recanalisation, in the seventh week, if incomplete, results in atresias or stenoses, particularly at the site of origin of the bile and pancreatic ducts. Rotation of the gut starts during the fourth week. At this time the structures that will form the rectum and anus are present as a hindgut ending in the cloaca. The cloaca then divides into an anterior urogenital sinus and a posterior anorectum. Division between the bladder and the rectum should be complete by the seventh week. In the female, any anomalies in this region are complicated by the interposition of the Müllerian duct system which may lead to a rectovaginal fistula.

Sucking and swallowing are established in utero and the term fetus may take in 500 ml of amniotic fluid per day. Meconium is usually passed within 24 hours of birth, and often in the first few minutes. It consists of swallowed amniotic fluid, mucus, bile, intestinal secretions and desquamated cells, and is dark green and soft.

Over the next few days meconium is gradually replaced by green or yellow, more formed, stools. The character of infant stools is very variable and depends on the type of feeding. Breast-fed babies tend to have soft, mustardy-yellow stools, whereas babies fed on artificial milk usually open their bowels less frequently and have firmer stools. Constipation without a specific cause is quite uncommon in breast-fed babies.

Voluntary bowel control is usually achieved before the second birthday but there are considerable variations, much as with the development of bladder control (pp. 30–31). There is often a phase of great self-interest in eliminations and lavatories, and this behaviour can be a particular source of pleasure for the child by manipulating the parents who become frustrated and anxious. If this phase is not successfully resolved, long-term problems with bowel control may ensue (Fig. 1).

NEONATAL CONSTIPATION

Hirschsprung's disease

Failure to pass meconium in the first day of life may suggest Hirschsprung's disease. This is due to an absence of ganglion cells in the inhibitory myenteric plexus innervating the large bowel. The length of bowel affected by this defect is variable: in 'short-segment' disease the problem is confined to the rectum. Failure of the internal anal sphincter to relax in response to rectal dilatation leads to a degree of obstruction. In other cases (long segment), the sigmoid colon and more proximal colon are also involved.

Boys are affected more commonly than girls and the disease can be familial. Most cases present in the first week of life with bowel obstruction: the abdomen becomes progressively distended, often with visible peristalsis. Rectal examination can be diagnostic by the rapid expulsion of faeces or meconium on withdrawal of the finger. Bile-stained vomiting occurs if obstruction continues. Plain X-rays show absence of gas in the rectum and dilated loops of bowel above the lesion. The definitive diagnosis depends on rectal biopsy demonstrating the absence of ganglionic cells in the affected segment.

Treatment is surgical; usually a diverting colostomy is performed initially, with removal of the aganglionic segment and anastomosis of healthy bowel at a later stage. A small number of children with quite extensive Hirschsprung's disease go through infancy with minimal symptoms and present later with constipation and soiling. There is, however, usually a history of delay in passage of meconium even in these children. The mortality in late-diagnosed cases, whether in the neonatal period or later, is significant, with bowel perforation, sepsis and shock, all recognised complications.

Other causes

Other causes of bowel obstruction presenting in the neonatal period include:

- intestinal atresias or stenoses
- imperforate anus
- malrotation
- meconium ileus.

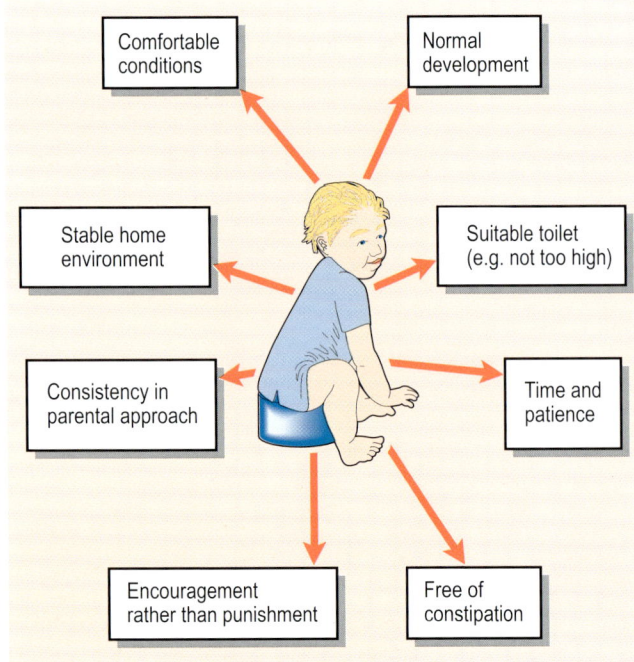

Fig. 1 **Some elements for successful toilet training.**

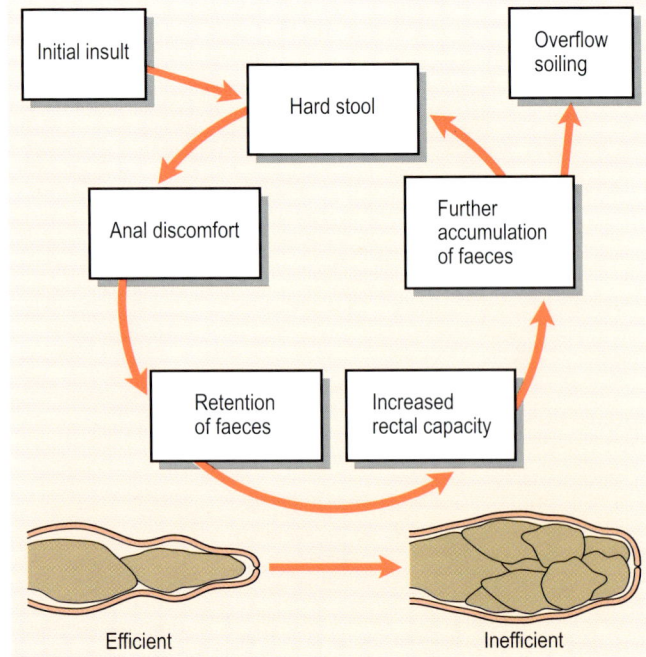

Fig. 2 **Vicious cycle of constipation.**

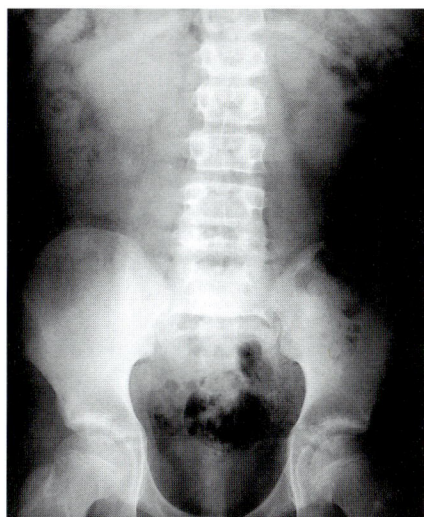

Fig. 3 **Plain abdominal film showing faecal loading.** Although not necessary to diagnose constipation, X-rays can be useful in evaluation and to show the child the problem.

CONSTIPATION AND SOILING IN CHILDHOOD

Many factors can lead to constipation. Often the cause is obscure but sets off a vicious cycle which exacerbates the problem (Fig. 2). In particular, even one hard stool may cause an anal tear which hurts the child so that the further normal passage of stools is withheld. This leads to further constipation and eventually to overflow faecal incontinence and soiling. When established, it is often very difficult to break this cycle.

Plain X-rays are of value in assessing the degree of constipation (Fig. 3).

Causes

Causes of constipation include the following:

- **Dietary factors.** Although plenty of roughage is now more generally recognised as an important dietary constituent, poor diet is still frequently a major factor. Too much milk is often included in the diet of a toddler. However, a good fluid intake in combination with adequate roughage is important in relieving constipation.
- **Anal anomalies.** Mild degrees of anal stenosis may resolve spontaneously. Anal malposition (usually anterior displacement) can be clinically overlooked.
- **Neurological.** Loss of voluntary control leading to soiling may occur in the severely subnormal. Even in very severe neurodevelopmental delay it is constipation that is commonly the major problem rather than the expected faecal incontinence: the combination of chronically poor gastrointestinal tone and motility and poor diet leads to very prolonged food transit times.

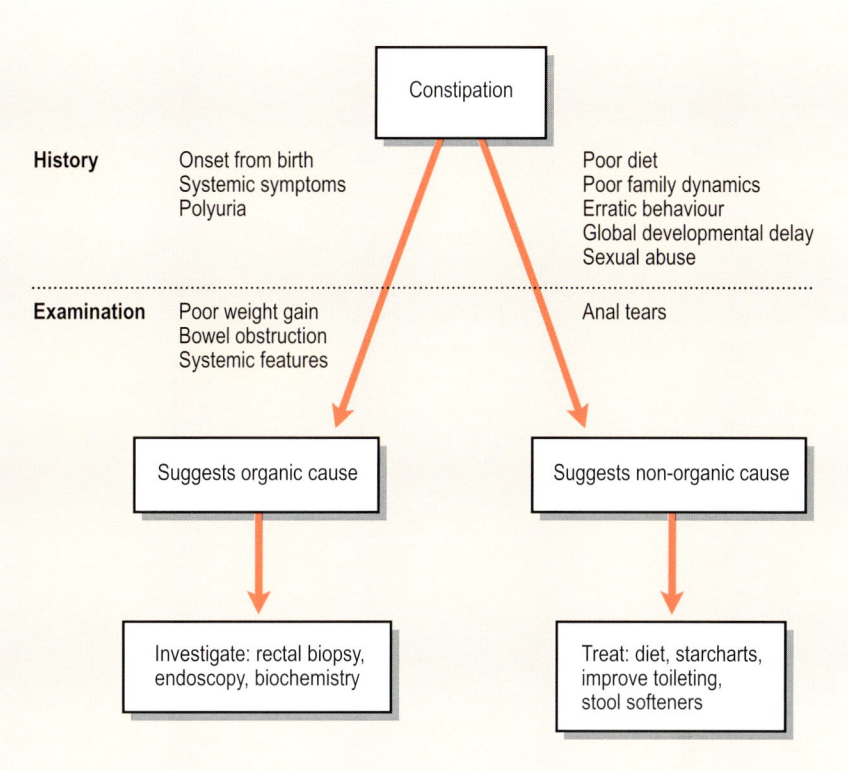

Fig. 4 **Simple approach to constipation management.**

- **Metabolic causes.** Hypothyroidism, hypercalcaemia and any cause of polyuria are rare causes of constipation.
- **Chronic disease.** Cystic fibrosis and inflammatory bowel disease are two chronic diseases which may present in this way. In less Westernized areas, 'common' constipation is rare, presumably related to lifestyle and diet, even in childhood, but chronic infections can cause severe gastrointestinal problems. In American trypanosomiasis (Chagas' disease), the initial acute phase of infection by *T. cruzi* is usually asymptomatic and unrecognised in infants and children, but the chronic phase, perhaps 10 years afterwards, can involve the heart, CNS, and gastrointestinal tract with destruction of ganglia, particularly in the oesophagus and large bowel. Millions are affected in Latin America.
- **Sexual abuse.** This should be considered particularly when the onset of constipation is acute or if there are signs of trauma.

TREATMENT

Apart from addressing the causative factors as above, the most important aspect of management is to realise that chronic constipation requires long-term treatment (Fig. 4). Stool softeners such as lactulose are helpful, but some children also need stimulant laxatives like senna, as the voluntary retention of stools tends to persist even after the stools have become looser.

Suppositories and enemas have a very limited role in paediatrics as they are physically and psychologically traumatic. It is important to be able to discuss bowel function easily with children, and the family will need explanation and support to continue with prolonged medication

ENCOPRESIS

Whereas soiling is caused by the involuntary passage of loose stool, and usually associated with constipation, encopresis refers to inappropriate opening of the bowels, often in inappropriate places, but certainly not in the toilet, in the absence of physical disease. It is usually related to a significant psychological problem. There are often other features of aggression in the child, and a disordered parent–child relationship. Treatment is usually geared towards family therapy.

Constipation and soiling

- Babies usually pass meconium in the first 24 hours after birth.
- Constipation in childhood often requires long-term treatment and family support.
- Overflow soiling is often confused with diarrhoea.
- Encopresis should be distinguished from soiling and constipation.

SLEEP

Variations in sleeping pattern are common in children. Unusual sleeping patterns may not in themselves cause a problem, but disorders of sleep can often cause significant stress to all the members of a family and have a deleterious effect on a child's educational achievements as well as, in some cases, the parents' jobs. Despite this, problems with sleep are frequently referred late for a medical opinion and often only after considerable conflicting advice from relatives and friends. Even when they are referred, the management is often inadequate. The development of sleep is related to age and as children become older, they need fewer hours of total sleep and have less rapid eye movement (REM) and non-REM deep sleep (Fig. 1).

The sleep cycle is accompanied by various hormonal rhythms that occur during sleep: growth hormone (GH) is released just after the start of a phase of deep sleep, prolactin is maximally secreted in the early morning, followed by corticosteroid secretion. The causes of sleep problems are varied (Table 1). In many cases they are a result of particular child rearing practices but they may also be associated with organic disease either in children who are acutely unwell or in those with psychiatric and/or mental handicap (Table 2). In this last group, although the sleep problem may be caused by poor sleep habits, some specific sleep disorders are also well recognised such as obstructive sleep apnoea in Down's syndrome. Most sleep problems can be assessed on an outpatient basis (Table 3). For some of these patients, physiological sleep recordings are helpful and in others

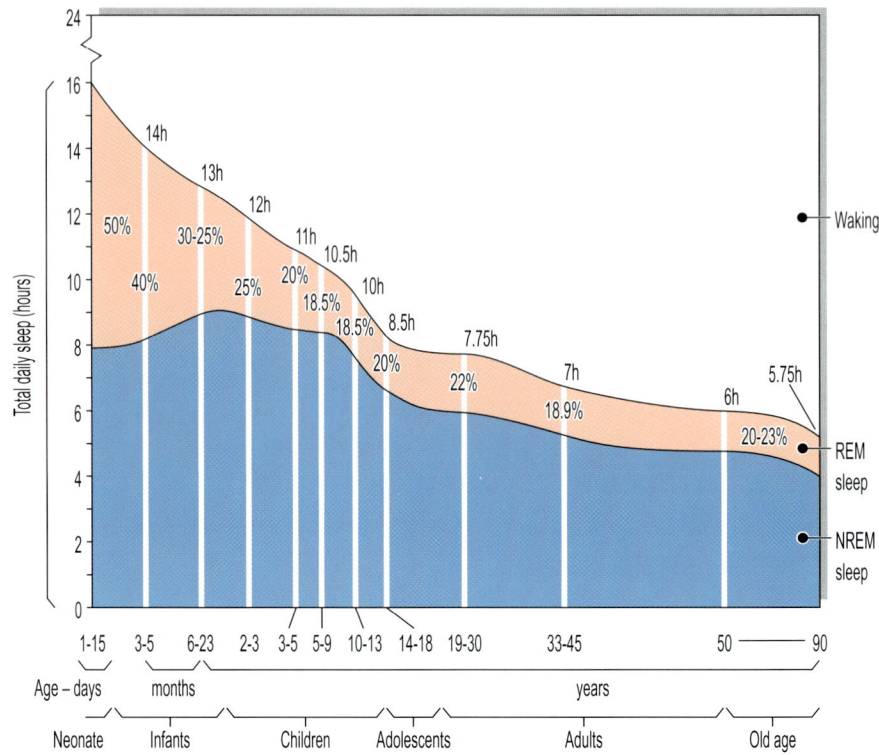

Fig. 1 **Amount of sleep required according to age.** (Modified from Roffwarg *et al* 1966 Science 152: 604–619)

home video assessments of their sleep can be useful.

SLEEPLESSNESS

This can refer to many different situations and a careful history must be obtained in order to define the nature of the problem. There may be a reluctance to go to sleep at the time expected by the parents or just difficulty in getting to sleep. Sometimes the problem is of repeated waking during the night, or it can be that the child wakes too early for the parents in the morning. Some children only need a very small amount of sleep: this may not suit their parents. The

age of the child must always be taken into consideration when the cases are assessed.

In some babies, night-time waking may be because they are in the habit of regular night feeds. In most circumstances night-time feeding should be reduced or stopped once it is no longer needed to try to promote longer night-time sleeps. Young children with no routine to their bedtime are often reluctant to settle into night-time sleep in a regular way. This can be exacerbated if there are extra daytime sleeps, irregular meals and generally if their days lack routine. Older children have more fears and may be frightened to go to bed or to sleep. They may fear the dark or being alone or have vivid imaginations; for example, believing there to be snakes under the bed. If an adolescent is having sleeplessness problems, there may be genuine emotional problems, e.g. quarrelling parents or teasing at school causing anxiety. As with adults, coffee, alcohol and 'drugs' can all result in sleep problems.

For many of these situations a regular bedtime routine, and reassurance so that the child feels safe at night, is all that is necessary to resolve the problem. Although sedatives can be prescribed, they are rarely recommended and should never be more than a short-term measure. Psychological factors need to be attended to and in some cases behavioural programmes can be used.

Table 1 **Types of sleep disorder**

Sleeplessness	Problems with settling into sleep
	Recurrent waking
	Early waking
	Short duration sleep
Night-time attacks	Headbanging
	Night terrors and sleepwalking
	Nightmares
	Nocturnal seizures
Excessive sleepiness in the day	Insufficient night-time sleep
	Sleep pathology, e.g. sleep apnoea and narcolepsy

Table 2 **Causes of increased risk of a sleep disorder**

- Physical illness — fever, pain, dyspnoea, (e.g. asthma), nocturia
- Medications, e.g. anti-asthma treatment and anticonvulsants
- Hospital admission — upset sleep patterns, anxiety
- Mental handicap
- Psychological disturbance, e.g. anxious children, depressed adolescents, conduct disorder children

Table 3 **Investigation of sleep problems**

- Full history, in particular
  — bedtime routine
  — nature of sleep, length of sleep
  — nature of events during sleep
  — waking pattern
  — activity and mood when awake, any extra daytime sleeps
  — medications
  — family history of sleep disorders
  — family dynamics
- Sleep diary
- X-rays of pharynx, chest, airways
- Physical examination
- Physiological sleep studies, EEG, oximetry while asleep
- Overnight video recordings (if indicated)

NIGHT-TIME ATTACKS

There are different episodes which occur during the night and they should not all be labelled as nightmares. These different attacks happen at certain stages of sleep. At the start of sleep headbanging or other rhythmic movement disorders can occur and are common in children under 3 years. Parents need to be reassured that the repetitive movements help the child to get to sleep and they almost always grow out of it. If the headbanging occurs in the daytime, the behaviour is more worrying and may imply an underlying condition such as developmental delay or autism.

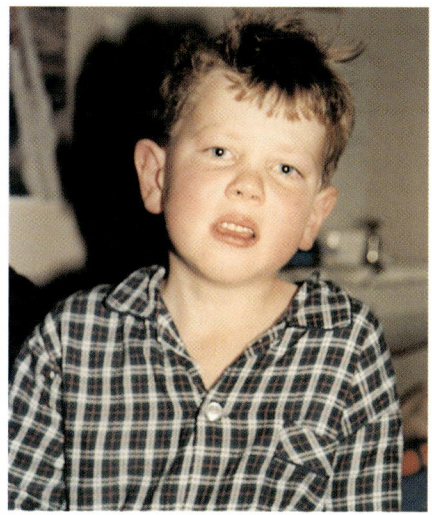

Fig. 2 **A child having a night terror.**

Once a child has gone into deep non-rapid eye movement (NREM) sleep, night terrors and sleepwalking episodes can occur in which the child does not usually wake up. A child who is having a night terror seems to wake up (but does not), cries and appears very distressed, then after a period of about 10 to 15 minutes settles down and returns to peaceful sleep (Fig. 2). During this period the child resists cuddling and consoling and does not recognise anyone (because he/she is asleep). If these attacks are very regular, the cycle can sometimes be broken by waking the child completely just before the parent thinks an attack is about to occur. In sleepwalking, the child again does not wake up but walks around the house purposefully. The usual age for this is between 4 and 8 years. Fortunately, children grow out of both of these types of attack and treatment with drugs is usually not indicated.

Nightmares are frightening dreams that occur in rapid eye movement (REM) sleep, which happens later on in the night. The dream can always be recounted and the child wakes and needs to be comforted. Fears from real life can contribute to nightmares, either from reading, television or from personal experiences.

All of these non-epileptic attacks are fairly common and they improve and stop as the child gets older and are rarely associated with psychological problems.

Nocturnal seizures are unusual compared to all the above night-time attacks. If children have seizures during the day, there should be a higher index of suspicion that they might suffer from night-time attacks as well. Nocturnal seizures can occur at any time of night and are usually complex partial seizures. EEG recordings may be needed to determine the diagnosis in consultation with a neurologist.

EXCESSIVE SLEEPINESS IN THE DAY

This is often misdiagnosed as boredom or laziness and children may present with learning difficulties. The most common treatable cause is obstructive sleep apnoea when enlarged tonsils and adenoids cause obstruction to breathing, particularly at night, which results in snoring and restless sleep. If the tonsils and adenoids are removed, there is usually a dramatic resolution of the symptoms and, in some cases, better performance at school (the improved sleep pattern improving concentration).

Narcolepsy, pathological sleepiness, is rare. Most excessively sleepy children are just lacking adequate sleep for reasons both social and psychological. The main difficulty in these children is the recognition of this problem.

TREATMENT OF SLEEP PROBLEMS

A number of possible remedies of sleeplessness and other problems are summarised in Figure 3.

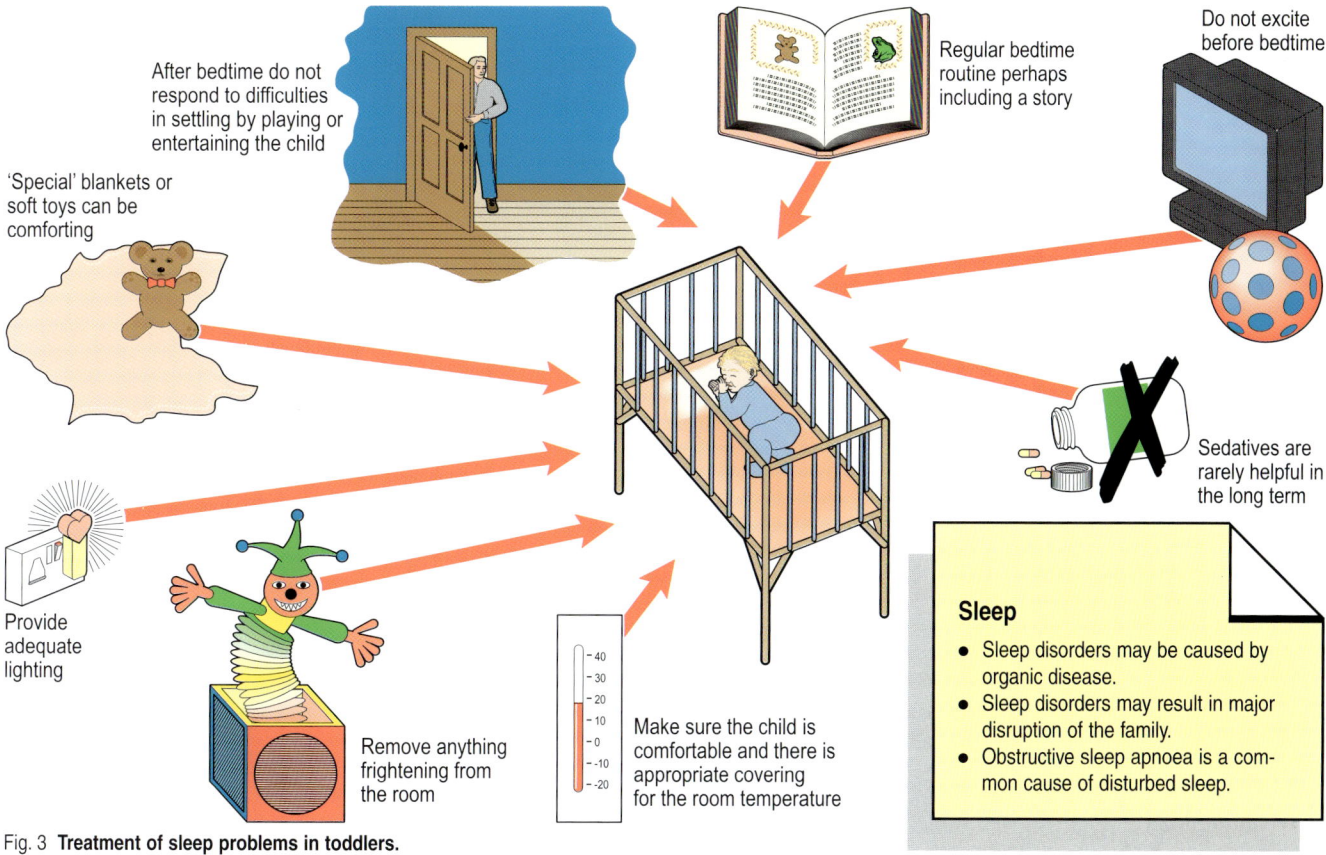

After bedtime do not respond to difficulties in settling by playing or entertaining the child

Regular bedtime routine perhaps including a story

Do not excite before bedtime

'Special' blankets or soft toys can be comforting

Sedatives are rarely helpful in the long term

Provide adequate lighting

Remove anything frightening from the room

Make sure the child is comfortable and there is appropriate covering for the room temperature

Sleep
- Sleep disorders may be caused by organic disease.
- Sleep disorders may result in major disruption of the family.
- Obstructive sleep apnoea is a common cause of disturbed sleep.

Fig. 3 **Treatment of sleep problems in toddlers.**

FEEDING

Feeding problems in childhood are a common cause for concern; however, the term covers a multitude of situations. Some of these reflect a lack of knowledge by the child's carers (e.g. the amount of milk a baby needs), others represent normal variation (the fact that some babies open their bowels during every feed) and a minority are 'pathological' or at least merit investigation.

INFANTS AND TODDLERS

Figure 1 summarises the normal feeding recommendations in the first year of life.

MILK FEEDING

The breast-fed infant

Clearly at one time all infants were breast-fed. However, the introduction of formula milks and the tendency for extended family networks (in the Western world) to be stretched over many miles has led to a general loss of skills and support available to new mothers. As a result, management problems are common. However, there is no doubt that there are advantages to the infant from breast feeding:

- correct biochemical composition (e.g. low sodium, low solute load)
- specific anti-infective properties (e.g. antibodies against bacteria identified in the mother's gut)
- non-specific and anti-infective properties (e.g. low free iron content — inhibits division of *E. coli*)
- maternal infant bonding is enhanced.

At birth the breasts contain only small amounts of protein-rich milk called colostrum. Significant amount of milk are not made for perhaps 48 hours in a first baby, less for subsequent deliveries. In the interval, the hungry baby sucks frequently and this is important in enhancing the supply of milk that will become available. However, this demanding behaviour can cause great distress to a tired mother. In particular, the frequent sucking can make the nipples very sore if the baby is not properly 'fixed' to the breast (Fig. 2). Similarly, during this time the nipples may crack allowing the baby to swallow significant amounts of maternal blood. Haematemesis and melaena may follow and cause great alarm.

Once the milk supply is established, frequency of feeding is very variable and it is impossible to define 'the norm'. However, if the baby is feeding very frequently, it is important to consider whether the milk supply is inadequate, i.e. is the baby hungry?

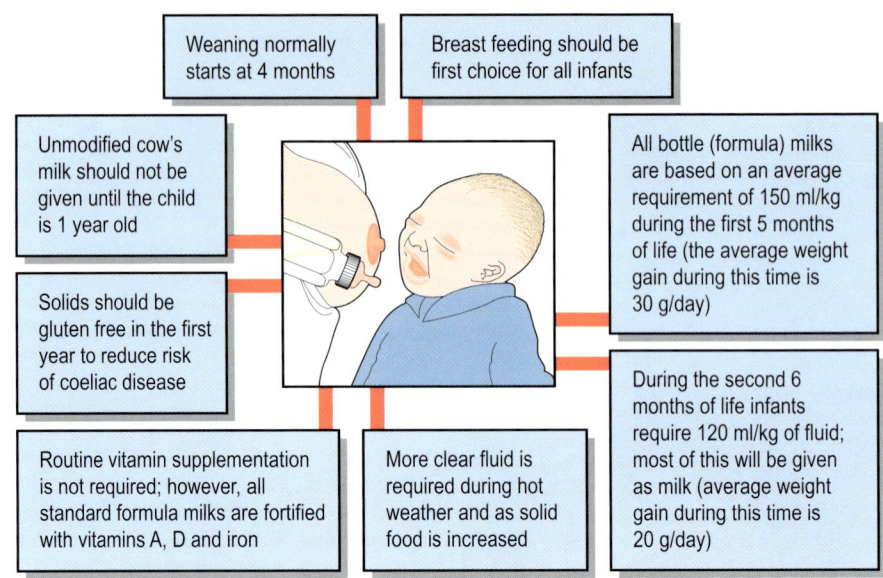

Fig. 1 **Normal feeding recommendations in the first year of life.**

Weaning normally starts at 4 months

Breast feeding should be first choice for all infants

Unmodified cow's milk should not be given until the child is 1 year old

All bottle (formula) milks are based on an average requirement of 150 ml/kg during the first 5 months of life (the average weight gain during this time is 30 g/day)

Solids should be gluten free in the first year to reduce risk of coeliac disease

During the second 6 months of life infants require 120 ml/kg of fluid; most of this will be given as milk (average weight gain during this time is 20 g/day)

Routine vitamin supplementation is not required; however, all standard formula milks are fortified with vitamins A, D and iron

More clear fluid is required during hot weather and as solid food is increased

Stools of the breast-fed baby are typically golden yellow and smell of cottage cheese (due to the presence of lactobacillus). The consistency is normally soft and most breast-fed babies will open their bowels several times a day. If the milk supply is poor, stools tend to become harder and green.

The bottle-fed infant

In many ways bottle feeding is a more straightforward option. Modern formula milks are now so highly modified that all of the known risks associated with the biochemical differences from breast milk have been eliminated (Table 1). Mothers know that if they feed their baby the correct amount the baby should achieve the same growth as a breast-fed infant without the uncertainty over intake. Many mothers also prefer the freedom of not being the sole person able to provide milk for the baby (it is possible for mothers to express milk to be given later by bottle). However, bottle milk is relatively expensive (this is of crucial importance in underdeveloped countries), constipation, obesity and gastroenteritis are more common, and the 'bonding effect' of breast feeding is lost. *Therefore, breast feeding should always be seen as the method of first choice.* Mothers who wish to

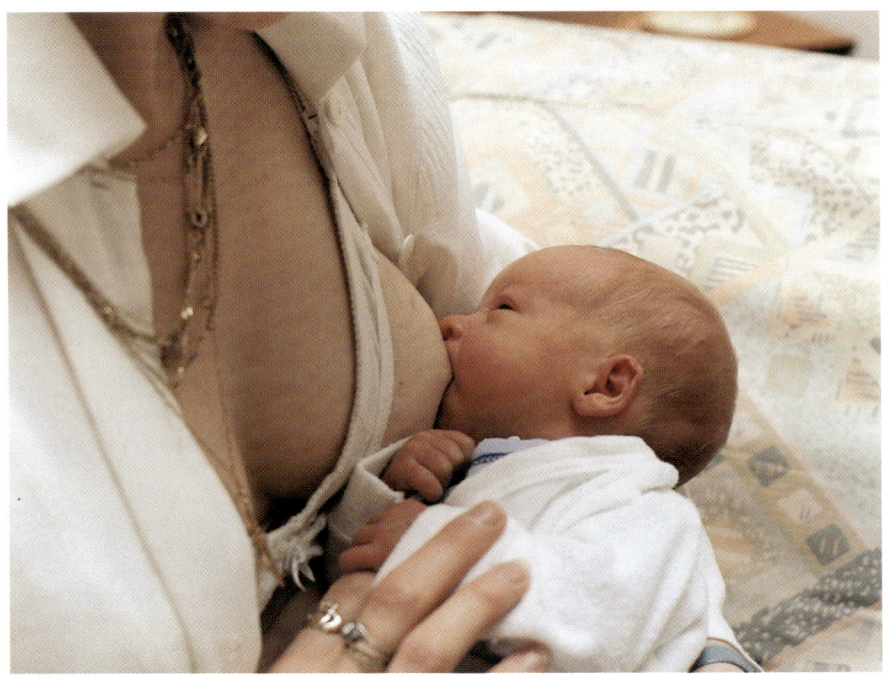

Fig. 2 **Baby properly 'fixed' to the breast.** Note that babies feed by taking the whole areola into the mouth.

breast feed but who, for whatever reason, fail often find this a huge psychological blow which should not be underestimated.

It is important that all the equipment used in bottle feeding is sterilised adequately (sterilising solution or boiling water). Feeds must be made correctly (1 level scoop to 30 ml or 1 fl oz) if the child is to get adequate nutrition.

Normal stool colour for a bottle-fed baby varies with the brand but most are yellow/green.

Vomiting

Small vomits are common after feeding (breast or bottle) and frequently accompany the process of winding. Vomitus often contains milk turned solid by the effect of renin and smells strongly acidic. These findings are of no consequence, although parents are frequently alarmed. Frequent small vomits are most likely the result of gastro-oesophageal reflux, whilst large intermittent vomits are more typical of pyloric stenosis (see pp. 68–69). Bile-stained vomits are frequently associated with intestinal obstruction and need investigation.

Constipation

It is important to understand that constipation refers to difficulty in defaecation not irregularity. It is more common in bottle-fed infants and it is important to ensure that the feeds have been made properly, i.e. not too concentrated. In breast-fed as well as bottle-fed babies it is important to ensure that the child has been given adequate clear fluid especially in hot weather. Where this fails, medication (e.g. lactulose) may be used but, if simple interventions are ineffective, the possibility of an organic cause should be considered.

Diarrhoea

Gastroenteritis is rare in the totally breast-fed baby because of the potent anti-infective properties of the milk. Maternal diet (e.g. eating hot curry or too much fruit) may cause diarrhoea. The development of loose stools in a bottle-fed baby may be the result of viral gastroenteritis or, more rarely, cow's milk allergy.

WEANING

This term refers to the introduction of solid food to a baby's diet, and should take place at about 4 months of age. The process is usually initiated by offering the child a small amount (5 ml) once a day of a 'sloppy' food. In the first instance it is sensible to use simple foods (e.g. baby rice) in order to reduce the risk of food allergy occurring. Slowly, the amount, consistency and variety of solid foods are increased.

Occasional 'choking' episodes are common at this stage and rarely of any significance unless they become a persistent problem. There is a great deal of natural variation in the ease with which babies cope with weaning and some may reject solids until 6 or 7 months of age.

COLIC

Infant colic is a very ill-defined condition; however, it is common and causes great distress to families. Affected babies usually develop symptoms soon after birth but problems peak at around 2 to 3 months of age. Each attack consists of apparent abdominal pain and inconsolable crying, often of very acute onset. Attacks can occur at any time but are most common in the early evening. No clear pathophysiology has been established and there is no consistently effective therapy. The condition normally resolves spontaneously by 6 months of age.

Colic is a diagnosis of exclusion and can only be made when other conditions (e.g. oesophagitis, milk sensitivity and intermittent intestinal obstruction) have been ruled out.

FEEDING TODDLERS

A large number of feeding problems occur in children aged 1–3 years. These tend to centre around a variety of parental concerns. However, certain themes are common: the child does not eat enough; the child will only eat snacks and not meals; the child will only eat a very limited range of foods (e.g. just yoghurt). Because parents are often very worried that their child

will come to harm, they may indulge in peculiar rituals to get the child to eat (e.g. dancing on a chair). In reality, children very rarely induce significant nutritional deficiencies by their behaviour. However, relative iron deficiency may occur especially if the milk content of the diet is inappropriately high. Certain principles should be explained to parents:

- the child is unlikely to suffer harm
- regular meals should be offered with the rest of the family, without bribery or distraction
- portions should not be too large
- snacks between meals should only be allowed when family meals have been eaten
- never force feed
- ensure that excessive milk (or other fluid) intake is not suppressing the child's appetite.

OLDER CHILDREN

OBESITY

Obesity results from overeating; however, familial factors also seem to play a part. In addition, it is more common in bottle-fed babies and those weaned early. Help from a dietician may be very useful in order to review both the child's intake and the feeding practices of the family as a whole.

ANOREXIA NERVOSA

This is a strange but sometimes fatal condition that affects adolescents. Girls are more commonly affected than boys. Affected children either starve themselves by not eating or use various techniques to vomit back food or give themselves diarrhoea. The wasting that occurs leads to a number of secondary effects, e.g. amenorrhoea. It appears that a fear of maturity may be important in the aetiology. Inpatient care and psychiatric support are required for the most serious cases.

Table 1 **Special milks**

- **Soya-based milks:** contain no cow's milk protein and hence can be used in cow's milk protein allergy. Most brands are also low in lactose and can be used in lactose intolerance (a common short-lived sequel of severe gastroenteritis)
- **Preterm formulas:** contain extra calories, protein, calcium and phosphorus. They are used to optimise growth in preterm infants during the first few weeks of life
- **'Elemental milks':** made of simple sugars, peptides and amino acids, and medium chain triglycerides. They are used in infants who have suffered extensive bowel damage or disruption (e.g. gut resection) since absorption is easily achieved
- **Goat's milk** is sometimes used in infants with a strong family history of allergy. The high solute content makes it unsuitable for infants under 6 months of age. Goats milk allergy may occur

Feeding

- Always exclude organic disease before concluding that any feeding problem is caused by parental anxiety.
- Bile-stained vomiting is always significant.
- Where problems exist, watching a breast/bottle-feed can be very helpful.
- Subtle congenital abnormalities (e.g. small posterior cleft palate) can present with feeding problems and, where appropriate, must be excluded.

GROWTH

Other sections in this text deal with situations where children present with signs and symptoms which require investigation and where the growth pattern is a very important part of the overall assessment. Many children present where the dominant parental concern is their growth. Slow growth may first be noted by health professionals. Occasionally the question of the growth of the child is raised by Social Services as part of their work with children in need. Because of its significance, growth measurement is a standard part of child health surveillance (pp. 14–15). Weight is measured at key ages and opportunistically when indicated. Length (children less than 2 years) or height (after 2) and head circumference are measured less often but particularly when indicated by other concerns.

NORMAL GROWTH

Stature varies in different populations and ethnic groups. Each child has an individual inherited genetic potential for growth, usually reflected in parental stature. From conception onwards, growth can be affected by genetic, environmental and endocrine factors, and significant chronic illness. Children that are born extremely prematurely needing long-term intensive care are often affected by inevitable undernutrition, permanently affecting growth potential. Similarly, gene or chromosome disorders such as achondroplasia (Fig. 1), Down's (Fig. 2) and Turner's (Fig. 3) syndromes are associated with small stature.

Growth is a vital indicator of the general health and well-being of children. It is a dynamic process with a rate and pattern which changes significantly with age. Growth is at its fastest in the first few months of life. It slows a little in mid-childhood before accelerating in the growth spurt around puberty. Final height is achieved after puberty.

Any assessment of the health of a child must include an evaluation of both the rate and pattern of growth. A child's growth at one point in time is plotted on centile charts and compared with:

- the child's previous growth
- the growth of the normal population of children at the same age.

Children who are crossing centiles (growing faster or slower than average) need closer attention. Those who fall 2–3 standard deviations outside the mean are more likely to have a medical or social causation requiring intervention. However, the majority of children below the 2nd centile (2% of the population by definition) are normal albeit small children.

Apparent abnormalities in growth may take various forms (Table 1) .

THE YOUNG CHILD WITH SLOW GROWTH: FAILURE TO THRIVE

This is the most common growth problem requiring medical attention. Failure to thrive (FTT) means a failure to achieve a normal rate of growth over time. A child may fall from 75th to 25th centiles, remaining above the 2nd centile: that child is nevertheless failing to thrive. One useful definition states: 'A child is failing to thrive if weight has deviated two or more major centiles below the maximum weight achieved between 4 and 8 weeks of age, and for a period of a month or more'. The 4–8th week of age is a more useful baseline from which to assess growth as birth weight is subject to many influences not related to growth potential.

Small stature means height (length before 2 years) below the 2nd centile.

The most significant causes of abnormal growth worldwide are poverty, malnutrition and diarrhoeal diseases. In the developed world, inadequate feeding, for whatever reason, is the most common cause. Social and emotional deprivation are also important aetiologies, emphasising that growth reflects the overall well-being of the child. Any prolonged period of ill-health (e.g. severe asthma, chronic renal failure, congenital heart disease or malabsorption) may lead to undernutrition and secondary growth failure. Where the underlying cause of failure to thrive can be corrected, the child's growth potential usually reasserts itself with a full catch-up in growth. In other cases, optimal nutrition and health care will substantially improve the growth of children with chronic illness such as cystic fibrosis or Crohn's disease.

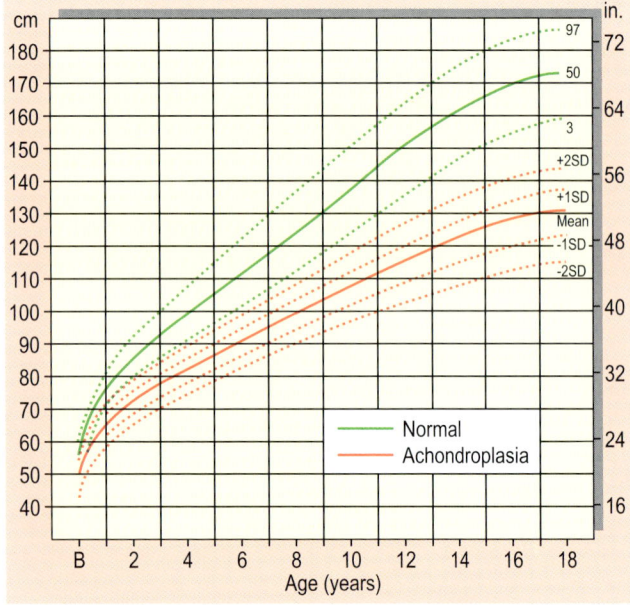

Fig. 1 **Height in male with achondroplasia compared with normal.**

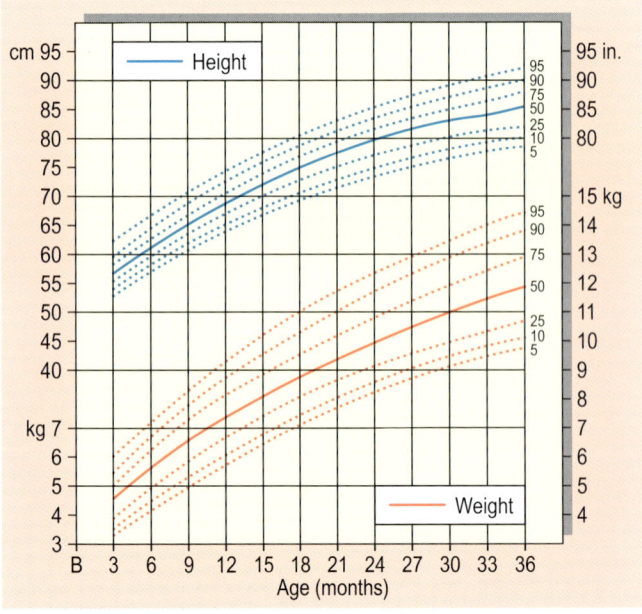

Fig. 2 **Height and weight in Down's syndrome child during period of 3–36 months of age.**

Table 1 **Patterns of presentation with growth abnormalities**

Presentation	Differential	Management/Investigations
Normal stature infant with period of poor weight gain, relative sparing of length	Feeding problems Organic illness: heart, renal, respiratory, malabsorption (coeliac/milk allergy) Social problems including emotional, physical neglect Poverty	Full assessment: history, examination, and dietary intake Look for systems-related signs Investigate including UTI, malabsorption & FTT screen Consider admission to observe feeding Consider social assessment if no organic reason found
Baby/child with short stature from birth	Familial short stature Low birth weight conditions: intrauterine growth retardation Congenital infection Maternal toxins Genetic anomaly, e.g. Russell–Silver syndrome, achondroplasia	Assessment as above Family stature/history Chromosomal analysis TORCH screen if other signs Targeted investigation
Child with small stature following normal stature in infancy	Chronic illness, e.g. coeliac disease Rickets Severe neglect Turner's syndrome (girls) Growth hormone deficiency: 1 per 3000	Assessment as above Bone metabolism and bone age Chromosomes in girls Endocrine investigations
Child with fluctuating weight loss	Recurrent illness Child in need	Social assessment if medical causes excluded
Child with excessive weight for height	Usually nutritional: often relatively tall stature Rarely endocrine cause: hypothyroid	Dietary advice Thyroid function if relatively small stature cf. weight
Child with large stature	Familial Some syndromes: Sotos', Marfan's,	Investigate height over 98th centile if outside parental target range Investigate if premature sexual development
Child with abnormal head growth: shape/symmetry	Plagiocephaly common Craniosynostosis	No action Refer to specialist craniosynostosis team skull X-ray/CT scan to demonstrate sutures
Child with small head or slow growth	'Microcephaly': below 2nd centile Familial Commensurate with general small stature	Investigate if delayed development, if head circumference is crossing centiles, if neurological signs or systemic symptoms
Child with large head or rapid growth (beware head growth crossing centiles)	Hydrocephalus Intra-cranial tumour Familial macrocephaly Some cerebral malformations and syndromes	Urgent neurology referral and imaging if growth across centiles Full examination and developmental assessment

ASSESSMENT

The following should all be considered in a child who is failing to thrive:

- **Family and social history:** parental stature and familial conditions affecting growth, economic status, emotional security and level of care.
- **Antenatal and perinatal history:** maternal health and pregnancy; the child's birth history, and exposure to maternal toxins (smoking, drugs, alcohol).
- **Infancy and childhood:** feeding history, bowel function and developmental milestones; an assessment of general health, nutritional status and level of care.
- **Examination** should include inspection for dysmorphic features, accurate plotting of length/height, weight and head circumference on centile charts, developmental progress and thorough system examinations.

SPECIFIC CAUSES OF GROWTH FAILURE

These are listed in Table 2.

Table 2 **Causes of growth failure**

Genetic	Familial short stature Chromosomal disorders
Environmental causes	Poverty and poor nutrition Other causes of poor nutrition Emotional and physical abuse
Systemic disease	Cystic fibrosis Coeliac disease Chronic renal disease
Endocrine disorders	Growth hormone deficiency Hypothyroidism
Normal variant	Constitutional delay of growth and puberty

Growth

- Growth and development are dynamic factors in children.
- Assess the rate and pattern of growth, plot on centile chart and assess nutrition.
- A small, well child growing at an appropriate rate is likely to be normal: note parental stature.
- The most common non-familial causes of small stature are environmental, e.g. poor nutrition.
- Chronic illness affects children's growth.
- Growth hormone replacement is effective in GH deficiency but not in other causes of small stature.

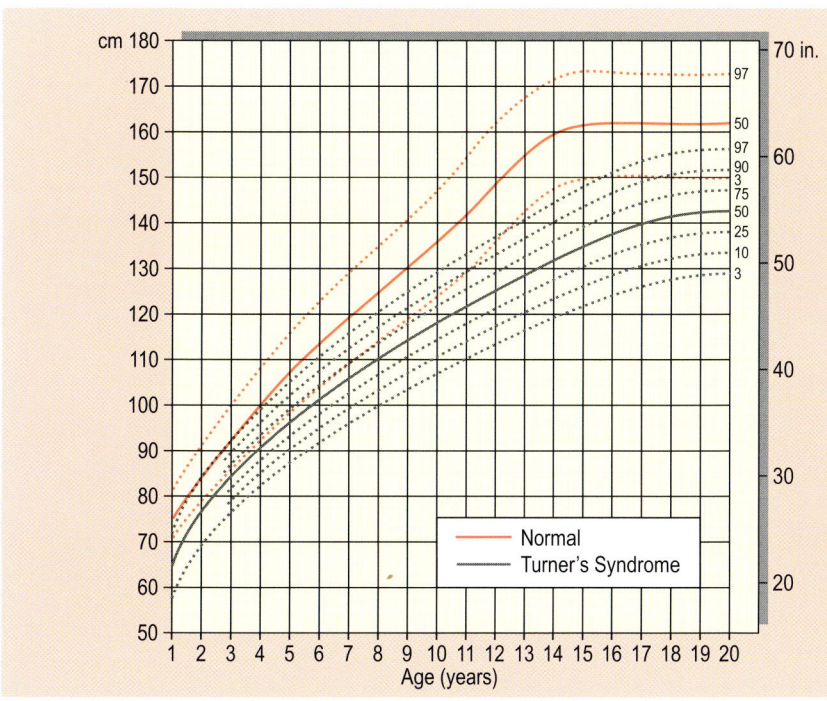

Fig. 3 **Height in female with Turner's syndrome compared with normal.**

ILLNESS ASSOCIATED WITH TRAVEL

Travel is increasingly common either for pleasure or because of a permanent change of country of residence. Although illness from foreign travel can be minimised with appropriate preparation and taking precautions (Table 1), the risk of illness can be increased because of unfamiliarity with local conditions, prevalence of local infections and failure to take advice seriously.

The risk of becoming ill also depends on nutritional status, any genetic tendency to disease and the geographical area visited. People from different cultures may also have attitudes to illness, for both prevention and treatment, which increase the risk of developing illness by failing to take appropriate precautions or delaying seeking medical advice.

Children who present with symptoms after entering the UK from overseas will come from one of two groups:

- healthy UK residents who acquire minor or serious illness, usually infection, while temporarily abroad (Table 2)
- new arrivals who may bring locally acquired illness with them, or have genetic conditions common to their country of origin (Table 3).

ASSESSMENT OF THE UNWELL CHILD

The incubation period of imported infection varies considerably (Fig. 2), although most acquired infection will present within 6 weeks. Many illnesses are readily diagnosed and treated, but unusual diseases or those with public health implications (e.g. legionnaires' disease, haemorrhagic fever,

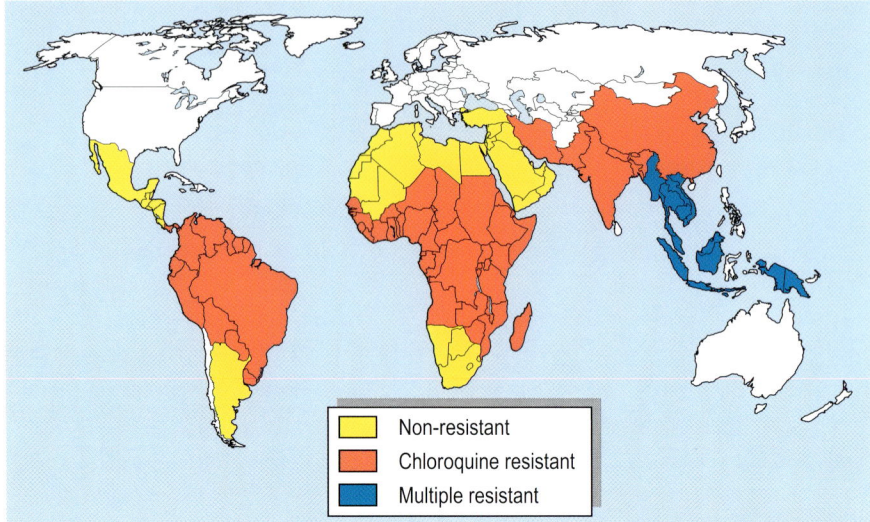

Fig. 1 **Areas where malaria prophylaxis is recommended.**

Legend:
- Non-resistant
- Chloroquine resistant
- Multiple resistant

typhoid) may need referral to a tropical diseases unit for diagnosis or advice.

The normal process of assessment must be carried out thoroughly:

- a full history and details of regions visited
- ethnic background, attitude to the illness and likely local diseases
- reasons for travel
- family illnesses
- immunisation status
- contact with animals, insects, etc.
- diet
- symptoms, in particular:
  — vomiting and diarrhoea
  — rashes
  — fever
  — jaundice
  — fits and rigors
  — bleeding and bruising
  — weakness and paraesthesiae
  — weight loss
- physical examination including height and weight, temperature and hydration status.

COMMON PRESENTING FEATURES: ASSESSMENT

Diarrhoea

Diarrhoea with minor abdominal symptoms is common and is usually caused by a gastroenteritis with a virus or *E. Coli*. It is usually self-limiting, but if symptoms are prolonged or are associated with bloody stools and mucus, other organisms are more likely, e.g. *Salmonella*, *Shigella*, *Campylobacter* or *Yersinia*. Profuse watery diarrhoea may be due to cholera; more chronic symptoms with abdominal pain or nausea suggest *Giardia lamblia* or amoebae.

Investigation should include stool culture and microscopy of a fresh specimen, a blood culture, blood count and electrolyte estimation.

Treatment is usually supportive and may include intravenous fluid replacement, or oral glucose–electrolyte solution. Antibiotics are only indicated in septicaemia or if the illness is prolonged (Table 4). In unresponsive conditions, a non-infective cause should be excluded, e.g. lactose intolerance, malabsorption (tropical sprue), TB, or infection outside the bowel, e.g. malaria.

Fever

While fever may be associated with minor illness, a persisting high fever associated with generalised symptoms demands the exclusion of serious infection, in particular malaria, typhoid, haemorrhagic fever, TB and HIV. Less usual infection may need

Table 1 **Precautions and preparation**

Routine immunisation
- DTP
- polio
- Hib
- MMR
- BCG

Specific immunisations (depending on the area to be visited)
- typhoid
- hepatitis A
- yellow fever
- cholera
- plague
- meningococcus

Malaria prophylaxis (depending on area to be visited) (Fig. 1)

Avoid contaminated water and food
Avoid contaminated swimming areas
Good personal hygiene
Avoid bites and stings (clothing, repellents, mosquito nets)
Avoid sunburn
Take appropriate medication (first aid kit, etc.)

Table 2 **Acquired infection during travel**

Minor	Gastroenteritis – *E. coli*, *Salmonella*, *Campylobacter*, *Shigella*, *Giardia* Hepatitis A Minor malaria
Serious	Severe malaria Cholera Typhoid Intestinal worm infection Bilharzia Rabies TB Amoebiasis Meningococcal meningitis Haemorrhagic fever
Rare	Polio Tetanus Plague Yellow fever

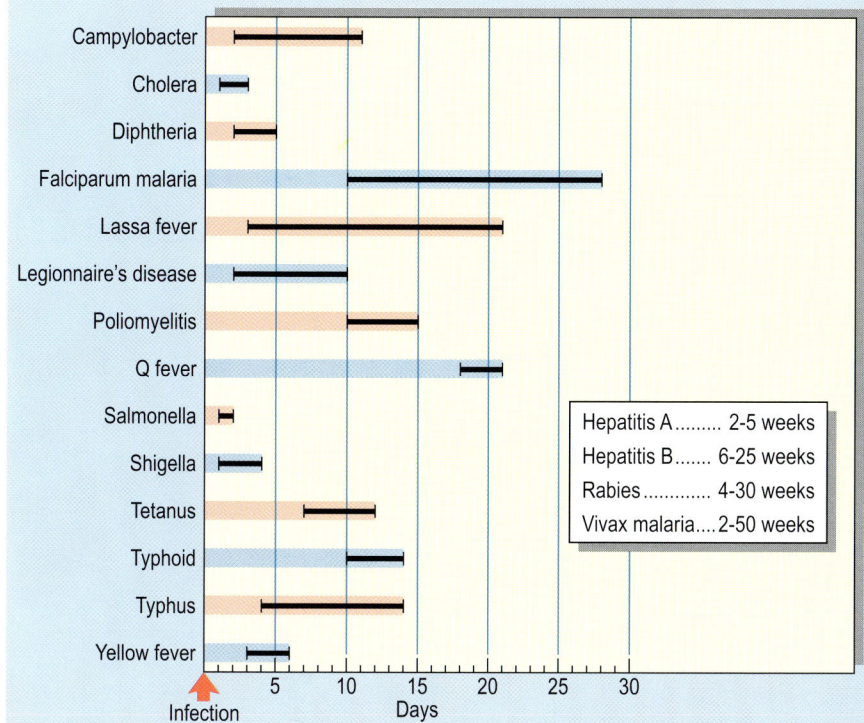

Fig. 2 **Incubation periods for common infections associated with travel.**

Table 3 **Medical problems of new immigrants**

Malnutrition
Iron deficiency anaemia
Positive hepatitis B carrier status: common in SE Asia but also sub-Saharan Africa and the Mediterranean area
Sickle cell disease: west and central Africa, south Asia and the Mediterranean area
Alpha thalassaemia: SE Asia
Beta thalassaemia: Asia, Mediterranean area
G6PD deficiency: Africa, Mediterranean area, Far East
TB
HIV
Malaria (Fig. 1)
Protozoal infection
Lactase deficiency

excluding, e.g. leishmaniasis, brucellosis, and non-infective causes such as inflammatory bowel disease, lupus and malignancies. Investigations include:

- thick and thin blood films for malaria
- Mantoux test
- blood cultures
- serological tests.

If there is any suspicion of rare serious disease, advice must be sought from a tropical diseases laboratory.

Treatment for malaria depends on the causative parasite and the likely sensitivity to drugs. Chloroquine is appropriate for *P. vivax*, but falciparum malaria requires urgent treatment with quinine.

Jaundice

This sign indicates liver disease or occasionally haemolysis. Most commonly jaundice will be due to malaria or hepatitis (usually hepatitis A in children unless they have been given blood products contaminated with hepatitis B or have acquired this infection prenatally). Liver abscesses (either pyogenic or amoebic) do not usually cause jaundice. More rarely yellow fever and leptospirosis (Weil's disease) may present with jaundice. Investigations include:

- thick and thin blood films for malaria
- liver function tests
- serological tests
- blood and urine cultures
- liver scan: either ultrasound or CT.

Treatment for hepatitis is supportive; leptospirosis is treated with penicillin and liver abscesses require surgical drainage.

Nutritional deficiency

The nutritional status of children who have been living abroad may be compromised because of poverty and an inadequate diet, dietary beliefs and customs and underlying disease which may be aggravated by nutritional deficiency.

Common nutritional problems include:

- rickets
- iron deficiency

- chronic intestinal infection (amoebiasis, giardiasis, worm infestation, in particular, roundworm, hookworm and tapeworm).

Children presenting with chronic diarrhoea, weight loss, slow weight gain, bone deformity, pallor or abdominal pain require additional investigation:

- blood count and iron estimation
- liver function
- calcium, phosphate, electrolytes.

Skin problems

Skin infections are frequent and many will be common conditions perhaps aggravated by a different climate. However, other skin diseases may also represent serious systemic disease or infection, e.g. HIV, and successful treatment will depend on correct diagnosis. Such conditions include:

- TB (either local skin involvement or manifesting as erythema nodosum)
- secondary infection of bites, etc.
- urticarial response to insect bites or protozoal infection
- hypopigmentation and local anaesthesia in leprosy
- local infection, e.g. scabies, fungus.

Table 4 **Treatment of diarrhoeal disease**

Fluid replacement • intravenous • oral (glucose–electrolyte solution)
Salmonella, Shigella — co-amoxyclav
Campylobacter — erythromycin
Cholera — co-trimoxazole
Giardia — metronidazole
Amoebiasis — metronidazole

Table 5 **Sources of further information**

Books ABC of Healthy Travel (BMJ) Travel with Children (Lonely Planet Publications) Publications on travel available from Dept of Health hotline 0800 555 777
Advice Hospital for Tropical Disease

Illness associated with travel

- Immigrant children may have disease not frequently seen in the UK.
- Diseases common to all children may have an unusual presentation in children from abroad.
- Nutritional deficiency is common in immigrant children.
- Much illness acquired during travel abroad can be prevented by immunisation and prophylaxis.

ACCIDENTS

Accidents are the single largest cause of death in children age 1–14, with two deaths every day in the UK as a result of accidental injury. Every year, one in five children attend an A&E department following an accident, and 150 000 children each year are admitted to hospital. The World Health Organization European region 'Health for All' project has set a target to reduce death as a result of accidents by 25% by the year 2000.

The type of accident is dependent on the age, sex, social circumstances and intelligence of the child and carer. Over 60% of accidents occur in the home (Fig. 1). However, road accidents are the most common cause of death, followed by drowning and burns. Toddlers tend to be fearless and inquisitive, but confined to home. They are at risk from falls, burns and accidental ingestion. Older children are more adventurous, and most at risk outside the home, especially boys.

ACCIDENT PREVENTION

The Department of Trade and Industry Home Accident Surveillance System in the UK collects nationwide statistics from selected A&E departments in order to monitor 'risk'. The Child Accident Prevention Trust determines the types of accidents that occur, and (with the help of many different agencies) implements methods to reduce their number and severity. Three types of prevention are defined:

- primary prevention aims to stop the accident happening
- secondary prevention aims to prevent injury during an accident
- tertiary prevention aims to optimise treatment of injuries sustained, and hence minimise morbidity.

Methods of accident prevention can also be considered in three main categories:

- education (e.g. making sure parents are aware of the dangers of hot drinks to toddlers; encouraging parents to learn first aid)
- enforcement of legislation (e.g. cycle helmets, speed restrictions)
- environmental change (e.g. stair gates).

FALLS

These are the most common cause of accidental injury. Morbidity is usually minor but severe morbidity or mortality may occur if the accident is associated with a head injury.

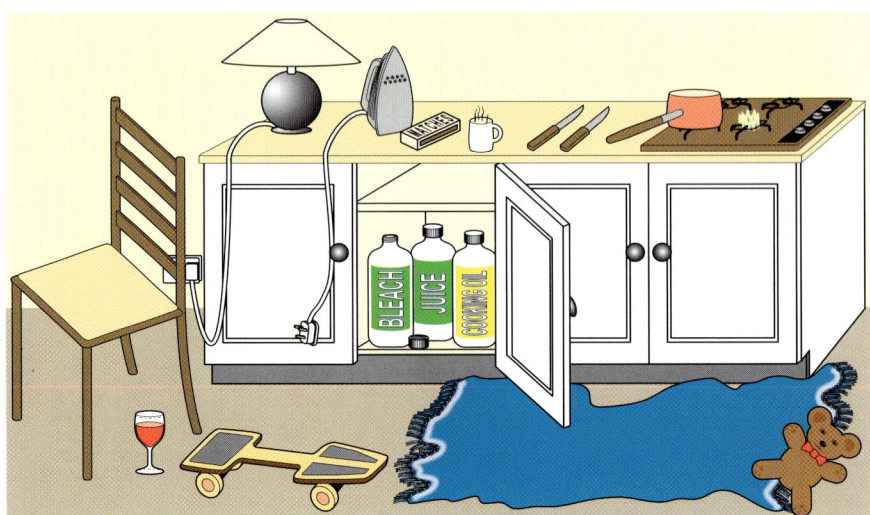

Fig. 1 **A dangerous kitchen.** Diagram illustrates the various means by which accidents commonly occur in the home.

Prevention

Stair gates and window locks can be used in the home to prevent falls occurring. Babies and young children should always be strapped into their high chair, pram or carrycot, and should never be left unattended on a raised surface. Secondary prevention, to reduce the trauma caused by a fall, is achieved with the use of protective helmets and limb pads, for example, when riding a bicycle or roller skating, and by making playground surfaces from softer materials.

ROAD ACCIDENTS

Road accidents are the most common single cause of death in childhood, accounting for 16% of all deaths in the age range 1–14 years. They are also the most common cause of severe head injury, and the major single cause of acquired neurological handicap. Boys age 5–8 years are most at risk. The child is a pedestrian in 50% of road accidents.

Prevention

Primary prevention is achieved by educating children and drivers on road safety, improving visibility at night with lights and reflective clothing, by reduction of traffic speed, and by separation of pedestrian areas from traffic. Secondary prevention involves using age-appropriate restraints for car passengers, and appropriate protective clothing for cyclists.

BURNS

14% of accidental deaths are due to burns with fatal burns usually being the result of a house fire.

Diagnosis of burns is not usually a problem. They are most common in the toddler age range when the child is mobile and inquisitive but has little sense of danger. Splash injuries from boiling water are the most commonly seen.

Prevention

The most important means of prevention is by educating children and their carers. Fire and cooker guards can be used to protect an inquisitive toddler. Smoke alarms reduce both the morbidity and mortality associated with house fires.

MANAGEMENT OF BURNS

Primary survey

Immediate assessment of airway, breathing, circulation, with appropriate intervention should be undertaken.

Secondary survey

Assess body surface area involved using surface area chart (Fig. 2) (a child's palm and closed fingers cover approximately 1% of body surface area). Assess depth of burn:

- superficial: only the epidermis is damaged, the skin is red and there is no blistering
- partial thickness: damage to dermis, with pink and blistered skin (Fig. 3)
- full thickness: damage to the epidermis and dermis, with or without damage to deeper structures. The skin is white or charred, painless and leathery to touch.

Initial burn care

Analgesia involves i.v. morphine 0.1 mg/kg as a bolus, with a continuous

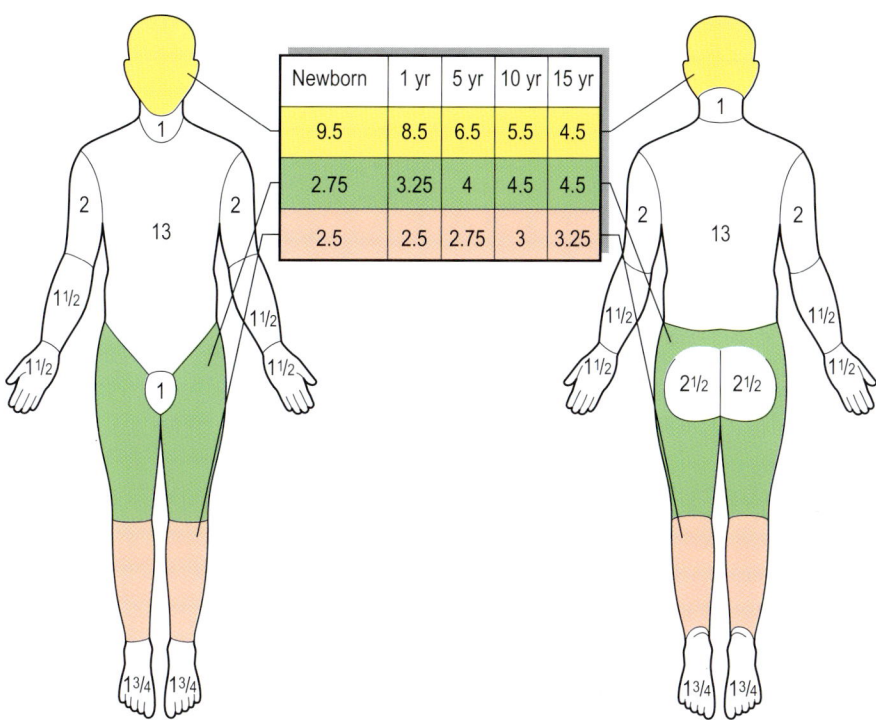

Fig. 2 **Chart to calculate percentage body surface area.** The table provides percentages that change with increasing age.

	Newborn	1 yr	5 yr	10 yr	15 yr
	9.5	8.5	6.5	5.5	4.5
	2.75	3.25	4	4.5	4.5
	2.5	2.5	2.75	3	3.25

infusion being set up if required. An older child may manage to use Entonox. **Fluid therapy** is important if the child is shocked. 20 ml/kg of a colloid is given immediately. If the burn covers more than 10% of the surface area, additional fluids are required. The additional volume required per day is calculated from the formula:

total % burn × weight (kg) × 4

Half the volume is given in the first 8 h, usually as 4.5% albumen. Normal maintenance requirements must also be given.

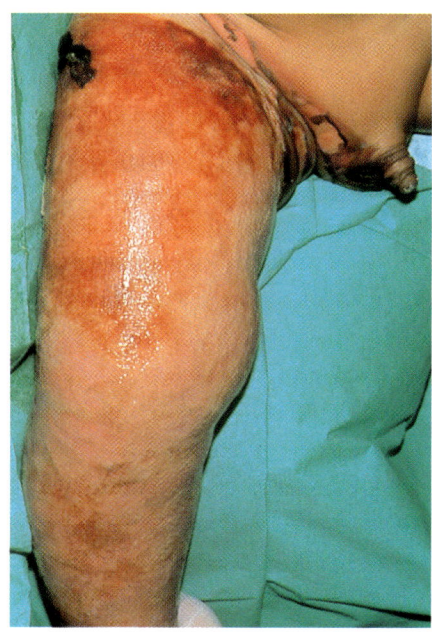

Fig. 3 **Scald burn.** Note lack of damage in skin fold.

Criteria for transfer to a burns unit

10% partial thickness burns, or 5% full thickness burns or burns to special areas such as face and hands require treatment at a burns unit.

DROWNING

Drowning most commonly occurs in inland waters, swimming pools and baths. The site usually depends on the age of the child, with a baby more likely to drown in the bath, and an older child more likely to drown in inland water or a domestic swimming pool. Boys have a higher incidence of drowning.

Prevention

Educating children on the dangers of water and teaching them to swim from an early age are the best forms of prevention. Swimming pool areas should be kept enclosed, so a child cannot have unsupervised access. Appropriate safety equipment, such as inflatable life-jackets, should be used for water sports.

POISONING

Poisoning is rarely fatal, but accounts for 40 000 A&E attendances annually. Toddlers, because of inquisitive behaviour, are most at risk, with the peak incidence at 2.5 years. Paracetamol is the most frequently ingested drug, but tricyclic antidepressants are the most common cause of fatality. General management principles are summarised in Table 1.

Prevention

Careful storage of medicines and household substances, using child-proof locks on cupboards and child-proof lids on drugs and household products, is advised.

Paracetamol ingestion

With a significant ingestion, early symptoms are nausea and vomiting. Later problems include acute hepatic failure, maximum at 3–4 days post-ingestion, and acute tubular necrosis.

Management

Induce vomiting if within 4 hours of ingestion. Measure blood paracetamol level at least 4 hours post-ingestion, and compare with the nomogram of level against time from ingestion (published in the BNF). Less than 200 μg/ml at 4 hours does not require treatment, but levels above the nomogram line usually require active intervention. Oral methionine or i.v. acetylcysteine treatment can prevent liver toxicity, but both agents must be given within 12–24 hours of ingestion for maximum benefit. Monitor prothrombin time and liver function tests for 3–4 days if initial paracetamol level is high.

Table 1 **Management of ingestions**

Establish what poison has been taken and always ask advice from the local Poisons Information Service

Induce vomiting with ipecac (a centrally acting emetic) unless contraindicated

Activated charcoal reduces absorption of some poisons

Gastric lavage is rarely indicated, but uses include iron and paraquat poisoning

Children should be admitted if they are symptomatic, or if they have ingested a substance with late effects, e.g. iron, tricyclics or digoxin

Contraindications to emesis
More than 4 hours since ingestion (except aspirin, lomotil, tricyclics, opiates)

Corrosive substances

Volatile substances such as paraffin, with a risk of inhalation and chemical pneumonitis

Decreased consciousness and absent gag reflex

Accidents

- Childhood accidents remain a major cause of morbidity and mortality.
- 'Risk taking' in early childhood and adolesence are the times of peak incidence.
- Most ingestions are trivial but each must be assessed with the help of the local Poisons Centre.

CHILD ABUSE

Child abuse is the description given to actions towards children which violate acceptable practices of parenting or child caring in a given culture at a given time. Child abuse is a major problem and in Britain approximately four children a week die as a result of abuse or neglect; double that number are left disabled and around 10 000 children are placed on the Child Protection (At Risk) Register each year (4:1000). Children suffer abuse in many different ways and some do not present to hospital. A proportion of abused children, particularly those suffering from emotional deprivation, may not be diagnosed until after childhood when as adults they present with psychiatric symptoms. Boys and girls suffer child abuse equally. It occurs more commonly in young children, those less than 2 years are most at risk of physical abuse and it is those under 1 year in whom death occurs most frequently (Table 1).

It is important to differentiate between abuse, deliberately inflicted injury, and an accident — a lapse in the usual protection given to a child which sometimes is associated with inadequate or negligent parenting (Table 2).

Table 1 **Risk factors for abuse**

Parents who were abused themselves or had a
  'disrupted' childhood
Parents with psychiatric histories, particularly depression
Young parents or single parent families
Stress in a family, e.g. unemployment, poor housing,
  alcohol or drug abuse, marital disharmony
Unplanned or unwanted pregnancy
Separation of mother and baby at birth

Table 2 **Types of child abuse**

Physical
Neglect
Emotional deprivation
Sexual
Munchausen syndrome by proxy

PHYSICAL ABUSE/NON-ACCIDENTAL INJURY

Features which suggest non-accidental injury (NAI) include a delay in presentation, an inconsistent story, a story not compatible with the injury or an injury found by chance, and multiple or different aged injuries. Poor hygiene and tatty clothing alone may reflect poverty and not abuse.

Bruises

It is common for healthy and normal children to have bruises on their shins, knees, elbows and foreheads but not on their abdomen, buttocks, thighs, inner aspects of arms, mouth or genitalia. Abnormal bruising can be sustained from pinches, punches, slaps, beating and even biting (Fig. 1). However, it is important not to misdiagnose abuse (Fig. 2). Any child who presents with suspicious bruises must have a full blood count and clotting screen performed to exclude haematological causes (pp. 90–91) such as leukaemia or idiopathic thrombocytopenic purpura.

Fractures

Some fractures such as rib and long bone and especially spiral fractures (resulting from a twisting injury) are particularly suggestive of NAI. It is very hard for a child aged less than 1 year to fracture a femur 'alone', so in these cases a diagnosis of NAI must be excluded. Osteogenesis imperfecta is a rare inherited condition and affected children can suffer multiple fractures and occasionally it can be confused with NAI. Children with osteogenesis imperfecta typically have blue sclerae and often have a positive family history.

Burns

Burns and scalds that occur as a result of child abuse are usually serious injuries from sadistic and violent punitive emotions in the abuser, e.g. 'I'll teach him a lesson'. They are found in 10% of physically abused children and account for up to 16% of all children presenting at hospital with burns. However, the diagnosis can be difficult as it is sometimes hard to differentiate between an accident and deliberate scalding in toddlers. Scalds are caused by hot water, e.g. drinks or baths (Fig. 3). Contact dry burns can be caused by hot objects, e.g. electric fires or irons. The injury site in these cases is sharply demarcated. Cigarette burns are relatively rare and leave circular marks often with a crater (Fig. 4). If there is a scald-like lesion and no history of a burn, skin diseases/infections must be considered as conditions such as epidermolysis bullosa, impetigo, papular urticaria, contact dermatitis and severe napkin rash can all mimic burns.

Abdominal injuries

These follow direct blunt trauma to the abdomen and occur in seriously abused children. More common injuries include a duodenal haematoma and ruptured viscera, e.g. bowel, liver or spleen.

Head injuries

Head injuries result from violent physical abuse including uncontrolled shaking and

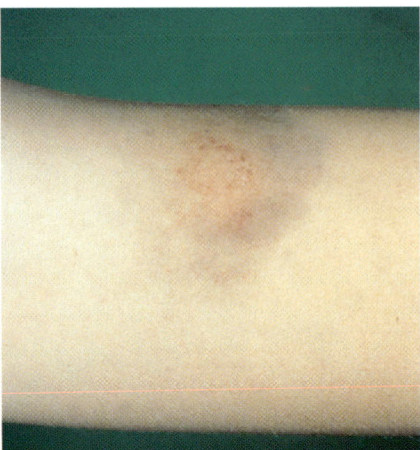

Fig. 1 **Bite mark on forearm.**

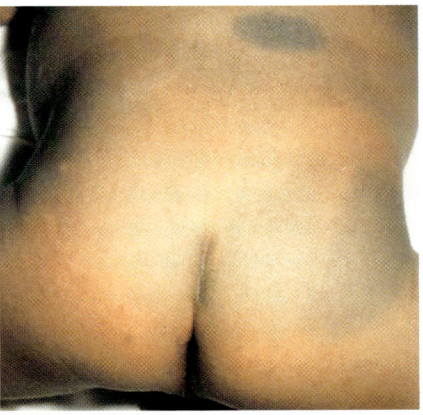

Fig. 2 **Mongolian blue spot in an Asian baby (not to be confused with bruising from abuse).**

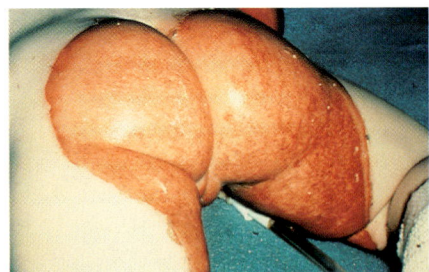

Fig. 3 **Scalded buttocks from hot bath.**

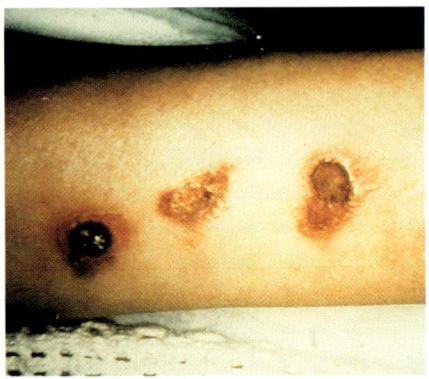

Fig. 4 **Cigarette burns on skin.**

swinging and direct trauma to the head. The majority of deaths from physical abuse follow head injuries and occur in children under 1 year. The injuries sustained include skull fractures (often extensive, multiple and depressed) and cerebral contusion (resulting from shaking and swinging injuries). A subdural haematoma in a young child with no adequate explanation strongly suggests physical abuse. Presentation in such cases can be immediate or delayed, with symptoms including fits, poor feeding, lethargy and drowsiness or increasing unconsciousness. Clinically there may be evidence of increasing head circumference: neuroradiology will confirm the diagnosis.

Retinal haemorrhages should always be looked for in suspected cases of NAI and if present (without an adequate explanation) are strong presumptive evidence of physical abuse.

NEGLECT AND EMOTIONAL ABUSE

This can take many forms from lack of care for physical needs through failure to love and nurture to straight rejection of a child. In infants, neglect of physical care leads to failure to thrive and recurrent and persistent minor infections often associated with frequent accident and emergency attendances. Emotional neglect means social and psychomotor skills will be affected resulting in general developmental delay. Preschool children treated in this way often suffer growth delay and delayed language skills. They have a limited attention span and may be overactive. In the child who has reached school age, the effects of long-term neglect and abuse are major learning problems at school because of poor concentration and physical overactivity. Relationships with peers are poor and they are either 'bullies' or totally withdrawn. Some of these children have major problems with nocturnal enuresis, soiling and encopresis. In adolescence they can turn to truancy, glue sniffing, 'drugs' and other criminal activities.

SEXUAL ABUSE

Child sexual abuse (CSA) is any use of children for the sexual gratification of adults. The abuser is usually a male known to the family, although it is a female in about 10% of cases. It can occur in any part of society but more commonly occurs in poor families. Children of all ages and either sex may be sexually abused. Retrospective studies interviewing adults report that the incidence of child sexual abuse is in the order of 1 in 10 children. Child sexual abuse can be:

- non-contact when the child is exposed to indecent acts, pornographic photography or sexual talk
- contact/non-penetrative when there is genital or anal touching, masturbation or fondling
- penetrative with oral, vaginal or anal intercourse.

Risk factors for child sexual abuse include previous incest or sexual deviation in the family, a new male in the family with a history of sexual offences, loss of inhibitions from alcohol and loss of maternal libido, e.g. the recent birth of a child. Symptoms often present after a long period of abuse and are due to:

- local trauma, e.g. vaginal discharge, anal bleeding, perineal soreness, constipation
- secondary to emotional effects, e.g. deteriorating school performance, enuresis, encopresis
- evidence of inappropriate sexual knowledge in a young child.

When child sexual abuse is suspected, the local multidisciplinary team specialising in this area should be contacted. Further interviews with the family and examination of the child can then be undertaken by the relevant members of the specially trained team which usually consists of a paediatrician, a psychiatrist, a police officer and a social worker.

MUNCHAUSEN SYNDROME BY PROXY/ FACTITIOUS ILLNESS

This is rare but very serious. A parent, almost always the mother, fabricates illness in her child or children by producing a history of symptoms and/or signs. Common presentations include apnoeas and epileptic seizures. In some cases children are deliberately poisoned, e.g. with sodium chloride.

MANAGEMENT

Management strategies in cases of child abuse are summarised in Table 3.

Table 3 **Management of a child in whom child abuse is suspected**

Details	Name Address Date, time and place of visit Who brought child — name, address
History	Details of injuries and how caused Previous injuries and medical history Social history Family history/full details of all family members
Examination	Drawings of all injuries Weight and height on centile chart Developmental skills
Investigation	Check if child on Child Protection Register Photograph injuries Full blood count, clotting screen Skeletal survey Contact Primary Health Care Team, other involved teams, e.g. school, social worker
Plan	Current safety of child — may need hospital admission Legal help if needed, emergency protection order ensures 7 days safety for child Arrange case discussion/conference
Action	At discussion/conference include medical team, primary health care team/GP and health visitor, teacher/counsellor (if involved), social worker, police. Decide: • Can child return/remain at home? • Should care proceedings be pursued? • Identify key worker and plan supporter. • Should child be on the Child Protection Register?

Child abuse

- NAI and sexual abuse have to be suspected before they can be diagnosed and appropriately managed.
- Presentation of child abuse can be to any members of the Primary Health Care Team, hospital, educational and social services team.
- The most common cause of death from physical abuse is following head trauma in children less than 1 year.
- Always check the full blood count and clotting in a patient with unexplained bruising before diagnosing physical abuse.
- All causes of definite NAI and sexual abuse must be handled by a well trained and experienced multidisciplinary team.

THE TERMINALLY ILL CHILD

Terminal care begins once it is realised there is no longer any possibility of cure and death is inevitable. This situation can be reached:

- at the end stages of a chronic illness, such as cystic fibrosis or malignancy
- acutely, for example after a road traffic accident or sudden illness.

The duration of terminal care varies greatly, from hours to months and, in some cases, may be extended for years. The approach to terminal care must be an individual one, tailored specifically to the child and family, in order to provide the best possible quality of the child's remaining life.

TERMINAL CARE AFTER CHRONIC ILLNESS

The transition from treatment aimed to cure, to palliative care is a difficult step for the child, the family and health professionals involved (Fig. 1). The exact circumstances show great variation. The child may have been born with a non-curable disease such as cystic fibrosis, a metabolic disorder, or HIV infection. Alternatively, the child may have had only a few months or years of chronic illness, such as a malignancy, that has either not responded to treatment or has relapsed after maximum treatment has been given. Children who are immunosuppressed, either due to their illness or as a result of treatment, may die of intercurrent infections. For these children, although they have a chronic illness, the transition from curative treatment to one of terminal care is often very rapid.

Initiating terminal care

The decision that there is no longer any chance of cure must be made by a senior member of the medical team. It is essential that everything is discussed openly and honestly with the parents. Involving the child may be appropriate, depending on maturity, involvement in the illness and ability to cope. Talking to the parents again about their child's disease, treatments they have had and why there is no longer a realistic possibility of cure can be helpful. Positive decisions should be made as early as possible regarding where the child is to be cared for and who should be involved in that care. It is important that any decisions made at this stage are flexible, as the situation may change according to the child's health and the family situation.

Aim of terminal care

The aim of terminal care is to maintain the best possible quality of life for the child and family for as long as possible. This may

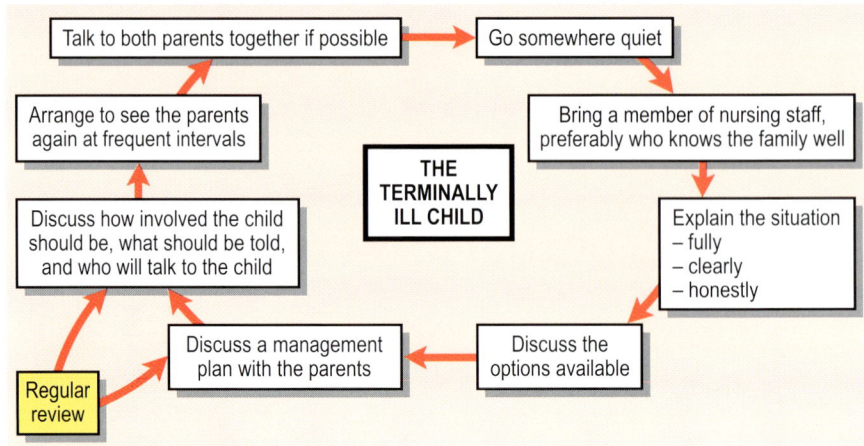

Fig. 1 **Breaking bad news.**

mean enabling the child to attend school, or go on a family holiday.

Where should terminal care take place?

In all situations it is important to accommodate, as far as possible, the wishes of the child and family. Most parents and children prefer the death to be at home. The ability to do this will depend on the home situation and the support services available, both from the hospital and the community. Many oncology units and district general hospitals have their own community liaison team who can be involved. This type of additional aid may permit general supportive measures, such as blood products and intravenous drugs, to be given at home. If available, a local paediatric hospice should be considered as a place for respite or terminal care. The general practitioner will have a vital role in the delivery of care at home and effective communication between the hospital and the GP is vital.

Palliative care

Palliative treatment is an attempt to delay or relieve symptoms caused by an illness, with no expectation of cure. In the case of malignant disease, this usually takes the form of a specific anti-tumour therapy, aimed at reducing the speed of disease progression. The treatment should be as non-invasive as possible, preferably given orally and with minimal requirement for hospital visits or blood tests. If there is no obvious benefit, or unacceptable toxicity, treatment should be discontinued.

Symptom control

A whole variety of symptoms, depending on the underlying condition, may trouble the child during the terminal phase of an illness. In order to maintain the highest possible quality of life it is important that these are controlled effectively.

Pain
- Usually the main concern of the parents and child.
- Often caused by local tumour growth or bone and bone marrow invasion.
- Always assess fully for simple (treatable) causes, such as constipation.
- Pain from local tumour growth may respond to local radiotherapy or palliative chemotherapy.
- Start with simple analgesia and build up stepwise through paracetamol, codeine, non-steroidal anti-inflammatories, oral morphine and continuous morphine infusion.
- Parents often find the transition to morphine difficult, as they see this as the 'beginning of the end'.

Nausea and vomiting
- May be caused by raised intracranial pressure, compression of the stomach by a tumour mass, intestinal obstruction, or as a side-effect of the analgesia.
- Dexamethasone may reduce vomiting from raised intracranial pressure.
- Haloperidol can be given in a syringe pump combined with opioids.
- Metaclopramide is often used, but must be avoided in intestinal obstruction.

Bleeding and anaemia
- Can be due to thrombocytopenia caused by bone marrow invasion.
- Sometimes result from coagulopathy secondary to marrow invasion or chemotherapy.
- Platelet infusions are only given if there is active bleeding that reduces the child's quality of life.
- Tranexamic acid can be applied to achieve local control of bleeding.
- Blood transfusion may be appropriate if increased tiredness is occurring as a result of anaemia.

Seizures

- Often due to CNS involvement (primary or metastatic) or raised intracranial pressure.
- Parents should be shown how to administer diazepam at home.
- Where intractable seizures occur, hospital admission is usually necessary.

Intercurrent infections

- Infection may develop as the terminal event, or may be a less serious complication of on-going palliative care.
- The decision to treat, and how aggressively, will depend on many factors: the wishes of the child and family, the severity of the infection, the likelihood of recovery from this infection, the treatment involved and the stage of the child's illness.
- Oral antibiotics are usually the most appropriate form of treatment.

Constipation

- Causes include poor nutrition, analgesics, inactivity, intestinal obstruction or chemotherapy.
- Laxatives should always be given when codeine or opioids are used.

Anorexia

- May be due to nausea and vomiting, mouth ulcers, swallowing difficulty or general lethargy.
- Nasogastric feeding or parenteral nutrition are only appropriate if the child's quality of life is compromised.

Agitation and restlessness

- Cause is often unidentified.
- Can be relieved by haloperidol or chlorpromazine.

Alternative therapies

- Sometimes used by families either looking for a cure, or for symptom relief.
- Relaxation therapy, massage, aromatherapy, osteopathy, etc. may all have some benefit.

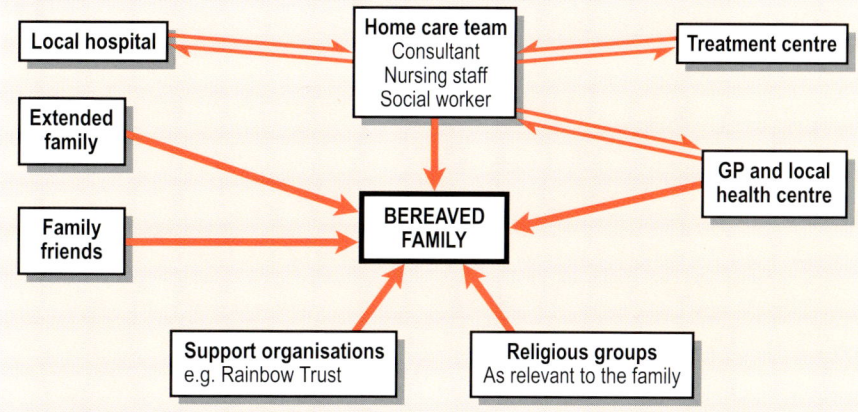

Fig. 2 **Support for a bereaved family.**

Psychological support

The child's concept of death and ability to cope will depend on his age, intellectual ability and experience of people dying. The child should be involved in decisions as much as possible, but within his or her level of coping. Even young children may have wishes to carry out before they die. Children are more likely to be frightened if they are excluded from discussions and providing children with the opportunity to discuss issues related to death will often reduce their anxieties. Brothers and sisters should also be included in discussions, where appropriate, for similar reasons. Medical staff should prepare the parents for questions the child may ask.

Spiritual needs of the child and family must be accommodated. This includes the desires of the family to seek alternative therapies, so long as this does not compromise the child's quality of life or ability to cope. Emotional support for the family must continue to be available well after the child has died (Figs 2 and 3).

TERMINAL CARE IN ACUTE ILLNESS

The situation in which a previously well child suffers a sudden illness or accident clearly presents different problems. There has been no time for the family to adjust to the possibility of the child's death. In addition there is no comfort for the parents in terms of 'release from illness' that they may feel when their child has been chronically unwell. In acute illness, terminal care usually only lasts a few hours or days and patients are unlikely to be cared for at home.

TERMINAL CARE IN THE NEONATE

The decision to withdraw active care is usually made by a senior member of staff, when it is thought that the child has little chance of survival, or has little expectation of a reasonable quality of life should he/she survive. The parents and appropriate family members should be involved in the decision. Where the decision involves the withdrawal of intensive care this can often be timed to permit close family members to visit and religious ceremonies to be completed. It may be appropriate for a ventilated baby to be extubated and held by the parents while he dies. Occasionally, for example with an untreated hydrocephalus, it may be possible for the child to be cared for at home.

As in older children, control of distressing symptoms is essential.

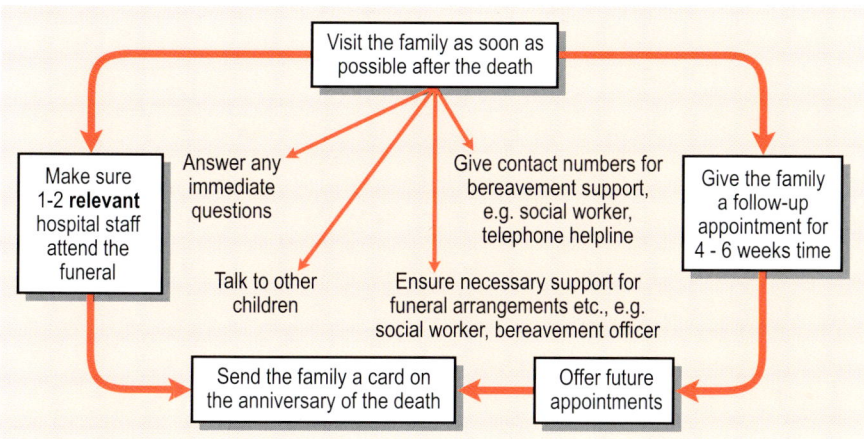

Fig. 3 **Good practice points after death.**

> **The terminally ill child**
>
> - Decisions that a child cannot be cured should be made by senior medical staff.
> - Parents must be fully informed; the child should participate in decisions.
> - Excellent communication between all those who care for the child is essential.

THE CHILD AND THE LAW

Children are clearly more vulnerable than adults and have particular needs, e.g. a caring environment and education. As a result, most developed countries recognise their position by a legislative framework which is intended to afford them a degree of protection within society. What follows is a review of the law as it applies in the UK and this is presented as an example. However, significant differences exist between countries.

THE CHILDREN ACT 1989

The Children Act was implemented in October 1991. The main aim was a restructuring of court proceedings regarding child protection and child welfare issues. The child's safety and place of residence were given increased importance. Where appropriate (i.e. if the child was old enough), the child's opinion was always to be taken into consideration. Key points of the Act include:

- The child's welfare is the most important issue and, wherever possible, the child should remain living with the family.
- Parents have responsibility for their child, but not 'rights' over their child. Wherever possible, parental responsibility is maintained, even if the child becomes the subject of a court order.
- A court order should only be made if it would positively contribute to the child's welfare.
- Delay in court proceedings relating to child protection issues is harmful and should be avoided.
- The wishes of the child should be given consideration. This includes consent to medical investigations and operations, within the limits of the child's understanding.

Emergency protection order (EPO)

This replaced the previous Place of Safety Order which was able to remain in place, unchallenged, for a longer period. An EPO is implemented when a child is felt to be at immediate risk of physical, sexual or emotional abuse. The order lasts for up to 8 days, but it can be challenged within 72 h of issue. Only one extension is allowed, which is for a further 7 days. Applicants for an EPO are usually social service officers or the NSPCC, although anyone can apply. Where possible, the child should remain in the home, and the source of risk (e.g. an abusing parent) should be removed.

Police protection provision

A child can be removed from the home by the police for up to 72 h if it is felt that the child may otherwise experience significant abuse. No court order is necessary. This was a new provision of the 1989 Act.

'Looked after by local authority'

This replaced the previous 'voluntary care order' and serves to provide accommodation for the child where the parent(s) is absent/ill or the child has been abandoned. The child can be removed by the parent at any time. The local authority is not prevented from seeking a Care order if this is in the child's best interests.

Care order

To implement a Care order, the court must be satisfied that the child has suffered, or is likely to suffer, significant harm, either because the standard of care provided is below that which is reasonable, or because the child is beyond parental control. Once such an order is in place, parental responsibility is shared jointly by the social services and the parents. A guardian 'ad litem' is appointed by the court to represent the interests of the child during the proceedings. The child is usually, but not always, removed from the home.

Interim care order

With an interim care order, the child is placed in the care of the local authority while the risks and needs of the child are assessed. The duration of care is limited to 8 weeks, but one extension is allowed for up to 4 weeks.

Supervision order

In this situation, a supervisor, usually a social worker or probation officer, is appointed to advise and assist the child and family. A 'responsible person' (usually a parent) is appointed by the court to inform the supervisor of the current address and to allow access to the child. The maximum duration is 3 years.

Education supervision order

This order is usually applied for in the case of children of compulsory school age who are not attending school. It lasts for 1 year, but can be extended to 3 years.

Child assessment order (CAO)

This allows assessment of the child's health and welfare where there is suspicion of harm, or when medical appointments have been refused or not attended. The order lasts only for 7 days, and only the local authority or NSPCC may apply. The CAO cannot override the wishes of the child, but it can override the wishes of the parents.

Family assistance order

This is usually applied during parental separation or divorce, and aims to give professional advice to the family. The duration is for up to 6 months.

Residence order

This specifies where the child is to live, and is usually applied in cases of parental separation or abuse.

Contact order

This order determines what contact the child is to have with other people. As with the residence order, it is usually implemented in cases of parental separation or abuse.

Prohibited steps order

This aims to prevent certain issues that may be detrimental to the child's welfare, such as unsupervised visits with a parent.

Ward of court

Where a child becomes a 'ward of court', the High Court takes legal responsibility for the child. This applies to all issues concerning the child, such as place of residence or medical treatment. It is used in a variety of circumstances not appropriately covered by other forms of legal intervention listed above. A child can only remain a ward of court until the age of 18 years, but wardship can be reversed earlier by the Court if it is considered appropriate.

ADOPTION

Adoption gives a person or persons parental responsibility for a child. The local authority social work department must be involved in deciding if the applicants are appropriate, and if adoption is the most appropriate step for the child and natural/legal parents. A reporting officer is appointed to ensure the natural parents give informed consent. Consent from the parents is not needed if they cannot be found, have persistently neglected or ill-treated the child, or are unlikely ever to be able to look after the child adequately. On reaching 18 years, the name and address of the natural parent(s), and or the birth record, can be obtained by the child.

ACUTE PAEDIATRICS

BLUE BABY AT BIRTH

Before birth the fetal circulation largely bypasses the lungs and oxygenation of the fetus takes place via the placenta. At birth changes take place in the circulation to adapt the baby for extra-uterine life, as shown in Figure 1.

If these changes do not take place successfully the baby will remain blue. This can occur through:

- failure to commence independent respiration
- pathology of the lungs
- pathology of the heart.

FAILURE TO COMMENCE INDEPENDENT RESPIRATION

In this situation the baby has normal heart and lungs but has not begun to breathe properly. The infant does not struggle for breath, but is simply not breathing. Problems arise immediately after birth.

The most important cause of this situation is asphyxia. There are many causes including feto-placental dysfunction, placental abruption and prolapsed cord. Each of these results in a fall in PaO_2 and acidosis in the baby. If the anoxic period is of short duration, the baby will respond rapidly to resuscitation. In prolonged anoxia, the baby will respond less quickly, and damage to vital organs such as the brain and kidneys can occur unless resuscitation is prompt and vigorous.

A newborn baby can survive up to 20 minutes with no oxygen because of large glycogen stores in the brain, liver and heart. Attempts at resuscitation are therefore always worthwhile.

In the early stages of asphyxia, recognisable by the baby being in reasonable condition and a heart rate >100, physical stimuli such as rubbing with a warm towel may be sufficient to stimulate breathing again. However, in the later stages of asphyxia, recognisable by extreme pallor, markedly reduced tone and a heart rate of <100, the baby will need full resuscitation, including artificial respiratory support.

PATHOLOGY OF THE LUNGS

In this situation the baby usually appears well at birth, with satisfactory onset of respiration. Soon after birth, difficulty in breathing arises, with signs of respiratory distress. These include tachypnoea, tachycardia, intercostal and subcostal recession, nasal flaring, grunting and cyanosis.

The history and the CXR give clues as to the cause of the problem. These include:

- respiratory distress syndrome
- congenital pneumonia
- meconium aspiration syndrome
- pneumothorax
- congenital abnormalities of the respiratory tract.

RESUSCITATION

Assessment of the non-breathing baby

Assessment is done by means of the Apgar score (Table 1). This gives the baby a score of 0, 1 or 2 for each of five clinical features. The scores are added to give a total score out of 10. The better the score, the better the condition of the baby. The first score is taken at 1 minute of age. Subsequent scores can be taken at 5, 10, 20 min, etc. to monitor the baby's progress and the effectiveness of resuscitation.

Action

The following steps should be undertaken immediately after delivery:

1. Warm and dry the baby.

2. Clear the airway with gentle suction.

3. Stimulate the baby if breathing is inadequate.

4. Give oxygen.

5. Provide artificial respiration, e.g. using bag and mask, if the above methods fail.

6. Consider giving naloxone to reverse the effects of any pethidine given to the mother.

7. Discontinue resuscitation once the baby is pink and active.

Table 1 **The Apgar score**

	0	1	2
1. Colour	Pale	Blue	Pink
2. Respiration	Nil	Gasps	Regular
3. Heart rate	Absent	<100	>100
4. Tone	Flaccid	Present	Good
5. Response to stimulation	Nil	Present	Brisk

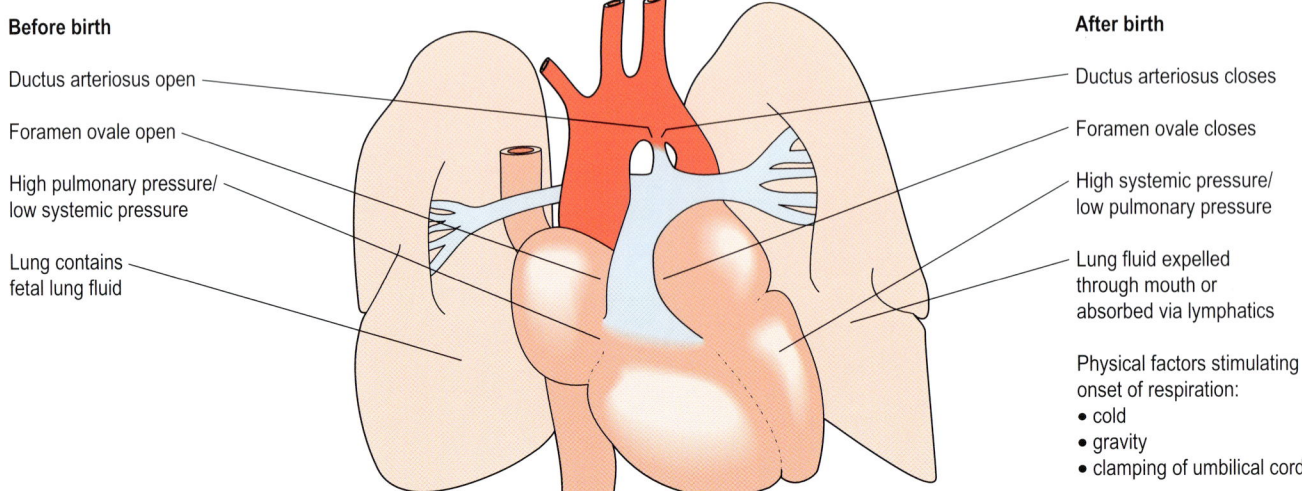

Before birth

Ductus arteriosus open

Foramen ovale open

High pulmonary pressure/ low systemic pressure

Lung contains fetal lung fluid

After birth

Ductus arteriosus closes

Foramen ovale closes

High systemic pressure/ low pulmonary pressure

Lung fluid expelled through mouth or absorbed via lymphatics

Physical factors stimulating onset of respiration:
- cold
- gravity
- clamping of umbilical cord

Fig. 1 **Anatomical and physiological changes after birth that allow independent respiration in a baby.**

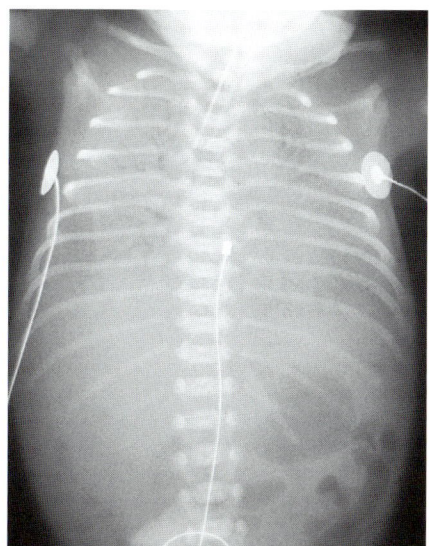

Fig. 2 **CXR of 'ground glass' appearance in respiratory distress syndrome.**

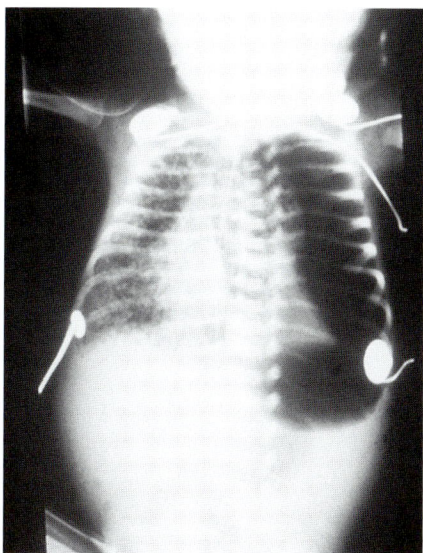

Fig. 3 **CXR shows a hyperlucent area on the left — a tension pneumothorax.**

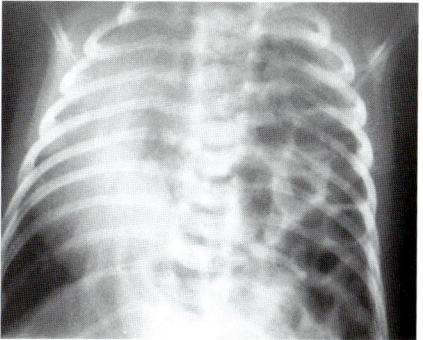

Fig. 4 **CXR of a diaphragmatic hernia.**

Respiratory distress syndrome

This tends to be a problem of premature infants since it is caused by lung surfactant deficiency. Surfactant is a complex lipoprotein consisting mainly of phosphatidyl choline, which lines the alveoli to reduce surface tension. It is synthesised in Type 2 pneumatocytes within the alveoli. Synthesis commences during the second trimester and is usually complete by 35 weeks. A baby born before this time may have insufficient surfactant, resulting in increased work of breathing and signs of respiratory distress. Acidosis, hypoxia and hypothermia further reduce surfactant levels; thus it is important to keep premature babies warm, oxygenated and well-perfused.

The CXR shows a 'ground glass' (Fig. 2) appearance because of poor aeration. Treatment is supportive until the baby's own surfactant is produced in adequate amounts. Oxygen is given by headbox or mechanical ventilation depending on the severity of the illness.

Congenital pneumonia

This is an ascending infection from the birth canal and, therefore, can occur in term or preterm infants. Affected babies show signs of respiratory distress. The risk of infection is increased by prolonged rupture of the membranes (>24 hours). Common organisms are those normally resident in the birth canal such as group B streptococcus and *E. coli*. The CXR shows patchy areas of collapse or consolidation. Treatment is with antibiotics and supportive measures.

Meconium aspiration syndrome

During labour, an asphyxiated term baby may pass meconium into the amniotic fluid and gasp because of sympathetic stimulation. As a consequence, meconium may be aspirated into the lungs. It is irritant, causing pneumonitis, and because of mechanical obstruction results in gas trapping. Resolution occurs with time, therefore treatment is supportive with oxygen, antibiotics and mechanical ventilation where necessary.

Pneumothorax

Pneumothorax (Fig. 3) can be spontaneous or secondary to other lung disease (see above). There is respiratory distress which may be very acute. The CXR shows a hyperlucent area. It is treated by inserting a chest drain.

Congenital anatomical abnormalities

A number of congenital conditions can lead to difficulty in breathing.

A *tracheo-oesophageal fistula* is a connection between the oesophagus and the trachea and is usually combined with oesophageal atresia. The baby presents with cyanosis and frothy oral secretions as it cannot swallow saliva. Treatment is surgery.

A *diaphragmatic hernia* (Fig. 4) is a defect in the diaphragm allowing abdominal contents to herniate up into the thorax in utero. The lungs and heart are compressed causing respiration to become distressed. The CXR shows bowel in the chest. The defect is repaired surgically.

Choanal atresia is an anatomical blockage to the nasal passages preventing the baby from breathing through the nose. Since babies are obligate nose breathers, the obstruction results in intermittent cyanosis.

'Pierre Robin' syndrome (Fig. 5) is the combination of a central cleft palate, a small jaw and a malpositioned tongue (because of the small jaw) which intermittently obstructs the airway. The condition improves as the child grows although the cleft requires surgical closure.

PATHOLOGY OF THE HEART

In these cases the baby commences respiration normally and the lungs are normal, but there is a structural cardiac anomaly preventing oxygenation. The baby is blue, but does not usually have signs of respiratory distress and breathes normally. The condition usually appears within a few hours of birth. There may or may not be a heart murmur or signs of heart failure. Causes and management are dealt with on pages 52–53.

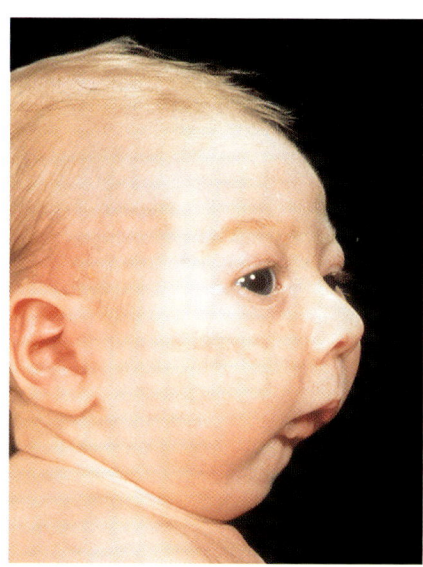

Fig. 5 **Pierre Robin syndrome.**

Blue baby at birth

- Oxygen is the most important drug in resuscitation.
- Central cyanosis is always significant.
- Check resuscitation equipment carefully before resuscitation begins.

CYANOSIS

Cyanosis is a blue coloration of the skin caused by an increase in deoxygenated haemoglobin in the circulation. It is clinically detectable when there is deoxygenated haemoglobin of > 5g/100ml and is, therefore, easy to see in a child with a normal or raised Hb, but difficult to detect in an anaemic child.

Peripheral cyanosis results from poor perfusion of the extremities. The hands and feet appear blue, but the mouth and tongue are pink. It is common in the newborn and in older children, when cold, and is of no significance.

In central cyanosis the mouth and tongue are visibly blue in colour (Fig. 1), indicating that deoxygenated blood is present in the systemic circulation. This is always significant. The discussion below deals primarily with central cyanosis of cardiac origin.

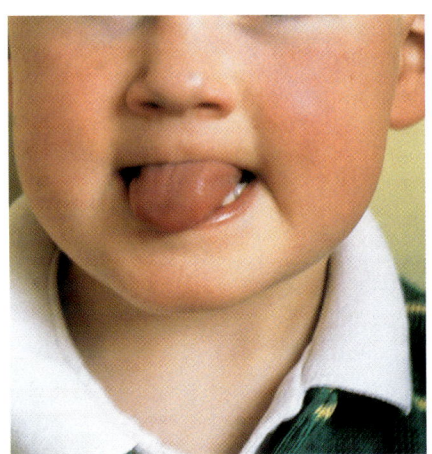

Fig. 1 **Central cyanosis in Fallot's tetralogy.**

CAUSES

Central cyanosis can result from a variety of causes (Table 1). Anatomical cardiac lesions can produce cyanosis by different mechanisms, for example:

- preventing oxygenated blood passing to the systemic circulation in adequate amounts (e.g. transposition of the great vessels)
- by limiting pulmonary blood flow and as a consequence preventing adequate oxygenation (e.g. pulmonary atresia)
- by preventing adequate pulmonary flow and encouraging deoxygenated blood to enter the systemic circulation (e.g. Fallot's tetralogy).

PRESENTATION OF CYANOTIC HEART DISEASE

The presence of significant cyanosis at or soon after birth should be sufficient to bring the infant to medical attention and lead to a diagnosis being reached. However, where cyanosis is not intense, other symptoms and signs become equally important. The combination of low oxygen saturation and reduced systemic blood supply (e.g. hypoplastic left heart syndrome) often leads to rapid collapse with marked hypoxia and acidosis. In less acute situations other symptoms may be present, e.g. respiratory distress, sweating, lethargy, poor feeding and even failure to thrive.

A number of additional signs may accompany the cyanosis (depending on the anatomical defect) and can include: poor peripheral perfusion, hepatomegaly and cardiomegaly. A murmur may be present but is not essential to a diagnosis of cyanotic congenital heart disease.

INVESTIGATIONS

CXR

The following signs may be visible on X-ray:

- Enlarged heart: increased strain on the heart may cause heart failure/dilatation, e.g. transposition.
- Increased lung markings: excess blood flow to the lungs, e.g. transposition.
- Reduced lung markings: insufficient blood flow to the lungs, e.g. tricuspid or pulmonary atresia, Fallot's tetraology (Fig. 2).

A chest X-ray is important to exclude pulmonary pathology, such as pneumonia or the respiratory distress syndrome (RDS).

ECG

The following signs may be seen on ECG:

- Left ventricular hypertrophy: present in lesions causing increased work load on the left ventricle, e.g. pulmonary atresia.

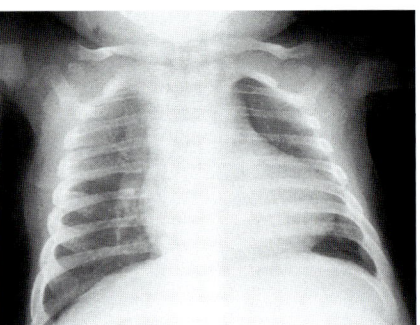

Fig. 2 **CXR in Fallot's tetralogy.**

- Right ventricular hypertrophy: as above but with strain placed on the right ventricle, e.g. Fallot's tetralogy (Fig. 3).
- Biventricular hypertrophy indicating overload on the heart, e.g. patent ductus arteriosus (PDA).
- Right axis deviation, e.g. Fallot's tetralogy.
- Left axis deviation, e.g. tricuspid atresia, pulmonary atresia.
- Other typical ECGs, e.g. huge P wave in Ebstein's anomaly.

Blood gases

Low oxygen (< 7 kPa) is indicative of all true cyanotic conditions. A normal $PaCO_2$ would be expected in uncomplicated cyanotic heart disease.

Nitrogen wash-out test

The baby is placed in 100% oxygen (using a headbox) for about 15 minutes. A blood gas is taken at the beginning and the end of this time. If the cyanosis is caused by a pulmonary problem, the PaO_2 will rise to at least 15 kPa at the end of the test. If, however, the cyanosis is due to cyanotic heart disease, the PaO_2 will not change substantially.

Anatomical diagnosis

Both ultrasound and angiography are used to demonstrate the precise anatomical details of the abnormality (Fig. 4).

Table 1 **The causes of central cyanosis**

Cause	Newborn	Older child
Heart disease	Congenital heart disease, e.g. transposition of the great vessels pulmonary atresia tricuspid atresia hypoplastic left heart Ebstein's anomaly	Congenital heart disease, e.g. Fallot's tetralogy
Pulmonary disease	Respiratory distress syndrome Meconium aspiration Congenital pneumonia Pneumothorax Anatomical abnormality e.g. diaphragmatic hernia	Acute asthma attack Pneumonia Bronchiolitis Epiglottitis Croup Cystic fibrosis
Cerebral depression	Birth asphyxia Septicaemia/meningitis	Raised intracranial pressure Septicaemia/meningitis

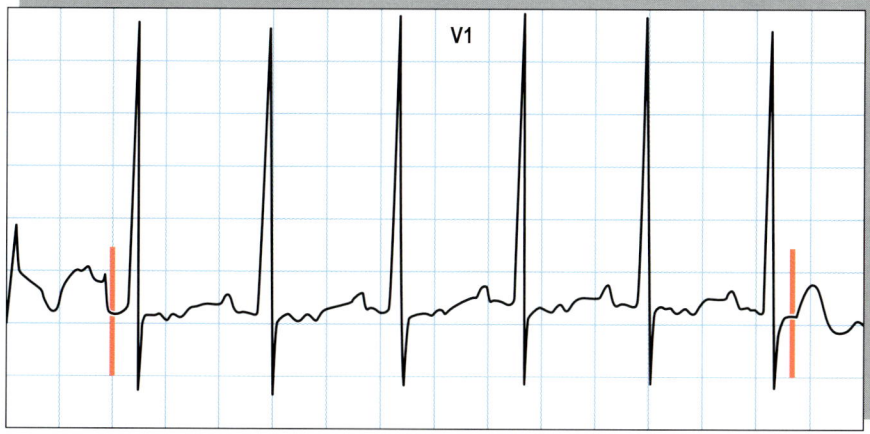

Fig. 3 **ECG in Fallot's tetralogy.** Right ventricular hypertrophy (R > 20 mm and flat T wave).

MANAGEMENT

Emergency treatment

Guidelines for resuscitation are as follows:

- Restrict fluids and give diuretics if the child is in heart failure.
- Give plasma if shocked.
- The blood flow to the lungs may be dependent on the presence of a patent ductus arteriosus, so this must be kept open. It is important to:
  — stop oxygen therapy (oxygen encourages closure of the ductus)
  — give intravenous prostaglandin which inhibits closure of the ductus.

These measures should be employed in a severely cyanotic infant in which the exact cardiac diagnosis is uncertain.

Long-term treatment

Surgical correction of the lesion is always the long-term aim and in most cases is possible. Increasingly, non-invasive techniques are being used in cardiac surgery but few are applicable to cyanotic lesions. In many cases it will be necessary to carry out a minor (palliative) procedure in order to allow the child to grow, total correction being postponed to a later stage.

COMMON CYANOTIC CONGENITAL HEART DISEASES

Transposition of the great vessels

This is the most common cause of cyanotic heart disease in the newborn. The aorta comes off the right ventricle and the pulmonary artery arises from the left ventricle. Desaturated blood enters the systemic circulation and oxygenated blood returns to the lungs. When the ductus arteriosus closes after birth, there is no connection between the pulmonary and systemic circulations, which is incompatible with life. This can be prevented by prostaglandin infusion whilst corrective surgery is planned. The switch operation, which restores normal anatomical connections, is the operation of choice and is performed within the first few days of life. The prognosis is generally good and children go on to lead normal lives.

Pulmonary atresia

In this condition there is an atretic pulmonary valve causing reduced blood flow to the lungs. Treatment is urgent surgery to create a temporary shunt between the left and right sides of circulation. Total correction using a graft can be undertaken later in childhood.

Hypoplastic left heart

In this condition part or all of the left heart is very poorly developed. There is increased blood flow to the lungs and very poor blood flow to the body. Deep cyanosis and severe heart failure are charateristic. Attempts at surgery remain experimental, and the baby usually dies at a few days of age.

Tricuspid atresia

In this condition there is an atretic tricuspid valve which causes reduced blood flow to the lungs. Treatment is surgery in later infancy.

Fallot's tetralogy

Fallot's tetralogy is characterised by four abnormalities:

- pulmonary stenosis (infundibular)
- hypertrophy of the right ventricle
- VSD
- aorta overriding the VSD.

Cyanosis does not occur until later infancy (as the infundibular stenosis develops) and is accompanied by increased tiredness. Some children have 'cyanotic spells' where the child suddenly becomes more deeply cyanosed. During these episodes, the child typically 'squats' on the haunches, which improves the cyanosis by reducing blood flow from the legs, decreasing venous return and improving cardiac function. The CXR shows a small boot-shaped heart (right ventricular hypertropy) with reduced blood flow to the lungs.

Treatment is with surgical correction before the child starts school. The prognosis is very good. Cyanotic spells are treated by putting the child in the knee–elbow position and giving oxygen, β-blockers and morphine.

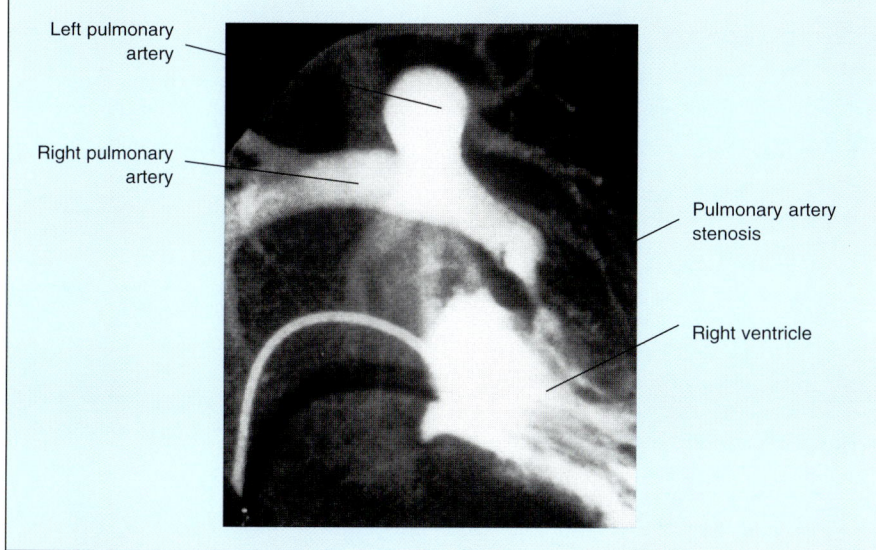

Fig. 4 **Angiogram of Fallot's tetralogy**

Left pulmonary artery

Right pulmonary artery

Pulmonary artery stenosis

Right ventricle

Cyanosis

- Central cyanosis is always significant.
- Oxygen can make cyanosis worse in congenital cyanotic heart conditions.
- Transfer of the cyanotic neonate to a cardiac centre must be done with the utmost care.

MURMURS

A murmur is an extra noise heard on auscultation of the heart. It is caused by turbulent blood flow and can occur in systole or diastole. A murmur can be innocent, when there is no abnormality of the heart, or pathological, when there is an underlying cardiac defect.

Assessment of heart sounds is, thus, important. The first heart sound is caused by the closure of the mitral and tricuspid valves. The second is caused by the closure of the aortic and pulmonary valves. The closure of these latter two valves is not synchronous. The pulmonary valve closes after the aortic, but the delay is variable since respiration can enhance (on inspiration) or diminish (on expiration) right ventricular filling.

Transient murmurs sometimes occur in the newborn because the natural changes that should take place at birth have not been completed (see pp. 50–51). Pathological murmurs can be associated with cyanosis (see pp. 52–53), or they may be acyanotic, as described in this chapter.

INNOCENT MURMURS

Many childhood murmurs are 'innocent'. About one-third of children will have an 'innocent' murmur at some time in their life, especially when there is increased cardiac output causing turbulent blood flow, e.g. during a fever, after exercise or in the presence of anaemia. On re-examination when the fever has resolved or the anaemia is corrected, the murmur will normally have diminished or disappeared. Some 'innocent' murmurs are present all the time, but alter in character on changing the position of the child, in contrast to a pathological murmur. A 'venous hum' is an 'innocent' murmur heard through systole and diastole, loudest below the right clavicle, caused by turbulent blood flow through the great vessels.

PHYSIOLOGY OF ACYANOTIC LESIONS

Abnormal communication in the heart

In these lesions, there is an abnormal connection between the two sides of the circulation. This can be at any level: atrial septal defect (ASD), ventricular septal defect (VSD) or patent ductus arteriosus (PDA).

In all these lesions, blood flows (shunts) from the left side to the right (because the systemic circulation pressure is higher than the pulmonary pressure) and creates a murmur. As a result, excessive blood flows through the lungs and, if extreme, reduces pulmonary function with consequent signs of respiratory distress. Symptoms include breathlessness, tachypnoea, tachycardia, sweating and reduced exercise tolerance, i.e. poor feeding.

Reduced pulmonary blood flow

Pulmonary stenosis

This lesion impedes pulmonary flow and creates a murmur. Depending on severity, symptoms vary from tiredness to cyanosis.

Reduced systemic blood flow

Aortic stenosis

This narrowing leads to reduced systemic flow and produces a murmur. Depending on severity, symptoms may include: breathlessness on exertion (secondary to left ventricular failure), angina (secondary to reduced coronary blood supply), and syncope (secondary to reduced cerebral blood supply).

Coarctation of the aorta

In this condition, blood supply to the lower part of the body is reduced by a narrowing of the aortic arch. Because of the consequent reduction in renal flow, hypertension occurs, however effects are only seen proximal to the coarctation. Secondary heart failure may result in cardiac enlargement, pulmonary oedema and signs of respiratory distress.

KEY POINTS IN THE EXAMINATION OF A CHILD WITH A MURMUR

- **Observe for breathlessness or cyanosis. (Fig. 1).**

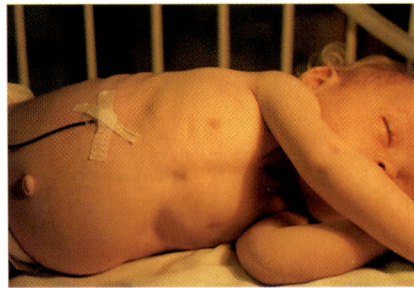

Fig. 1 **Breathless baby.**

- **Pulse:**
  — Palpable in arms, but not legs — obstruction to the aorta: coarctation.
  — Bounding — wide pulse pressure: persistent ductus arteriosus.
  — Weak at all sites — narrow pulse pressure: aortic stenosis.
- **Blood pressure:** lower in children than in adults. To obtain an accurate reading when taking the BP, the balloon must cover two-thirds of the upper arm and should wrap round two-thirds of the arm circumference.

- **Palpation:** palpate the suprasternal notch, and the four areas of the heart.
  — A 'thrill' denotes the presence of a loud murmur, e.g. a suprasternal notch 'thrill' often occurs in aortic stenosis.
  — A 'heave' denotes hypertrophy, e.g. left parasternal in right ventricular hypertrophy, apical in left ventricular hypertrophy.
  — Apex beat: outside midclavicular line and 4th intercostal space indicates an enlarged heart.
- **Auscultation:**
  — First heart sound: loud in anaemia, pyrexia, and after exercise.
  — Second heart sound: soft in pulmonary and aortic stenosis; widely split in ASD (does not vary with respiration because of constant right ventricular filling by the shunt); may be loud when there is pulmonary hypertension; may be single in aortic stenosis (because of late closure).
  — Systolic murmur — not always pathological.
  — Diastolic murmur — always abnormal.
  — Site of murmur: lower left sternal edge (VSD); aortic region (aortic stenosis); pulmonary area (pulmonary stenosis).
  — Timing of murmur: pansystolic (VSD); ejection systolic (aortic stenosis/pulmonary stenosis); through systole and diastole (patent ductus arteriosus).
  — Character of murmur: very harsh like tearing fabric (VSD).
  — Radiation of murmur: neck (aortic stenosis).

USEFUL INVESTIGATIONS

- **CXR:**
  — Enlarged heart: indicates failure or hypertrophy (Fig. 2).
  — Plethoric lung fields: significant left to right shunt, e.g. ASD, VSD, PDA.
  — Oligaemic lung fields: reduced pulmonary blood supply, e.g. pulmonary stenosis.

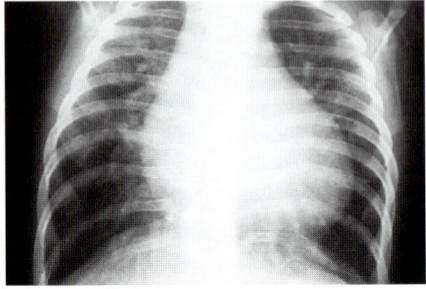

Fig. 2 **CXR showing enlarged heart in VSD.**

- **ECG:**
  — Demonstrates the electrical axis of the heart.
  — Can confirm hypertrophy of the right or left ventricle (Fig. 3).
  — Shows the rate and rhythm of the heart. NB sinus arrhythmia is naturally present more prominently in childhood than in adults and should not be mistaken for an irregular beat.
- **Oxygen measurement:** by arterial blood sample or transcutaneous saturation monitor (see p. 63).
- **Cardiac echo:** shows the precise anatomical abnormality of the heart. This investigation is particularly useful in children as it is not invasive (Fig. 4).
- **Cardiac catheter:** also shows the anatomical abnormality but is much more invasive than an echo. It is therefore only used to show features that cannot be obtained by echo, e.g. exact cardiac chamber pressure measurements.

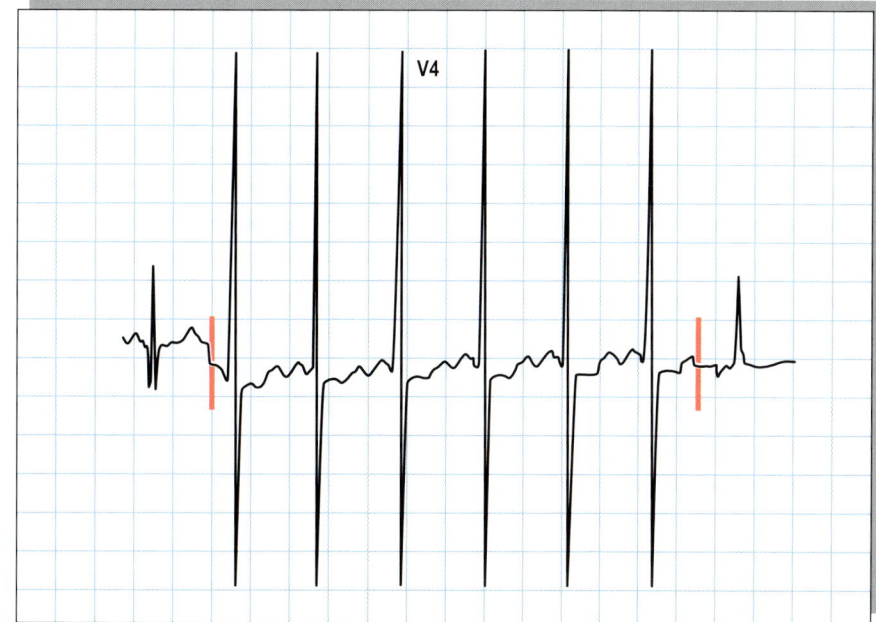

Fig. 3 **ECG showing biventricular hypertrophy in VSD.**

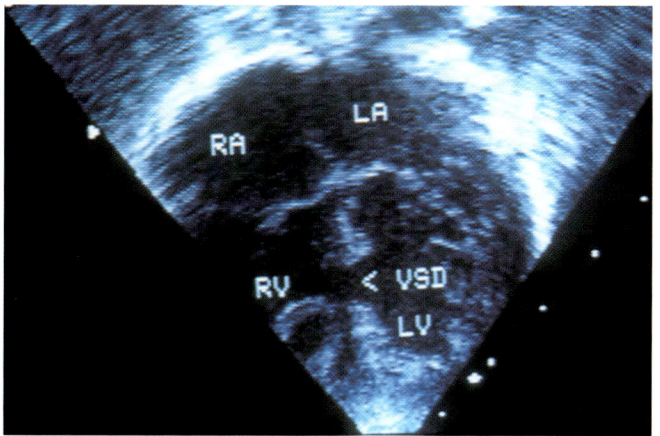

Fig. 4 **Echocardigram of VSD.**

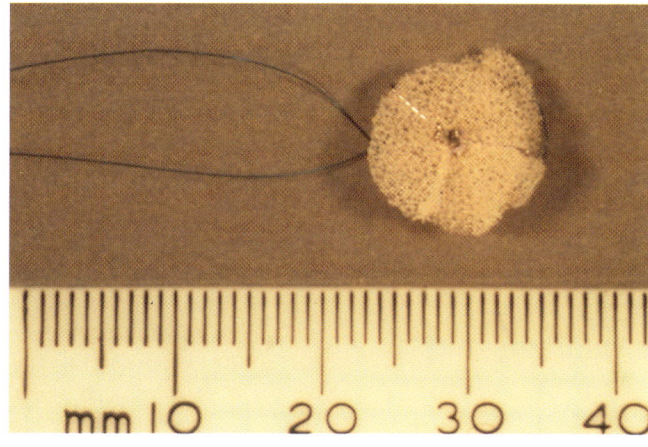

Fig. 5 **Umbrella used to close VSD.**

COMMON EXAMPLES OF CONGENITAL LESIONS CAUSING MURMURS WITHOUT CYANOSIS

VSD

This is the most common congenital heart lesion presenting in children. There is a hole between the right and the left ventricles. Blood flows from left to right ventricle in systole, causing a systolic murmur. There may be signs of heart failure at an early age if the hole is large. If the hole is small, there will be no signs of heart failure and the child will be well. If heart failure occurs, medical treatment and/or surgical closure will be needed. Surgery usually involves an open operation but, in suitable cases, an 'umbrella' can be inserted through a venous catheter (Fig. 5). Many VSDs close spontaneously as the child gets older. A symptomatic VSD left untreated will lead eventually to pulmonary hypertension (Eisenmenger's syndrome).

ASD

Here there is a hole between the right and the left atria, either through the septum primum (primum ASD) or through the septum secundum (secundum ASD). The murmur is not due to flow through the ASD, but due to the resulting increased flow through the pulmonary valve; thus it is heard best in the pulmonary area. As a consequence pulmonary valve closure is delayed, resulting in fixed splitting of the second heart sound. There are often no symptoms at all. Treatment is surgery: it does not close on its own.

PDA

This condition is common in premature neonates and is caused by the fetal connection between the aorta and pulmonary vessels remaining open. The murmur is initially in systole only, but as the pressure in the systemic circulation rises and that in the pulmonary circulation falls after birth, it becomes continuous through systole and diastole. All the pulses feel 'bounding', i.e. very full, because of the rapid fall in pressure as the blood escapes across the PDA, causing a wide pulse pressure. Unless the PDA closes spontaneously in the first few months of life, surgical closure is necessary.

Murmurs

- Many murmurs are innocent.
- Murmurs create great parental anxiety.
- Heart disease can exist without a murmur.
- Murmurs can be associated with other conditions, e.g. ASD and VSD with Down's syndrome, coarctation with Turner's syndrome.
- Abnormal heart sounds are important in the assessment of murmurs.

COUGH

Cough is an extremely common symptom and accounts for a large number of primary care consultations. The purpose of a cough is to protect the lower respiratory tract from inhalation of solid particles. The mechanism of cough involves:

- inspiration
- closure of the vocal cords (glottis)
- expiration against a closed glottis so pressure in the chest increases
- opening of the glottis.

The sudden acceleration of air out of the airways causes the characteristic noise of the cough. The respiratory tract is lined with a thin film of mucus and any inhaled particles tend to be held in the mucus. During a cough the high linear acceleration of the air column either pushes the particles up towards the glottis within the mucus film, or if they are a suitable size they are pulled into the air column and expectorated. Large objects in the airways may be difficult to cough up (Fig. 1). Cough is only useful at removing objects in the first few branches of the airways. Below that level, other mechanisms are needed (e.g. cilial movement).

THE COUGH REFLEX

A number of different stimuli can activate the cough reflex but the main receptors are irritant receptors in the larynx, trachea and large bronchi. They react to mechanical, chemical and inflammatory stimuli. As with other reflex arcs, there is a central nervous connection and an efferent pathway (via the respiratory and laryngeal muscles). The central control of cough is particularly important because coughing (and breathing) can also be partly affected by voluntary control.

A depressed or absent cough reflex is a serious cause for concern as it leaves the airway unprotected. It can be due to afferent, central or efferent pathway disruption (Table 1).

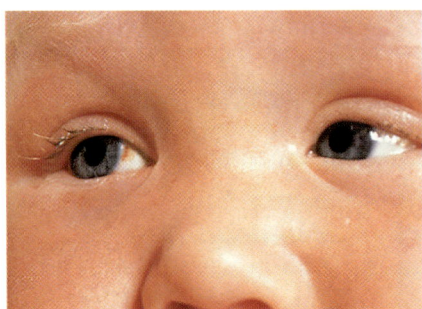

Fig. 2 **Sub-conjunctival haemorrhage.**

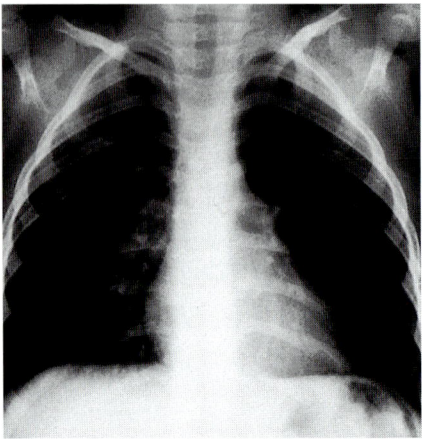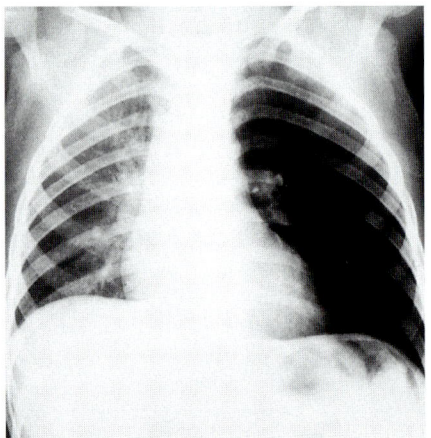

Fig. 1 **Chest X-ray showing the effect of a foreign body on inspiration (left) and expiration (right).** The left lung fails to deflate on expiration due to blockage by the foreign body.

TYPES OF COUGH

The sound and pattern of the cough can be helpful in distinguishing possible causes (Table 2) although some coughs are rather non-descript. Many children and parents find it difficult to explain what it sounds like but can recognise it when they hear it.

Barking cough

A barking cough is caused by oedema around the larynx. It is less explosive and more musical than a 'normal' cough and sounds like the bark of a sea lion. Because the larynx is involved, a barking cough is accompanied by a hoarse voice and, if the airway is narrowed sufficiently, stridor may also be present (pp. 58–59).

Paroxysmal cough

A paroxysmal cough occurs when there is particularly tenacious sputum which is difficult to expectorate. Essentially it is defined as a sequence of coughs without a breath between them. This results in the child becoming blue in the face (and often developing petechial haemorrhages) as maximum expiration approaches (Fig. 2). The subsequent inspiration may be noisy and is described as a 'whoop'. The whoop is unlikely to be heard in children under 6 months of age because of reduced muscle strength. At this age the cough may be associated with apnoea. Vomiting is often caused by the cough and fits may also occur. Whooping cough is a likely diagnosis even if the child has been immunised, but other viruses (respiratory syncytial virus, adenovirus and parainfluenza) are possible culprits.

In children under 1 year whooping cough is a frightening disease with a significant mortality from respiratory or neurological sequelae. Antibiotics (e.g. erythromycin) do not alter the clinical course once the child has progressed from the prodromal (coryzal) phase but may prevent transmission. For older children and adults the main problems associated with whooping cough are weight loss because of the vomiting and the prolonged nature of the cough. The coughing spasms gradually improve but may recur with subsequent colds for up to a year.

Wheezy cough

After the first sound of the cough, wheezes are heard. Although this is a common type of cough in asthma (pp. 62–63) it is also quite commonly heard in viral pneumonia and bronchiolitis.

Throat clearing cough

As might be expected, this sort of cough is a response to secretions in the pharynx. The usual source of the mucus is the nasal passages and is often described as a 'post-nasal drip'. The excessive mucus is usually caused by a viral upper respiratory infection but if other features are present further investigations or treatment may be warranted.

If the history is short with a high fever, a purulent discharge and pain, the child should be treated for sinusitis with antibiotics.

Table 1 **Depressed cough reflex**

Afferent nerves	Local anaesthetics
	Trauma to vagus nerve
Central	Depressed conscious level from any cause including anaesthetic drugs
	Congenital or acquired CNS damage
	Preterm babies (<32 weeks)
Efferent	Vocal cord palsy
	Decreased muscle power

Table 2 **Distinguishable types of cough**

Barking
Paroxysmal
Wheezy
Throat clearing
Productive
Dry/non-specific

Table 3 **History and differential diagnosis of chronic productive cough (bronchiectasis)**

Cause of underlying abnormality	Diagnosis	Features
Airway lumen	Inhaled foreign body (Fig. 1) Recurrent aspiration	Choking at start of symptoms Vomiting, choking on feeding, depressed cough reflex
Airway mucus	Cystic fibrosis	Loose stools, failure to thrive
Cilia dysfunction	Ciliary dyskinesia	ENT problems, dextrocardia
Airway immune deficiency	Variety of congenital or acquired problems	Recurrent proven chest infections, infections at other sites
Abnormal airway architecture	Congenital Post-infective	? other congenital lesions Previous whooping cough or measles

If the history is of persistent (perennial) or recurrent symptoms with clear discharge, sneezing, nasal blockage (often with snoring) and conjunctivitis, then allergic rhinitis is likely. The history may identify trigger factors (e.g. grass pollen, tree pollen, animal fur) and there may be the other atopic features of eczema, asthma and urticaria. Treatment with topical anti-inflammatory agents or oral antihistamines suppresses the allergic reaction.

Productive cough

Because small children swallow their sputum it may be difficult to get a sample to examine (Fig. 3). Gastric washings, vomit (children with cough often vomit) or cough swabs can be attempted if it is essential to obtain a sample.

An acute illness with a productive cough is associated with any number of organisms causing a lower respiratory infection. These include viral pneumonia, mycoplasma and bacterial infections. Contrary to popular belief, a productive cough is *not* a feature of lobar pneumonia in the acute stage, although it becomes productive as the pneumonia resolves and the alveolar exudate mobilises. Likewise, tuberculosis in children usually presents as a systemic disease with a dry cough and a history of contact. It is the adults with a breakdown of an old TB lesion who spread

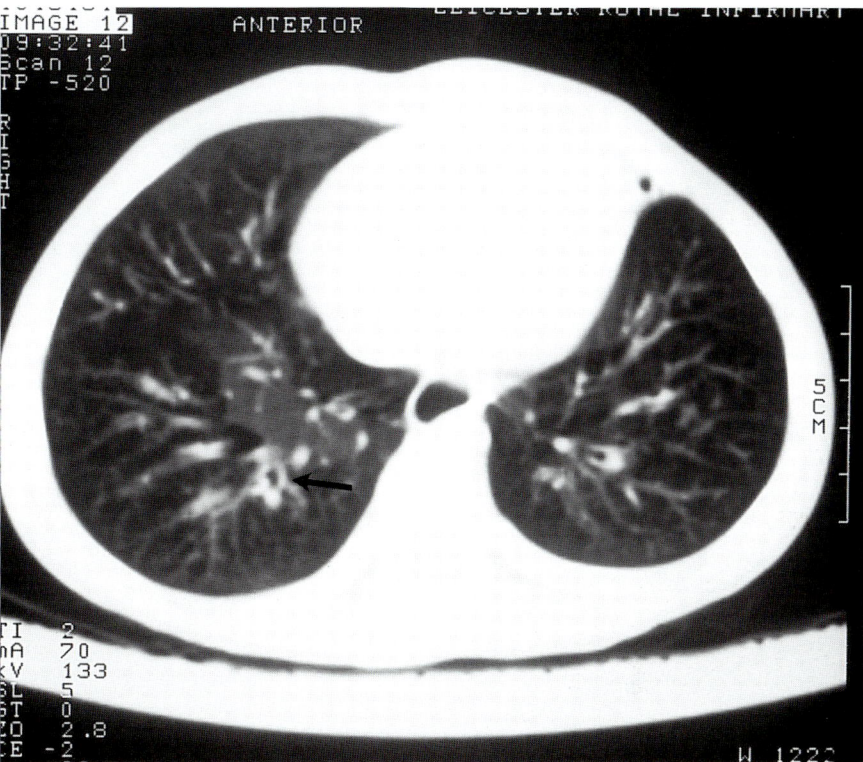

Fig. 4 **CT scan of bronchiectasis.** The arrow shows an enlarged airway with surrounding inflammation.

the disease and have a prominent productive cough.

A chronic productive cough is a worrying symptom and is usually equated with bronchiectasis. Bronchiectasis (Fig. 4) is a pathological term meaning dilated areas in the airways with walls weakened by chronic inflammation. Once the airways are damaged it is more difficult to clear secretions so stasis, infection and further airway damage occurs. Bronchiectasis is one of the main causes of clubbing and the differential diagnosis and appropriate questions in the history are given in Table 3.

Dry/non-specific cough

A dry cough is extremely common at the beginning of a cold and is not very helpful diagnostically. There are occasional children where the cough is psychogenic and if so it tends to disappear when the child is distracted and when asleep. A dry cough may be an

important finding in combination with other symptoms. The combination of a dry cough, high fever, tachypnoea and grunting respiration strongly suggests a pneumonia and if it is combined with chest (or sometimes abdominal) pain the diagnosis is almost certain even without a chest X-ray.

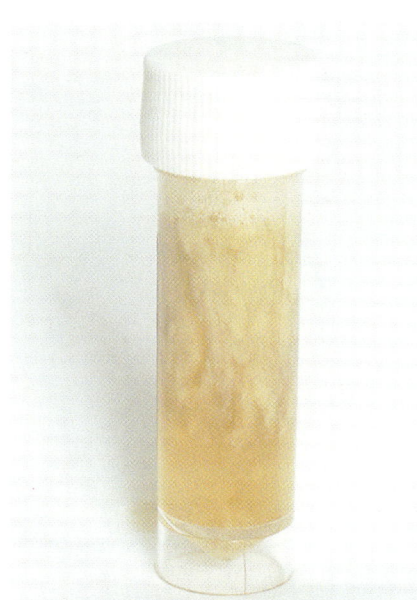

Fig. 3 **Purulent sputum, thick and yellowish in colour.**

Cough

- The type of cough may suggest the diagnosis.
- Upper respiratory infections and asthma are common causes of cough.
- Chronic sputum production (bronchiectasis) needs further investigation.

NOISY BREATHING

DEFINITIONS

There are a number of noises children can make while breathing. They are summarised in Table 1. Although it is often assumed that everyone knows what these noises are, in fact a lot of parents may not and, in particular, they often confuse stridor and wheeze.

SNUFFLES

Snuffly breathing is due to nasal secretions and blockage. It is almost always due to a cold. If it has been present since birth, a congenital nasal blockage (choanal atresia/stenosis) is possible and can be diagnosed by the inability to pass a nasogastric tube into the pharynx.

Colds in small babies are a cause of anxiety because they disrupt the baby's breathing and make feeding more difficult. A cold may also be the first sign of bronchiolitis in the winter season. In toddlers with snuffles and unilateral nasal discharge, a foreign body must be excluded. In older children with snuffly breathing, sinusitis or allergic rhinitis (see pp. 56–57) is likely.

SNORING

Snoring is so common that it is often not perceived as a problem by parents and not mentioned unless it is specifically asked about. Seven per cent of children are persistent snorers and during colds this rises to 50%. Persistent snoring, sometimes called obstructive sleep apnoea (OSA), can have significant adverse effects (Table 2) and may not be associated with much in the way of physical signs. The cause of snoring is a narrowed upper airway either physical

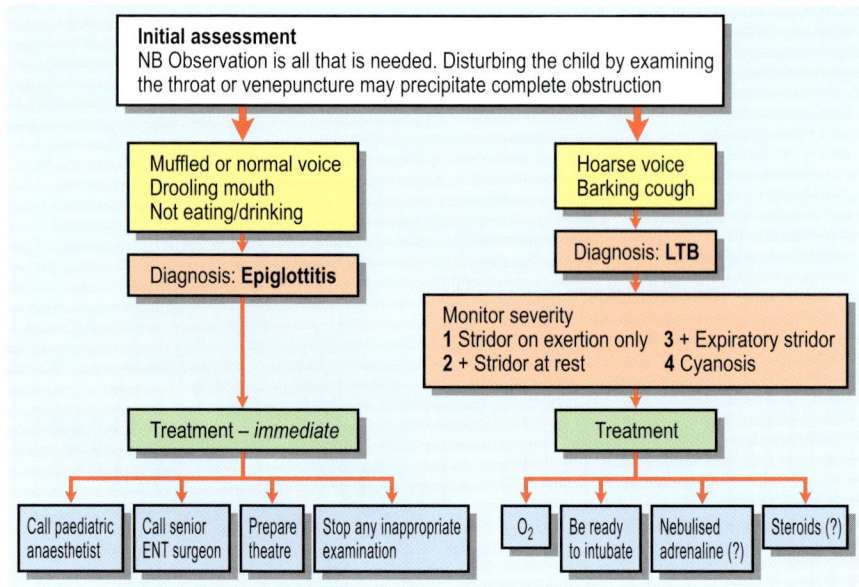

Fig. 1 **Emergency management of upper airways obstruction.**

(because of secretions, large adenoids, etc.) or functional (hypotonia or dysfunction of the muscles of the pharynx) or a combination of both. If the snoring is severe and does not respond to medical treatment adeno-tonsilectomy is usually performed to enlarge the airway.

STRIDOR

Stridor commonly presents acutely in a previously well child. Narrowing of the larynx or trachea is a potential emergency (Fig. 1). It is important to assess the severity of the obstruction and distinguish between

epiglottitis, viral laryngotracheobronchitis (LTB) and inhaled foreign body.

An inhaled foreign body should be suspected if there is a sudden onset of symptoms, especially if the child (usually a toddler) has been in contact with a source of small objects (e.g. peanuts, small toys, splinters of wood chewed off a cot). Often there is a history of choking at the onset of the inhalation. Differentiating epiglottitis from LTB depends on their relative anatomical positions and functions. Epiglottitis is now rare, particularly where Hib vaccination is routine (it is usually caused by *H. influenzae*) but is still important because it

Table 1 **Definition of respiratory noises**

Type of noise	Definition
Snuffles	Noise when breathing in and out, coming from the nose or throat. Sounds 'bubbly' and generally applied to infants
Snoring	Low pitched rumbling noise on inspiration or expiration while asleep
Stridor	Noise of uniform pitch nearly always on inspiration coming from the trachea, larynx or posterior pharynx
Cough	Expiratory noise with explosive start arising from the larynx (see pp. 56–57)
Wheeze	Musical noise with descending pitch usually heard in expiration and often multiple, coming from the lower respiratory tract. Often described as like a seagull's cry
Grunt	Expiratory noise from the larynx, similar to a cough but with vocalisation making it softer

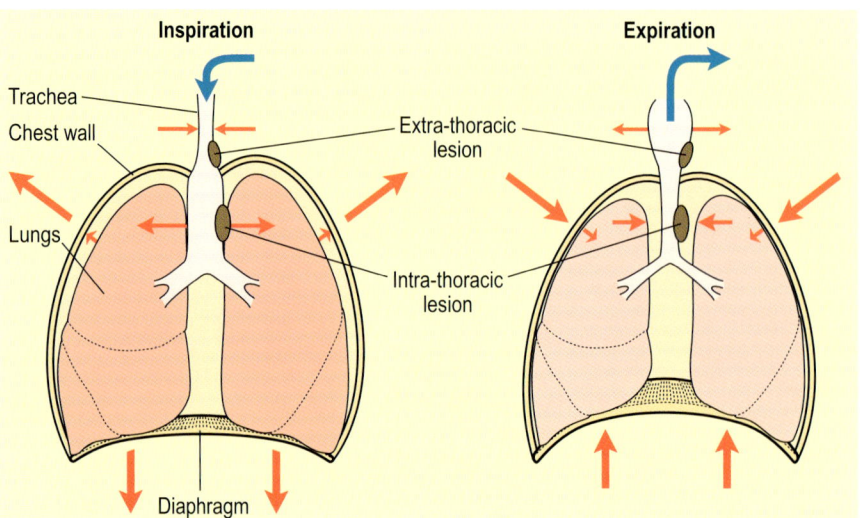

Fig. 2 **Mechanism of dynamic airways compression.** In inspiration the diaphragm moves down and the lungs inflate pulling open the intrathoracic airways. The extrathoracic trachaea tends to be sucked in. The reverse happens in expiration. In the presence of respiratory disease this effect is accentuated because of greater respiratory effort and hence bigger pressure gradients across the airway. Noise from the respiratory tract arises when the airway is narrowed sufficiently, i.e. in inspiration for extrathoracic and expiration for intrathoracic lesions.

Table 2 **Obstructive sleep apnoea**

Symptoms	Snoring
	Disturbed sleep
Consequences	Tiredness and falling asleep during the day
	Developmental delay
	Failure to thrive
	Heart failure
Examination findings	Usually nil
	Large tonsils
	Signs of cor pulmonale
Investigations	Low overnight oxygen saturation
	Right heart strain on ECG

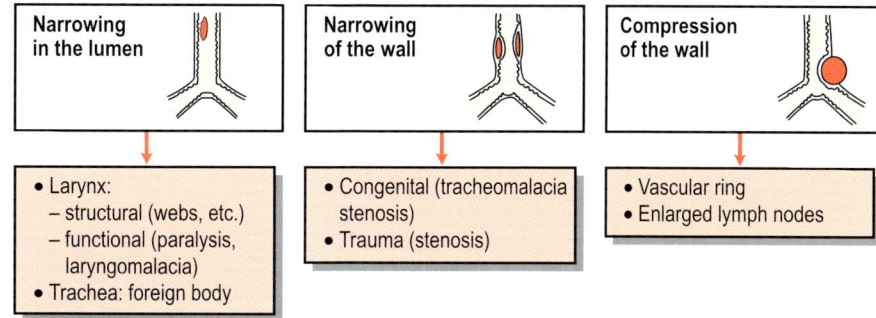

Fig. 3 **Causes of chronic stridor.**

is treatable and may result in sudden complete airway obstruction if managed badly.

The term 'croup' is often used to mean LTB but is also used to describe the symptom of stridor or even a barking cough. Once LTB has been confidently diagnosed, the treatment is supportive and intervention depends on the degree of respiratory distress.

Some children have recurrent episodes of stridor. Many of these seem to have a form of asthma and have other features of atopy. Alternatively, where there is a history of neonatal intubation, a sub-glottic stenosis may be present which only gives rise to symptoms when the airway is further narrowed by a cold. Stridor is usually heard on inspiration. The presence of expiratory stridor caused by an extrathoracic lesion indicates marked narrowing of the airway. The mechanism for this is shown in Figure 2. If the lesion is *intra*thoracic expiratory stridor predominates. Chronic or congenital stridor can be caused by a variety of lesions narrowing the airway (Fig. 3).

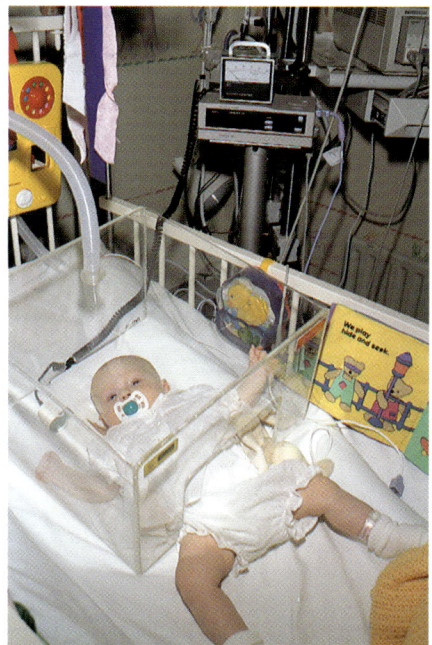

Fig. 4 **Baby with bronchiolitis.** The baby is in additional humidified oxygen from a headbox. This is monitored by an oxygen saturation monitor applied to the child's hand.

COUGH

Cough is an important symptom which is dealt with on pp. 56–57.

WHEEZE

The noise of a wheeze is caused by lower respiratory airway narrowing and may be heard with or without the stethoscope (auscultatory or auditory). Wheeze is *not* synonymous with asthma, although it is the most common cause in older children.

Infants

In infants (<1 year of age) the important features in the history are the pattern of the wheezing (first attack, chronic or recurrent symptoms) and the season of the year. The loudness of the wheezing does not give any idea of the severity, but associated features of respiratory distress (poor feeding, cyanosis or apnoea) are helpful.

An infant who starts with symptoms of a cold progressing to a first episode of wheeze in the winter months probably has bronchiolitis. Most cases are caused by the respiratory syncytial virus (RSV) and it varies in severity from a mild cold to severe respiratory failure requiring ventilation. The usual features on examination are a cough, respiratory distress, crepitations on auscultation and often a wheeze. The most severe cases occur when the baby is very young (<6 weeks) or has bronchiolitis complicating an underlying lung problem. Therefore, it is always important to check for clinical evidence in the history and examination, of neonatal chronic lung disease, cystic fibrosis, heart failure and congenital lung anomalies (see other sections for details). For this reason it is routine to X-ray the chest of all children with significant bronchiolitis admitted to hospital. Treatment is supportive with oxygen (Fig. 4), nasogastric feeds or i.v. fluids and mechanical ventilation if necessary.

The relationship between infantile asthma and bronchiolitis is confusing because both have clinical definitions which overlap. Moreover, a significant minority of children

who have had RSV positive bronchiolitis go on to have further wheezing episodes indistinguishable from asthma. This does not make any difference to treatment but may be important for the child's risk of continuing with asthma into adulthood. Infants with features of 'post-bronchiolitis wheeze' tend to improve as they get older, whereas children with atopic features are more likely to continue to have respiratory illness.

Older children

Asthma is the major diagnosis in children with recurrent wheeze and is dealt with on pages 60–63. As with younger children, an acute presentation with no past history could be infective (e.g. viral or mycoplasma pneumonia) as well as a first attack of asthma. Children with more severe or persistent wheezing occasionally turn out to have bronchiectasis (see p. 57).

GRUNTING

The presence of grunting (breathing out against a closed glottis) indicates alveolar disease. The lungs remain at higher inflation for a larger proportion of the respiratory cycle and this appears to act as a compensatory mechanism to help gas transfer. In the newborn it is one of the signs of respiratory distress and in older children often indicates pneumonia.

Noisy breathing

- Ask specifically about snoring.
- Epiglottitis is diagnosed on history and observation only — distressing the child can be fatal.
- Not everything that wheezes is asthma, particularly in infants.
- Bronchiolitis may unmask other diseases.

ACUTE BREATHING DIFFICULTY

In order to function normally, the respiratory system needs:

- an adequate gas exchange surface (alveoli)
- a normal airway for air to move in and out of the alveoli
- a pump (diaphragm and respiratory muscles) to move the air
- a control system (consisting of receptors, afferent nerves, the respiratory centre in the medulla and the efferent nerves).

For normal function the blood and gas supply to the alveoli must be carefully matched. In the presence of inflammation (e.g. following infection), inadequate or excessive pulmonary blood flow, diminished gas exchange and respiratory distress may result.

The air passages are usefully divided into upper and lower. Anatomically, the division between upper and lower airways is at the larynx. However, in clinical practice the lower airways are defined as starting at the carina. This is because pathology in the larynx and trachea presents in similar ways and is easily separated from more peripheral lung disease.

In normal breathing the diaphragm is the major muscle of respiration. It is dome shaped and it flattens when it contracts, sucking air into the chest and displacing the abdominal contents. The abdomen always moves out in inspiration and observing this can be helpful in babies when it may be difficult to tell if a baby is breathing in or out.

The physiology of the control of breathing is complex, involving peripheral and central chemoreceptors and an input from the mechanoreceptors of the chest wall and lung. Integration of these signals in the respiratory centre results in very tight control of levels of pH, oxygen and carbon dioxide. Abnormalities of the respiratory centre or chemoreceptors are rare even with severe brain injury and usually result in reduced breathing efforts rather than breathing difficulty. However, immature responses (such as periodic breathing, Fig. 1) are seen in neonates and especially in preterm infants. It has been suggested that this immaturity is a factor in the sudden infant death syndrome (SIDS).

In clinical paediatrics, difficulty breathing is usually secondary to a pulmonary problem in the airways, but occasionally unrecognised neuromuscular disease or metabolic acidosis (Kussmaul breathing) presents in this way.

DEFINITIONS

There are a number of terms to describe breathing difficulty which tend to be used interchangeably, although they have slightly different but overlapping meanings (Table 1).

Table 1 **Terms relating to respiratory distress**

Term	Definition
Difficulty in breathing	Generic term covering almost any problem with breathing
Respiratory distress	Increase in the work of breathing with recession, tracheal tug and increased chest/abdominal movement
Tachypnoea	Raised respiratory rate
Breathlessness	Subjective feeling by the patient of inadequate respiration
Dyspnoea	Unpleasant feeling of respiratory difficulty

HISTORY AND EXAMINATION

Important causes of acute respiratory difficulty in childhood are:

- asthma
- viral croup (see pp. 58–59)
- bronchiolitis (see p. 59)
- epiglottitis (see pp. 58–59)
- inhaled foreign body (see pp. 56–57)
- whooping cough (see pp. 56–57)
- cardiac failure (pp. 54–55).

Bronchiolitis occurs as a seasonal epidemic each winter in babies. Outside this period, asthma and viral croup are the most common causes of acute breathing difficulty presenting to hospital. History therefore tends to focus on the exclusion of other conditions.

If the illness is not life-threatening, a history covering the presenting symptoms, the onset, and their severity can be taken. Sudden onset of symptoms, particularly with choking at the start, strongly suggests inhalation of a foreign body. This is most common in the toddler age group where children are mobile but still examine objects by putting them in their mouths. At this age the child himself is unable to give a clear history. Alternatively, a slower onset of symptoms after an upper respiratory infection or exposure to allergens like cat fur, grass, etc. suggests asthma as a likely diagnosis. Fever may be an indication of pneumonia (viral, atypical or bacterial) but many acute asthma attacks are also accompanied by a fever from an associated upper respiratory infection. Whatever the cause, it is important to know the degree of respiratory distress the child has suffered during the illness. This may be difficult for the parents to describe objectively, but useful questions are given in Table 2. Chest or abdominal pain may be a prominent feature of pneumonia.

General examination including conscious level and vital signs (temperature, pulse, respiratory rate, blood pressure) is clearly important in determining the severity of the child's overall condition. A diagnosis of an upper respiratory disease can often be determined from the noise made on breathing (pp. 58–59). Observation can indicate a prolonged expiratory phase of respiration with or without audible wheeze (small airway obstruction), panting or grunting (alveolar disease) or asymmetrical movement (lobar pneumonia, pneumothorax, effusion). A subjective assessment of the amount of respiratory distress can also be made by observing the use of accessory muscles of respiration and the degree of

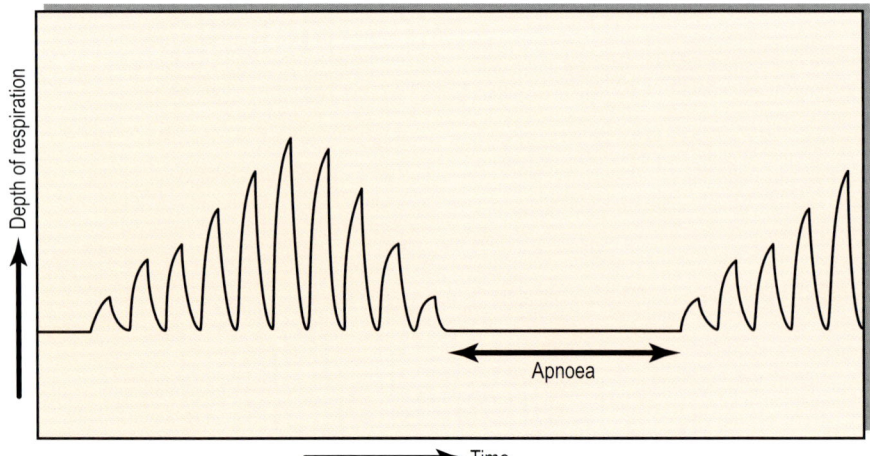

Fig. 1 **Periodic breathing.** The diagram shows overbreathing followed by apnoea caused by a lack of fine regulation of the breathing system. In an adult this 'Cheyne–Stokes' breathing implies severe neurological damage but it is a normal finding in term and preterm infants.

intercostal recession. Percussion is rarely helpful. Auscultation is often limited by the transmission of upper airway rattle. However, it may be possible to identify wheeze (airway obstruction), crepitations (alveolar disease) or bronchial breathing (collapse/consolidation). A silent chest denotes severe obstruction or a pneumothorax.

INVESTIGATIONS

The most important investigation in children with difficulty in breathing is measurement of oxygen saturation. Oxygenated and deoxygenated haemoglobin differ in their ability to absorb particular wavelengths of red light. Oxygen saturation monitors measure this difference and estimate the proportion of blood that is saturated with oxygen. Because they are non-invasive, they are much more practical than measuring blood gases. A graph of SaO_2 against PaO_2 gives the oxygen dissociation curve (Fig. 2). It can be seen that at high saturations (>95%) it is difficult to infer very much about PaO_2. However, ability to maintain 90% saturation is an indication that adequate oxygenation of the blood is occurring in the lungs. To be sure that tissues are adequately oxygenated, both cardiac output and haemoglobin level must also be satisfactory.

The chest X-ray is mainly useful in confirming a clinical diagnosis, e.g.

Table 2 **Questions to determine disease severity**

Questions	Comment
Can he speak in sentences? (for infants, does he struggle to breathe when feeding?)	Gives an idea of the degree of respiratory distress and tachypnoea
How much can he move about?	Is he in bed all the time? Can he get up to go to the toilet; can he climb stairs; can he manage to get to school? This gives information on the child's functional disability
Has he been blue?	Acute cyanosis is a sign of serious respiratory embarrassment
How much bronchodilator (reliever) has he taken?	For known asthmatics

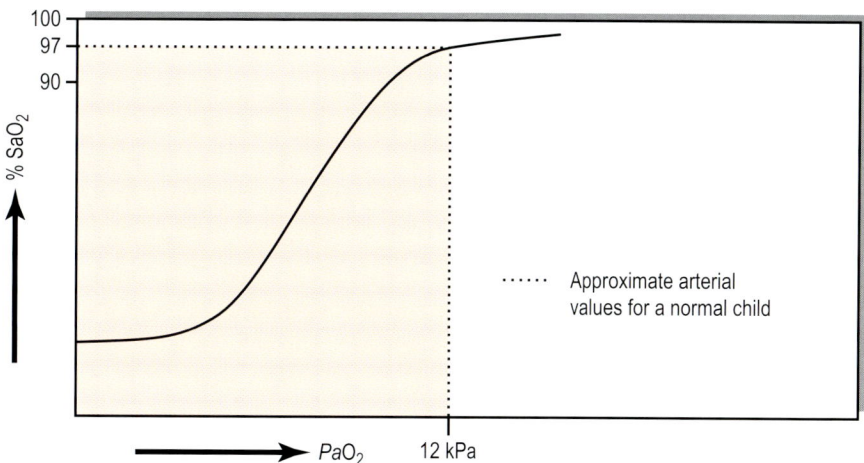

Fig. 2 **Keeping SaO$_2$ >90% ensures that arterial blood is at the top of the dissociation curve and indicates that adequate oxygenation is occurring in the lungs.** At high saturations (>97%) monitors are relatively inaccurate.

pneumonia, and, on first presentation, excluding an unsuspected anomaly. In asthma it may show hyperinflation, bronchial wall thickening, or small areas of collapse (atelectasis) due to mucus plugging but is quite often normal. Known asthmatic patients do not necessarily need an X-ray every time they have an attack.

TREATMENT

The treatment of acute asthma is as given in Figure 3. A short course (3–5 days) of oral steroids combined with regular bronchodilator is usually enough to settle acute symptoms but airway hyper-responsiveness may persist for up to 3 weeks after an attack. Antibiotics are used to treat lobar (bacterial) pneumonia and atypical pneumonia (commonly caused by *Mycoplasma pneumoniae*) but there is no specific treatment for viral pneumonia.

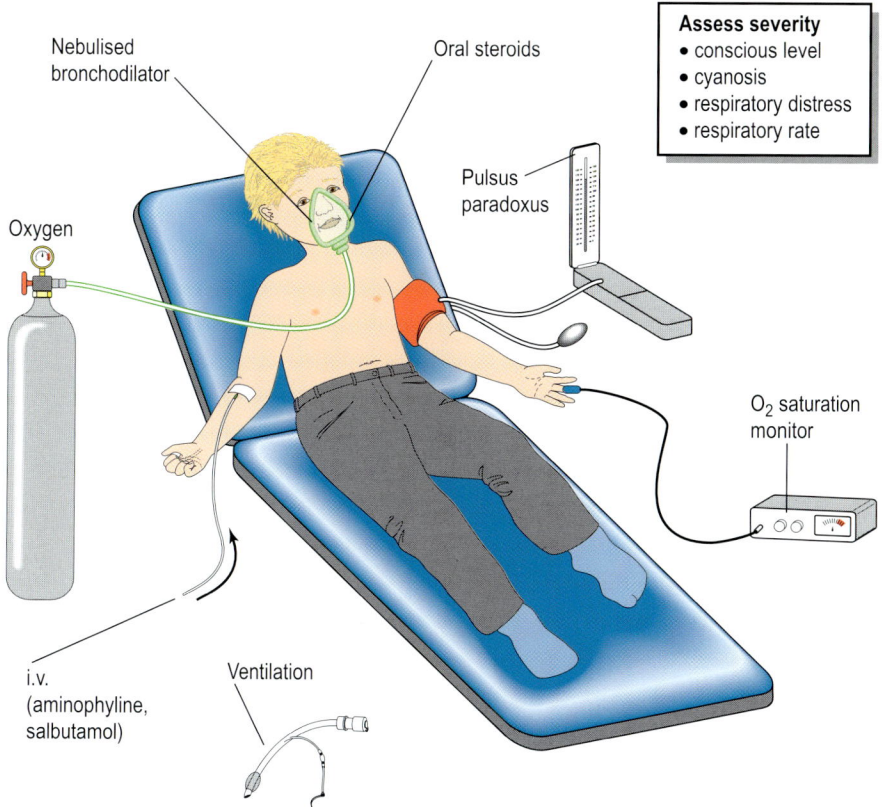

Assess severity
- conscious level
- cyanosis
- respiratory distress
- respiratory rate

Fig. 3 **Emergency management of asthma.** Ventilation should be reserved for those patients not responding to less invasive means of therapy.

Acute breathing difficulty
- Difficulty in breathing is almost always due to pulmonary disease but metabolic acidosis and neuromuscular disease are occasional causes.
- In an acute attack of respiratory distress, give oxygen and measure SaO$_2$ immediately while organising more definitive treatment.

CHRONIC BREATHING DIFFICULTY

Difficulty in breathing is a common symptom. Much of it is acute and related to upper or lower respiratory infection. Even so, a large number of children have episodic or persistent breathing difficulties. The prevalence of chronic respiratory symptoms in the childhood years is 10–15% and the vast majority are children with asthma. There is also evidence that the prevalence of asthma is increasing and various factors (changing allergen exposure, particulate or chemical air pollution) have been suggested as causes. In the hospital or tertiary referral centre, other, rarer diseases also present with breathing difficulty as a major symptom. The most common of these in the UK are cystic fibrosis and neonatal chronic lung disease (broncho-pulmonary dysplasia). Worldwide, TB is the leading cause.

PRESENTATION

History

As symptoms tend to fluctuate in severity, children may present with an acute exacerbation of a chronic illness. It is important to consider an underlying chronic condition in all children presenting with an acute respiratory problem (pp. 60–61). However, most chronic illness will present in the clinic or surgery as an outpatient. In the history, questioning should establish the pattern of symptoms, the severity and how the condition interferes with the child's life. Asthma is extremely common, but it is difficult to diagnose with certainty after only one episode of wheeze because viral or atypical pneumonias have similar features. A history of previous attacks is therefore essential. Because asthma is so common, the usual approach to making a diagnosis is to exclude other diagnoses and to focus on associated features (e.g. atopy). A list of important questions and their significance is given in Table 1.

Examination

In the outpatient clinic, examination of a known asthmatic is often normal. Severe asthma and other chronic lung disease can stunt growth, so height and weight should be plotted on a growth chart. Hyperinflation of the chest indicates persistent small airway obstruction. It can be recognised by an increase in the anteroposterior diameter of the chest; however, children normally tend to have barrel shaped chests making this sign more difficult to assess than in adults. Displacement of the liver is a better clinical sign of hyperinflation. This can be determined by percussing the upper border and palpating the lower border. A Harrison's sulcus indicates chronic hyperinflation with increased work of breathing. It is common in children with any form of obstructive airways disease because the relatively soft bones of the rib cage are easily distorted by the diaphragm.

In younger children the presence of a congenital anomaly also has to be considered. General examination may exclude heart failure, scoliosis or muscular disorders.

Asymmetry of the chest and its movement may give a clue to an underlying disorder such as a congenital lung anomaly. The presence of clubbing indicates cystic fibrosis or other suppurative lung disease. Conversely, the presence of eczema makes asthma a more likely diagnosis. However, it must be remembered that many children with cystic fibrosis (for example) also have asthma.

Assessment of the asthmatic patient in clinic should include peak flow measurement (in children over 5–6 years) and review of inhaler technique. Peak flow can be measured before and 15 minutes after a dose of bronchodilator to test for reversible airway obstruction which may suggest asthma. Different inhalation devices are used for different age groups (Fig. 1) based on the ability of the child to be able to suck through a device and distinguish sucking from blowing.

MANAGEMENT OF ASTHMA

Management is based on:

- drug treatment
- allergen avoidance
- family education
- awareness of psychological factors.

Drug treatments play an important part in management. The most commonly used are inhaled bronchodilators (relievers) given when the patient has symptoms and, if necessary, regular inhaled steroids or cromoglycate (preventers). For the more severe asthmatics, additional treatments such as long-acting bronchodilators and theophyllines may be given as well. Regular oral steroids tend to be reserved for a small group with intractable or life-threatening asthma where the long-term steroid side-effects are worth risking for the improved quality of life. This is summarised in Table 2. Infants often fail to respond well to anti-asthma treatment making it particularly difficult to confirm the diagnosis.

It can be a problem for the doctor to know whether the patient is taking the prescribed medication. Detailed questioning of children about how and when they

Table 1 **Important questions in assessing patients presenting with breathing difficulties**

Questions	Comment
To examine the pattern of symptoms:	
• How many days a week/weeks per month are there symptoms?	Distinguishes continuous from intermittent symptoms
• How much time off school in the last term/year?	Good measure of overall impact of the illness
• Night-time symptoms?	Common but often not mentioned unless asked about specifically
• Better in winter or summer?	Distinguishes pollen sensitivity from infective precipitants
• Better at school or home?	May reflect the differing enviromental precipitants and give insight into psychogenic component of illness
Precipitants:	
• upper respiratory infection	
• exercise	
• animals	
• grass	
To estimate severity of previous attacks:	
• Ever ventilated?	A marker for serious asthma and a high chance of further problems
• Number of hospital admissions	These depend on other factors as well as disease severity
• Number of courses of oral steroids	
• Clinical features of attacks	See under acute attacks (pp. 60–61)
To look for diagnoses other than asthma:	
• Always unwell?	Identifies continuous symptoms which are more likely to be caused by bronchiectasis
• Sputum production?	There is often green sputum in acute asthma but chronic purulent sputum needs further investigation
• O_2 for >1 month at birth?	Neonatal chronic lung disease likely to be a factor
• Poor growth?	May be cystic fibrosis but can be a feature of severe asthma
• Serious infections elsewhere in the body?	Possibility of an immune defect
• Prominent ENT symptoms?	Possibility of a cilial disorder if recurrent sinusitis and otitis media
	Possibility of allergic rhinitis if nasal blockage and clear discharge
• Frequent choking and vomiting?	Possibility of aspiration (particularly in infants)
• Is he sweaty and breathless and failing to thrive?	Possibility of chronic heart failure (particularly in infants)

take their medication and how often they need a repeat prescription can be helpful. The underlying reasons for non-compliance are often complex and may need a detailed understanding of the family priorities, attitudes and relationships.

Table 2 **Stepwise approach to asthma management**

Stage 1: inhaled β_2-agonist (delivery system tailored to age)
Stage 2: Inhaled β_2-agonist plus sodium cromoglycate
Stage 3: Inhaled β_2-agonist plus inhaled steroids (delivery system tailored to age)
Stage 4: Inhaled long-acting β_2-agonist plus inhaled steroids (delivery system tailored to age)
Stage 5: Long-term systemic steroids

In some children it is possible to identify allergens which precipitate asthma (grass pollen, house dust mite and cat hair are the most common). It may be appropriate to test asthmatic children with skin tests or blood for total and specific IgE levels likely to be allergic triggers. Once diagnosed, allergen avoidance is often difficult to achieve. House dust mite can be reduced by damp dusting, vacuuming the mattress and covering it with plastic, and by using short-pile carpets or removing them altogether.

Education of the child and the family helps compliance and enables them to feel in control of the treatment. It is important that they recognise the symptoms of asthma and know how and when to change their own treatment and when to seek help. Many children are given diary cards to help them recognise symptoms and also have asthma cards which give them an individual treatment plan for acute attacks.

Asthma has a psychosomatic component which may be prominent in some patients. The most severe asthmatics commonly have major family problems. Treatment for children affected by parental separation, child abuse, etc. is very difficult and a combined medical and psychiatric approach to treatment may be necessary.

MANAGEMENT OF CYSTIC FIBROSIS

Clinical diagnosis of cystic fibrosis is suspected when one or more of the cardinal features are present (Table 3). Confirmation of the diagnosis is by gene probe of the patient's genetic material and/or a sweat

Table 3 **Cardinal features of cystic fibrosis**

Early features
Chronic suppurative lung disease
Steatorrhoea (including neonatal meconium ileus)
Failure to thrive
Later features
Cor pulmonale
Diabetes
Infertility (males)
Portal hypertension and cirrhosis

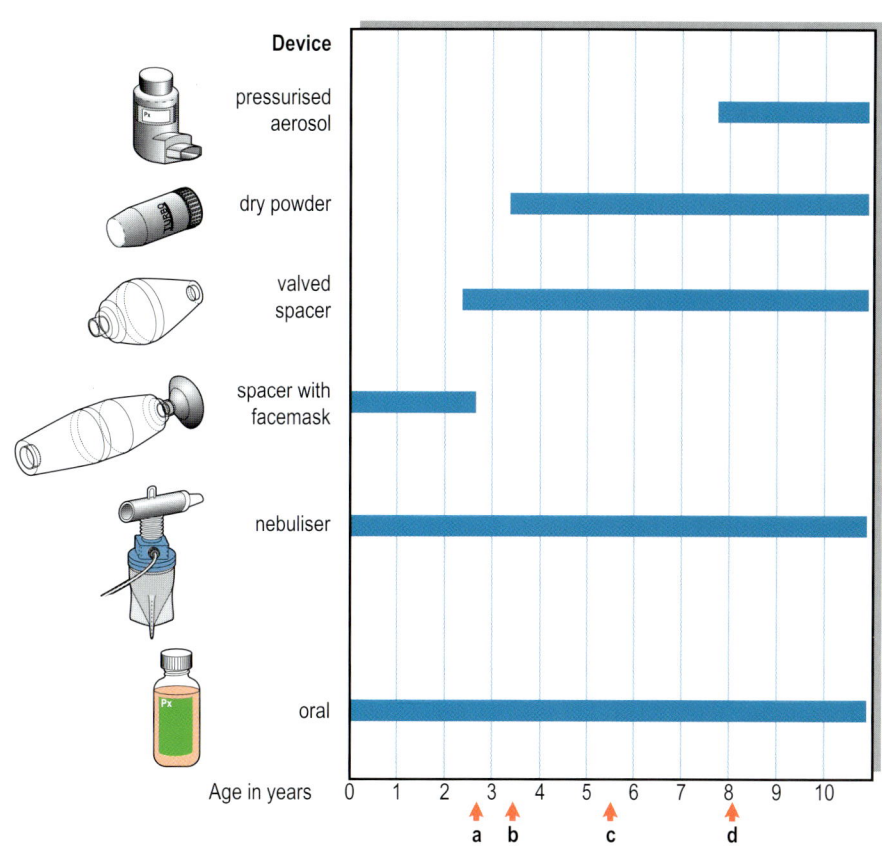

Fig. 1 **Selection of devices by age. (a)** First able to breathe through a device. **(b)** First able to suck but not blow. **(c)** Earliest age for using peak flow meter. **(d)** First able to coordinate breathing with actuating device. **NB** Ages are very approximate as there is marked variation from child to child.

test. Some children are now diagnosed soon after birth by population screening (see pp. 14–15).

Once the diagnosis is established, the long-term objectives of treatment are to prevent lung damage and to promote normal growth. In addition, there are the genetic implications for the family and the psychological effects of living with a chronic, ultimately fatal disease.

The mainstay of chest treatment is physiotherapy which helps to mobilise the pulmonary secretions. It is performed at least two times a day regardless of symptoms. Children at school should have a statement of special educational need to allow physiotherapy during school hours. Exercise is encouraged as it is a form of physiotherapy. Antibiotics are given for exacerbations and may be used prophylactically. Nebulised therapy to reduce the tenacity of the sputum can also be used in established cases and anti-asthma treatment is helpful for some.

The gut manifestations of cystic fibrosis are a result of pancreatic exocrine deficiency particularly the lack of protease and lipase. Replacement enzymes are given in concentrations to normalise the stools. In addition, fat soluble vitamins are added to the diet and aggressive nutritional support with a high calorie intake is promoted. The chance of the

parents having a further child with cystic fibrosis is 1 in 4 as it is recessively inherited. As with all inherited conditions there is some guilt felt by the parents that colours their relationship with the child and may need bringing out into the open.

With all the invasive medical management and pressure on the family, it is important for the child to have as normal a life as possible. This can be facilitated by educational, emotional and financial support for parents, school and other siblings.

Chronic breathing difficulty

- Look out for rarer diseases masquerading as asthma.
- The younger the child the wider the diagnostic possibilities.
- Check inhaler technique in all asthmatic patients in clinic.
- Be aware of the psycho-social effects of a chronic disease on child and family.

ABDOMINAL PAIN

Children of all ages frequently present complaining of abdominal pain; however, it is important to understand that young children are particularly poor at localising such discomfort. When asked 'Where does it hurt?', a toddler with pain anywhere will typically point to the periumbilical area and hence the symptom of abdominal pain always requires careful interpretation. When a young child does localise pain to a specific site other than the umbilicus it is likely to be of significance.

ACUTE ABDOMINAL PAIN

History and examination should be used first to establish the significance of the episode:

- Is the child's appetite normal (if normal is a sign of well-being)?
- Is the child able to move normally (not limited by pain)?
- Is the child showing a usual level of activity (does the child appear to feel unwell)?
- Has this happened before (not an acute problem)?
- Does the child appear in pain (difficulty in changing positions, dilated pupils)? This helps to judge the severity of the pain.

Secondly, it is essential to establish the nature of any underlying pathology:

- Is the pain localised?
- What is the time course: constant (e.g. appendicitis) or intermittent (colic is typical of obstruction to either the small bowel or renal tract)?
- Is there vomiting and does it contain blood or bile (bile-stained vomiting and large haematemeses are always significant whereas small haematemeses are common after frequent vomiting)?
- Have the bowels been open since the pain commenced (if not indicates constipation or obstruction)?
- What was the nature of the stool (an acute change to diarrhoea suggests gastroenteritis)?
- Are there any urinary symptoms, e.g. dysuria, haematuria (either points to a renal cause but alone neither is conclusive)?
- What is the child's temperature, pulse and respiration (raised temperature suggests infection but pain alone may cause a tachycardia and tachypnoea)?
- Is there abdominal distension or localised swelling (typical of obstruction)?

- Is there abdominal tenderness or guarding (characteristic of peritoneal irritation and commonly seen both in appendicitis and mesenteric adenitis)?
- Are there any masses (unless easily identifiable — e.g. indentable faecal mass — always requires further evaluation)?

Important pathologies which need to be considered include the following.

Gastroenteritis

This is considered in more detail elsewhere (pp. 66–67); however, severe colicky abdominal pain prior to the onset of vomiting and/or diarrhoea may initially make the diagnosis difficult.

Appendicitis

This is unusual in children under 5, but it is in that age group that the symptoms and signs are most non-specific, perhaps being limited to mild fever, anorexia and abdominal pain. Vomiting may be a feature. In young children, progress to perforation can be very rapid. The more typical symptoms and signs of appendicitis are seen in older children.

Mesenteric adenitis

This is an important condition since it mimics appendicitis in many respects. The pain occurs because of inflammation of the abdominal lymphatics usually as part of a generalised viral infection. Systemic upset (fever and headache) tends to be more marked than in appendicitis but with more diffuse abdominal pain. However, this distinction can be very difficult to recognise.

Intestinal obstruction

This is not a specific diagnosis since it can arise from a number of underlying pathologies but in general they share the characteristic symptoms (bile-stained vomiting, constipation and colicky abdominal pain) and signs (dehydration and abdominal distension). Malrotation may predispose to repeated episodes of volvulus (twisting of the gut on its mesentery) and, hence, repeated presentations with obstruction. Hernial orifices should all be carefully checked.

Intussusception

This is relatively common in young children where the passage of bloody mucus rectally and the finding of a mass in the abdomen point to the diagnosis.

Other surgical causes

Testicular torsion is seen most commonly in adolescence but can occur in the neonatal period.

Renal causes

These include urinary tract infection (where fever, dysuria, and haematuria suggest the diagnosis and pain may be diffuse or localised to the loin, back or either iliac fossa) and renal calculus (producing very severe episodic pain).

Constipation

Constipation commonly presents with abdominal pain (sometimes in combination with anorexia and vomiting). Parents may not be aware that the child has become constipated, the diagnosis being confirmed by the palpation of faecal masses in the abdomen or on abdominal X-ray.

Lower lobe pneumonia

Lower lobe pneumonia causing pleurisy may present with abdominal pain. Initially chest symptoms and signs may be absent, making the diagnosis difficult.

Henoch–Schönlein purpura

This is a vasculitic process which seems to be triggered by infection, but the exact mechanism is not clear. Sites involved include: skin (rash, Fig. 1), joints (arthralgia or arthritis), gut and kidneys (glomerulonephritis with haematuria). Organs may be affected in any order often with days or weeks in between. Abdominal manifestations usually take the form of severe abdominal pain sometimes accompanied by bloody diarrhoea. Perforation and intussusception are rare complications.

Other causes

Infantile colic is dealt with elsewhere (pp. 36–37). Other medical conditions which may present with abdominal pain include sickle cell disease and diabetes mellitus.

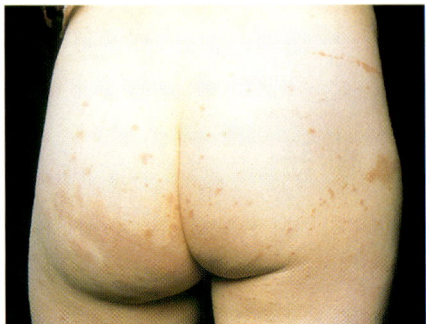

Fig. 1 **Rash in Henoch–Schönlein purpura.**

RECURRENT ABDOMINAL PAIN

Recurrent abdominal pain is common, affecting up to 10% of children. In approximately 90%, no organic cause is found. In children with no organic cause the pain represents a stress disorder, and other stress related phenomena may also be identified in the history, e.g. sleep disorders, enuresis and eating problems. A family history of recurrent abdominal pain is present in 10–20% of cases. Similarly, parents or siblings may have a history of migraine, peptic ulcer or irritable bowel syndrome. A careful history can be helpful in linking the onset of symptoms to a traumatic event (e.g. bereavement) or recurrent episodes to a particular activity (e.g. going to school). However, it is important to understand that for the child the pain is real. The child may scream, double up, vomit and look pale. Often there is associated headache; others may be sleepy after the attack. The pain varies enormously in timing and character but is usually periumbilical. In a situation where most children have non-organic disease it is essential to identify those children that do have a specific pathology.

Important points in the history and examination include:

- Is the nature of the pain compatible with non-organic disease? (Recurrent episodes of pain consistently localised away from the umbilicus do not support the diagnosis.)
- Are the attacks accompanied by vomiting? Whilst vomiting is of no specific importance bile-stained vomiting usually indicates organic disease. Blood-stained vomit may arise from mucosal tearing after forceful retching but may also be a sign of oesophagitis or peptic ulceration.
- Has there been a change of bowel habit? Loose stools are common in young children and may well be of no significance. Malaena or blood-stained stools are not compatible with a diagnosis of non-organic disease.
- Are there renal symptoms? Haematuria and or dysuria suggest renal pathology; repeated episodes of cloudy (Fig. 2) and/or strong smelling urine may indicate infection but may be of no significance.

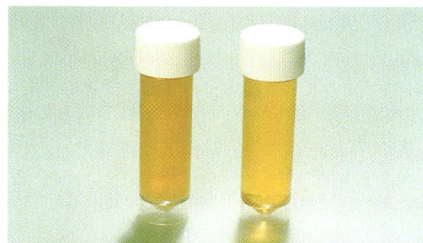

Fig. 2 **Cloudy but non-infected urine.** Colour and cloudiness of urine cannot be used alone to diagnose infection.

- Examination should focus on evidence of poor general health. Anaemia, evidence of weight loss, failure to thrive, abdominal distension or a mass suggest an organic cause is present.

Important conditions resulting in recurrent abdominal pain include:

Renal disease
Recurrent urinary tract infections may cause repeated episodes of pain without the more typical symptoms of dysuria and haematuria. Urine microscopy and culture should always form part of the assessment of such children (pp. 82–83).

Food intolerance
Both coeliac disease (Fig. 3) and cow's milk protein intolerance may present with abdominal pain, normally accompanied by other features of the disease. There is no evidence to suggest that other 'food allergies' present in this way.

Inflammatory bowel disease (Crohn's and ulcerative colitis)
This is not common in children. Presentation with episodes of abdominal pain may occur but other symptoms such as bloody stools and weight loss are usually also present.

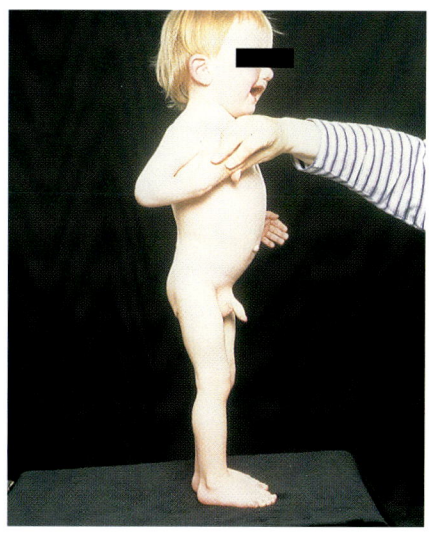

Fig. 3 **Child with coelic disease.**

Non-organic disease
For families with children affected by this condition reassurance that no serious pathology is present may be sufficient to break the cycle of anxiety. In other cases advice to take the pressure off the child at home or deal with a problem at school may be therapeutic. In a few cases in which the attacks are debilitating family therapy can be helpful in providing additional insight to the child's problems.

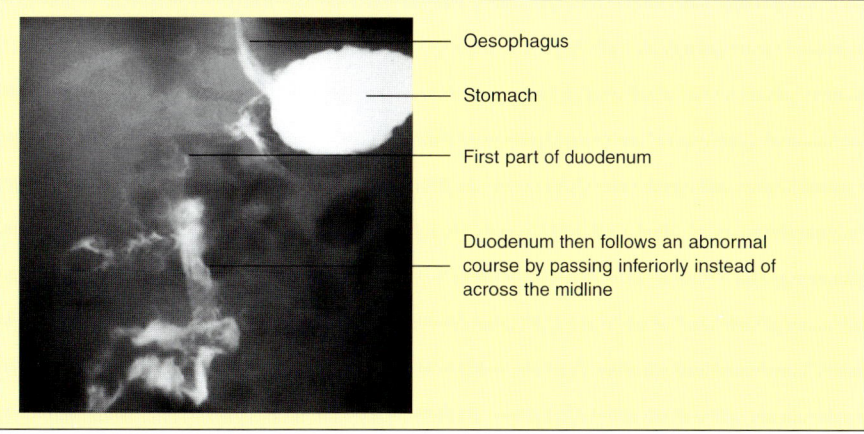

Oesophagus

Stomach

First part of duodenum

Duodenum then follows an abnormal course by passing inferiorly instead of across the midline

Fig. 4 **X-ray of malrotation.**

Peptic ulceration
This is an unusual but not rare cause of recurrent abdominal pain in children. Pain causing the child to wake at night is a particularly useful marker. *Helicobacter pylori* is an important causative agent in many children and adults and a serological screening test is available.

Malrotation
Malrotation, mentioned above as a cause of acute obstruction and pain, may also produce repeated episodes as the bowel twists and then untwists (Fig. 4). The presence of bile-stained vomiting on each occasion suggests the diagnosis.

Abdominal pain

- Appendicitis, although not common in children under 5, is frequently misdiagnosed.
- Non-organic recurrent abdominal pain should only be diagnosed after careful assessment.
- Food allergy is unlikely to be the cause of abdominal pain.
- Threadworms do not cause abdominal pain.

DIARRHOEA

Diarrhoea is a very common presenting complaint to Accident and Emergency departments, family doctors, and outpatient clinics. It can be defined as an alteration in stool frequency and/or stool consistency and usually includes an increase in stool water content.

Diarrhoea results when the normal absorptive capacity of the bowel is exceeded or when there is an imbalance between the secretory and absorptive roles of the gut (Fig. 1).

Many children presenting with diarrhoea are simply displaying normal variation. Breast-fed infants normally pass bright yellow, watery stools with every feed. Some toddlers pass frequent watery stools containing recognisable food items, especially peas and carrots, whilst continuing to thrive normally. This 'condition' is known as *non-specific toddlers' diarrhoea* and probably represents a functional immaturity of the bowel in association with a tendency to swallow food without adequate chewing. No treatment is required but advice to regulate excessive fluid intakes can be helpful.

ASSESSMENT

Children presenting with diarrhoea should be assessed for the following:

- length of history (most acute cases will be due to viral gastroenteritis)
- alteration in bowel habit (alternating hard and liquid stools suggest constipation and overflow)
- character of stool
  - watery (compatible with enteritis)
  - soft and bulky (suggests malabsorption)
  - fatty (suggests malabsorption)
  - bloody (seen in some bacterial gut infections, Crohn's and ulcerative colitis)
- effect on weight (weight loss always indicates significant pathology)
- accurate and complete dietary history (including drinks), and its relation to diarrhoea (may support a diagnosis of food intolerance)
- concurrent medication (drugs such as antibiotics may provoke diarrhoea)
- fever/constitutional upset/other symptoms (suggests diarrhoea is part of a systemic condition)
- known contacts/travel (see pp. 40–41)
- past medical history, e.g. frequent chest infections (suggests diarrhoea is part of a chronic disorder).

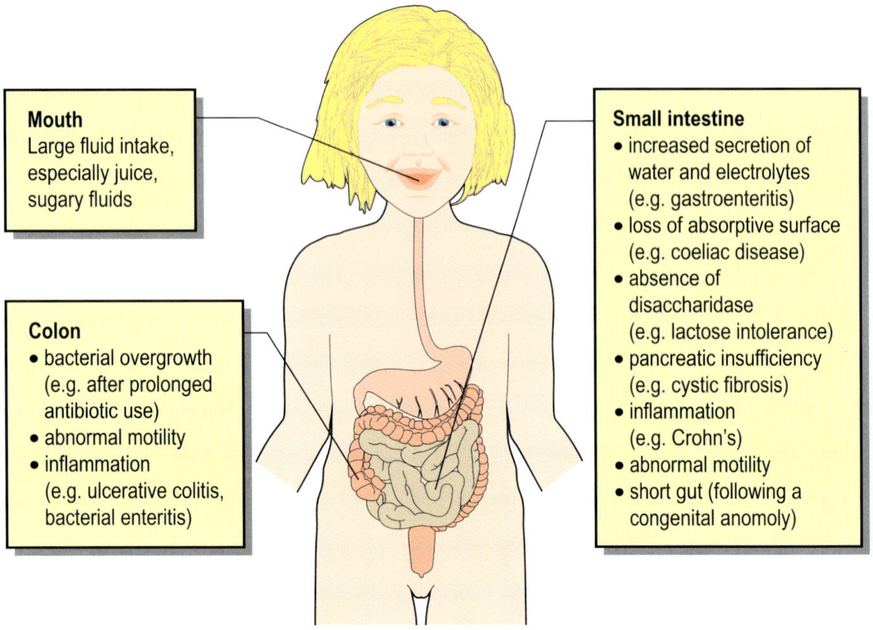

Table 1 **Dehydration table**

Percentage dehydration	0–3%	5%	10%	15%
Skin turgor	Normal	Slightly reduced	Reduced	Reduced
Mucous membranes	Normal	Slightly dry	Dry	Extremely dry
Fontanelle	Normal	Normal	Sunken	Sunken
Eyeball pressure	Normal	Slightly reduced	Decreased	Decreased
Tears	Normal	Normal	Normal	Reduced
Urine output	Normal	Reduced	Reduced	Reduced
Blood pressure	Normal	Normal	May be reduced	Reduced
Capillary refill	Normal	Normal	Reduced	Reduced
Level of consciousness	Normal/miserable	Thirsty/miserable	Lethargic	Moribund

Table 2 **Management of acute diarrhoea**

Percentage dehydration	0–3%	5%	10%	15%
Admit?	No	Usually no	Yes	Yes, extreme emergency
Mode of rehydration	Oral	Oral (occasionally NG)	Intravenous	Urgent intravenous resuscitation

ACUTE DIARRHOEA

Globally, acute infectious gastroenteritis is the most common cause of diarrhoea. It causes more than 10 million deaths per year in developing countries. The aetiology in most cases is viral with rotavirus accounting for 60–80%. It occurs predominantly in the autumn and winter months and can spread rapidly in crowded communities to produce epidemics. Children present acutely with profuse watery diarrhoea, low grade pyrexia and often associated vomiting and upper respiratory signs. The most serious consequence of acute viral gastroenteritis is dehydration. Management is, therefore, directed at recognising, preventing and alleviating this complication (Table 1).

Most children can be effectively rehydrated and treated with oral (or nasogastric) glucose electrolyte solutions, widely available as powder for reconstitution with boiled water. Very severely dehydrated children or those unable to tolerate oral or nasogastric fluids may require intravenous resuscitation before rehydrating. Once the child is rehydrated, normal feeds are reinstituted and supplemented with oral rehydration solution until the diarrhoea resolves. Antidiarrhoeal agents (codeine, loperamide, kaolin, etc.) and antibiotics are not indicated for acute childhood gastroenteritis (Table 2).

ACUTE BLOODY DIARRHOEA

Bacteria, e.g. salmonella, shigella and campylobacter, are also causes of acute diarrhoea. A history of cramping abdominal pain associated with small, frequent mucousy stools sometimes with visible blood is more suggestive of a bacterial enteritis. Management remains largely supportive, although antibiotics may be indicated for certain specific bacteria (e.g. erythromycin for campylobacter).

Necrotising enterocolitis is a serious

Mouth
Large fluid intake, especially juice, sugary fluids

Colon
- bacterial overgrowth (e.g. after prolonged antibiotic use)
- abnormal motility
- inflammation (e.g. ulcerative colitis, bacterial enteritis)

Small intestine
- increased secretion of water and electrolytes (e.g. gastroenteritis)
- loss of absorptive surface (e.g. coeliac disease)
- absence of disaccharidase (e.g. lactose intolerance)
- pancreatic insufficiency (e.g. cystic fibrosis)
- inflammation (e.g. Crohn's)
- abnormal motility
- short gut (following a congenital anomaly)

Fig. 1 **Mechanisms of diarrhoea.**

condition of unknown aetiology affecting preterm and occasionally term neonates. Infants present acutely with abdominal distension and the passage of bloody mucousy diarrhoea. X-ray of the abdomen is characteristic.

In an older infant or toddler, intermittent severe abdominal pain associated with 'redcurrant jelly' stool strongly suggests intussusception, a condition in which the bowel telescopes into itself. This is a surgical emergency (see pp. 72–73).

Rarely, bloody diarrhoea may herald the onset of haemolytic uraemic syndrome (HUS), a combination of diarrhoea, acute haemolysis and renal failure. Diagnosis is made with a combination of an abnormal blood film and deranged electrolytes. Children with this serious condition will need to be referred to a renal unit for further management.

CHRONIC DIARRHOEA

This is defined as diarrhoea persisting for more than 4 weeks. If associated with weight loss, it should be further investigated (Table 3).

Carbohydrate malabsorption

Diarrhoea resulting from carbohydrate malabsorption may be intermittent, associated with abdominal pain and excessive flatus and large, sometimes frothy stools. This may rarely be a primary condition, but more commonly follows viral gastroenteritis with damage to the brush border of the villi lining the small intestine. Lactase which is found at the tip of the microvilli is the most common disaccharidase involved and diarrhoea resolves after removal of lactose from the diet. Secondary lactase deficiency is usually a temporary condition, recovering in a matter of weeks. Deficiency of the other disaccharidases can also occur and diarrhoea resolves when the sugars are removed from the diet.

Protein malabsorption

Sensitivity to a variety of ingested proteins may also damage the lining of the upper small intestine, an example of this is coeliac disease or gluten sensitive enteropathy which involves the gliadin fraction of wheat protein. Treatment is by removal of wheat from the diet. Cow's milk protein sensitivity is another widely recognised example.

Fat malabsorption

Deficiency of pancreatic exocrine secretion results in fat malabsorption. This is seen most commonly in cystic fibrosis (pp. 62–63). Patients have frequent oily stools which are difficult to flush away and may stain the toilet bowl. Treatment is by replacement of deficient pancreatic enzymes.

Table 3 **Chronic diarrhoea**

Clinical features	Diagnosis	Mechanism	Investigation	Treatment
Bulky, frothy stools, +/– abdomen. pain, often post-gastroenteritis	Secondary lactose intolerance	Damage to small intestinal villi by virus causing loss of dissacharidases	Stool chromatography exclusion trial	Temporary exclusion of lactose from diet (in practice often exclusion of cow's milk)
Bulky stools +/– frothy +/– abdomen pain from birth	Primary lactose intolerance	Congenital deficiency of lactase	Stool chromatography	Permanent exclusion of lactose
Bulky stools after antibiotic usage	Bacterial overgrowth	Carbohydrate-induced osmotic diarrhoea	None specific	Spontaneous recovery when antibiotics stopped
Pale bulky stools, wasting, misery	Coeliac disease	Damage to small intestinal villi by immune response to gliadin fraction of wheat protein	Jejunal biopsy Antibody measurements	Exclusion of gluten
Pale bulky stools often postenteritis in small infants	Cow's milk protein enteropathy	Damage to small intestinal mucosa by cow's milk	Jejunal biopsy	Exclusion of cow's milk from diet
Pale, fatty stools, difficult to flush, may stain bowl, offensive ++ (+chest infections)	Cystic fibrosis (see pp. 62–63)	Pancreatic exocrine insufficiency causing fat malabsorption	Sweat test/ cytogenetic testing	Pancreatic enzyme supplements, high calorie diet
Pale fatty stool, difficult to flush, may stain bowl, offensive ++ (+neutropenia)	Schwachman's syndrome	Pancreatic exocrine insufficiency causing fat malabsorption	Cyclical neutropenia Characteristic hip X-ray	Pancreatic enzyme supplements
Bulky stools, +/– mucus, +/– weight loss, +/– upper abdomen cramps, travel	Giardiasis	Giardia present in duodenum and proximal jejunum	Stool microscopy Elisa test for giardia	Metronidazole
Watery or bloody stools, travel	Amoebic dysentery	Amoebae in small bowel	Stool microscopy	Metronidazole
Abdominal pain, bloody, mucousy stools, weight loss	Ulcerative colitis	Inflammatory damage to colon	Colonoscopy and biopsies Barium enema	Mesalazine, topical steroids
Abdominal pain, bloody stools, mucousy stools, weight loss, aphthous ulcers, rectal fissures	Crohn's disease	Inflammation at intervals throughout whole GI tract	Colonoscopy and biopsies Barium meal and follow through, ESR and CRP, full blood count	Elemental diet Steroids
Diarrhoea following major gastrointestinal resection	Short gut syndrome	Profound reduction in absorptive surface		Very slow introduction of feeds supported by intravenous feeding
Loose stools in immunocompromised child		Failure to clear common often low grade pathogens	Stool culture	Appropriate treatment for organism, supportive

Infections and inflammatory conditions

Infections with organisms such as giardia or amoebae may cause chronic diarrhoea, and this is especially important to consider where there is a history of travel to endemic areas.

Inflammatory conditions such as Crohn's disease and ulcerative colitis are increasingly recognised as a cause of bloody diarrhoea, abdominal pain and weight loss generally in older children and teenagers. Investigation and management of these conditions is as in adults, although particular attention to nutrition in these patients is essential to ensure normal growth.

Short gut syndrome

So-called short gut syndrome resulting from previous major intestinal surgery may

be a cause of intractable diarrhoea necessitating parenteral nutrition to maintain nutrition and normal growth.

Diarrhoea

- A detailed history will point to a diagnosis in most cases.
- 'Diarrhoea' may be normal.
- Acute viral gastroenteritis is a major cause of morbidity and should be managed symptomatically.
- Acute bloody diarrhoea may herald a surgical emergency or HUS.

VOMITING

Vomiting is a very common symptom in young infants and children; it may be a non-specific indicator of generalised illness or be due to a specific gastrointestinal problem. In order to reach a diagnosis it is helpful to consider the various mechanisms that result in vomiting (Fig. 1).

Where cerebral irritation is responsible, other symptoms and signs arising from the CNS may well be present, e.g. headache and neck stiffness in the child with meningitis. However, the exact combination of symptoms will vary with the underlying cause of the cerebral irritation. Children with gastro-oesophageal reflux have frequent, effortless vomits because of an incompetent cardiac sphincter. In consequence, their stomach contents move easily up into the mouth and hence the observed pattern.

Gastric irritation of any cause may result in associated vomiting. Accompanying pain and/or haematemesis would be typical.

Pyloric stenosis produces a characteristic pattern of vomiting (projectile) as the obstructed stomach forcefully empties itself.

Intestinal obstruction, at any site, will eventually prevent normal stomach emptying and cause retrograde passage of bowel contents into the stomach. This leads to both gastric distension and irritation. Vomiting results which, characteristically, is bile-stained.

VOMITING IN THE NEONATAL PERIOD

Gastro-oesophageal reflux (GOR)

Small, effortless vomits of semidigested milk are common in neonates and infants. Resting lower oesophageal pressure in infants is below that seen in older children and adults; this, plus the large volume liquid feed they consume and the fact that they spend large portions of the day lying flat, makes reflux of gastric contents up the oesophagus a common occurrence. Most infants with this problem do not come to medical attention. Of those that do, a clear majority continue to thrive and develop normally without intervention. Parents can be reassured that symptoms will improve as the child goes on to more solid food and spends more time upright. In some, GOR may be more troublesome and in these thickening of feeds, nursing the child at 30° rather than flat or the use of agents such as cisapride (which enhances gastric emptying) may improve symptoms.

There are a small number of infants with gastro-oesophageal reflux who present with

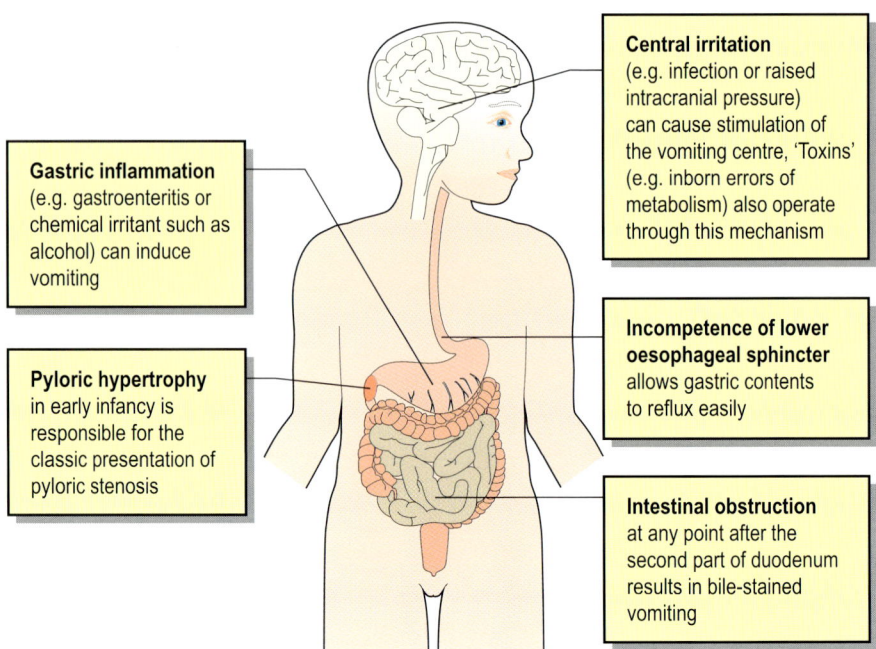

Fig. 1 **Mechanisms of vomiting.**

Gastric inflammation (e.g. gastroenteritis or chemical irritant such as alcohol) can induce vomiting

Pyloric hypertrophy in early infancy is responsible for the classic presentation of pyloric stenosis

Central irritation (e.g. infection or raised intracranial pressure) can cause stimulation of the vomiting centre, 'Toxins' (e.g. inborn errors of metabolism) also operate through this mechanism

Incompetence of lower oesophageal sphincter allows gastric contents to reflux easily

Intestinal obstruction at any point after the second part of duodenum results in bile-stained vomiting

life-threatening apnoea or recurrent chest infections due to aspiration of milk. Further investigation of these infants is indicated, ideally with 24-hour pH monitoring (Fig. 2) to document the severity of the reflux. Aggressive medical management is indicated with feed thickeners, and agents to increase gastric emptying. In some infants even this fails to control their symptoms, and in this small group surgical gastric fundoplication (tightening the sphincter) is indicated.

Acute onset of vomiting

Although vomiting is common in newborns, more profuse vomiting or vomiting associated with constitutional upset should prompt rapid and careful assessment. *Bile-stained vomiting must always be taken to indicate a significant disease.* In this age group it may be difficult to establish from history and examination alone the nature of the underlying pathology. Important surgical conditions resulting in intestinal obstruction may present at this time (Table 1).

Sepsis in newborns, at almost any site, readily results in septicaemia (and secondary paralytic ileus). Symptoms may be non-specific, e.g. apnoea, lethargy, crying and vomiting. Signs include temperature instability, pallor and hypotension. Investigations suggesting significant infection include: high white count, low white count, hypoglycaemia and thrombocytopenia. Therefore, where significant vomiting accompanies any of the above, the child

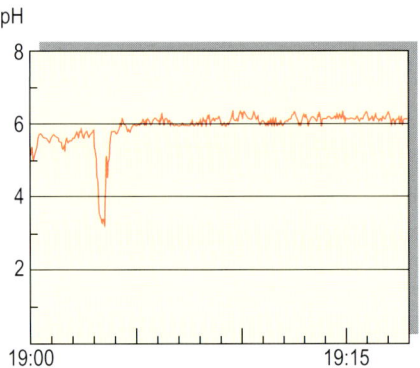

Fig. 2 **24-hour pH monitoring.** Section of printout from pH probe showing a sudden drop in oesophageal pH during an episode of reflux.

should be screened for infection and given broad spectrum antibiotic cover.

VOMITING IN OLDER INFANTS

Vomiting in this age group is often a sign of systemic infection, usually self-limiting viral gastroenteritis. Such children are managed with frequent small drinks of clear fluid. Occasionally, vomiting may be so severe that the child is unable to tolerate any oral fluids or becomes dehydrated, in which case intravenous fluids are indicated.

In children with a more profound systemic upset and no obvious focus of infection, a 'septic screen' is indicated and the child should be treated with broad spectrum antibiotics until a diagnosis is made.

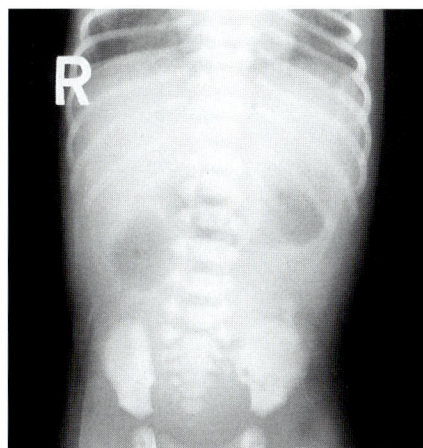

Fig. 3 **Double bubble X-ray of duodenal atresia.**

Bilious vomiting in this age group, as in the younger infant, should always prompt consideration of a surgical problem including malrotation and volvulus (pp. 64–65).

Pyloric stenosis

Projectile vomiting developing in an infant classically from 3–4 weeks of age should suggest a diagnosis of pyloric stenosis. In this condition infants have large, non-bilious vomits after every feed. Initially they appear hungry and will often take a second feed immediately after vomiting, although as the condition progresses they may become increasingly dehydrated and lethargic. Examination usually reveals an infant with signs of recent weight loss or dehydration, and in established cases a dilated stomach with visible peristalsis (Fig. 4). Palpation of the right upper quadrant, especially after a feed, may reveal the olive shaped 'tumour' of the hypertrophied pylorus. Diagnosis is confirmed by ultrasonography or occasionally barium meal. Infants with pyloric stenosis develop a characteristic biochemical picture (metabolic alkalosis, hyponatraemia, hypokalaemia and hypochloraemia), as a result of persistent vomiting of gastric acid.

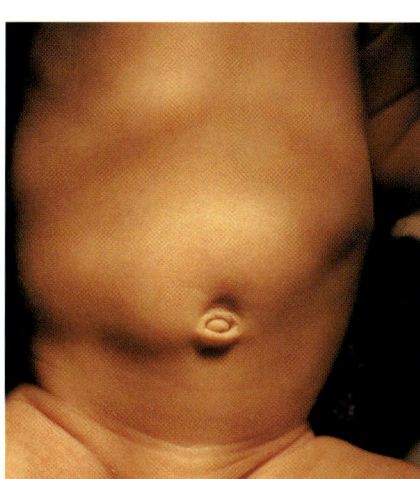

Fig. 4 **Pyloric stenosis showing gastric distension.**

Table 1 Surgical conditions resulting in intestinal obstruction

Condition	Clinical features
Duodenal atresia	Upper abdominal distension and vomiting (may or may not be bile-stained); characteristic abdominal X-ray (see Fig. 3)
Ileal atresia	Abdominal distension, bile-stained vomiting, and dilated bowel on X-ray
Meconium ileus	Abdominal distension, bile-stained vomiting, contrast enema reveals impacted meconium in the terminal ileum
Imperforate anus	Abdominal distension and vomiting; requires careful external inspection as some meconium may be passed via a fistula
Hirschsprung's disease	Delayed passage of meconium with either acute or sub-acute obstruction. Abdominal X-ray shows gas throughout small and most of large bowel
Necrotising enterocolitis	Typically, but not exclusively, a problem of sick preterm infants. Presents with signs of intestinal obstruction, bloody stools and evidence of sepsis

Table 2 Persistent vomiting and/or weight loss

System	Mechanism	Aetiology
CNS	Raised intracranial pressure (cerebral irritation)	Cerebral tumour Hypertension Blocked ventricular shunt
	Infection (cerebral irritation)	Encephalitis Labyrinthitis
CVS	Congestive cardiac failure (compression of oesophagus by large left atrium)	Congenital heart disease
Respiratory	Persistent coughing (raised abdominal pressure)	Pertussis Cystic fibrosis
Renal	Systemic upset	Urinary tract infection Renal colic
	Central stimulation/gastric irritation	Uraemia
Metabolic	Central stimulation	Diabetes mellitus Adrenal insufficiency Urea cycle defects
Gastrointestinal	Local gut inflammation	Food intolerance

Management is initially directed at resuscitation and correction of the metabolic abnormalities prior to surgical correction (Ramstedt's pyloromyotomy).

Persistent vomiting

Persistent vomiting always needs careful assessment. Of particular importance is the child who complains of early morning headache and vomiting. This is the characteristic presentation of a posterior fossa tumour where early hydrocephalus (caused by compression of the aqueduct) is exacerbated whilst the child is lying down overnight.

Appendicitis, although rare in preschool children, is notoriously difficult to diagnose and hence may be missed. A careful examination of the abdomen, possibly followed by ultrasound examination, may help to make the diagnosis.

Other conditions which should be considered are shown in Table 2.

Cyclical vomiting is an uncommon condition in which the individual presents with bouts of vomiting lasting several hours but which go on to resolve spontaneously. These bouts occur at variable time intervals and may be sufficiently prolonged to cause dehydration. Cyclical vomiting is thought to represent a form of migraine, and whilst often self-limiting may require anti-emetics or intravenous rehydration. Diagnosis is suggested by the typical cyclical picture and the absence of features of any other underlying condition. Cyclical vomiting usually disappears as the child matures, but may be replaced with more typical migraine.

In older children and teenagers a picture of recurrent vomiting and weight loss, especially if vomiting is concealed, should prompt consideration of conditions such as anorexia nervosa or bulimia. These typically affect teenage girls although boys may be affected. It is very important to exclude an organic cause for such symptoms before coming to a final diagnosis. Sufferers are often surprisingly unconcerned at the extent of their weight loss, and will often deny any problem at all.

Vomiting

- Vomiting may be a feature of a very wide range of paediatric conditions.
- A careful history and examination will often narrow the differential diagnosis.
- Management of vomiting is often symptomatic; medication is rarely indicated.
- Bilious vomiting should always prompt consideration of a surgical condition.
- Profuse vomiting in the neonate should always be promptly investigated and treated.

JAUNDICE

Jaundice is caused by the presence of bilirubin in the skin. It is a sign, not a diagnosis. The normal metabolic pathway for bilirubin is shown in Figure 1a.

The causes of jaundice differ between the newborn period and later childhood; as a result each requires separate consideration.

NEONATAL JAUNDICE

Mechanism

During intrauterine life the fetus is supplied with blood at a relatively low oxygen tension. The fetus adapts to this situation in two ways. The presence of fetal haemoglobin increases (compared to adult haemoglobin) the amount of oxygen delivered at low partial pressures. In addition there is a compensatory increase in red cell production in order to augment the amount of oxygen that can be delivered at tissue level.

After birth, with greater availability of oxygen, there follows a rapid reduction in red cell numbers and, as a consequence, an acute rise in unconjugated bilirubin. The hepatic enzyme systems for the metabolism of bilirubin have, in utero, been exposed to only small quantities and hence are slow in processing the load (Fig. 1b). Within a few days, red cell breakdown declines and bilirubin metabolism is more rapid. As a result, the transient backlog of unconjugated bilirubin in the circulation declines. This is a natural process and is the basis of physiological jaundice. It is apparent to some extent in all babies, but in many the level of bilirubin rises sufficiently to cause jaundice to appear. The timescale of the process means that physiological jaundice should never be apparent before day 2 of life and should reach a maximum around day 4.

Complications

During the first few days of life a number of diseases or mechanisms can intensify this process and result in a more dramatic rise in bilirubin (Fig. 1c). Clearly any such factors, if present, will need to be assessed (e.g. relative dehydration in a breast-fed baby). However, the level of jaundice must also be monitored closely.

Unconjugated bilirubin is fat soluble. When present in exceptionally high levels it can cross the blood–brain barrier and deposit in brain tissue, particularly the basal ganglia. This situation is called *kernicterus* and is associated with cerebral irritability. Both deafness and/or choreoathetoid cerebral palsy can result in the long term. Choreoathetoid cerebral palsy is a consequence of basal ganglia damage and shares many features with Parkinson's disease. The risk of long-term damage is greater when:

- the blood–brain barrier is poorly developed (e.g. in prematurity)
- when the baby is unwell (e.g. acidotic)
- when other substances are present which can dislodge bilirubin from its binding sites (e.g. lipid infusion).

Management

In order to avoid the risk of kernicterus, babies with jaundice which appears significant are monitored using capillary bilirubin measurements. Where intervention is indicated, management is as follows:

1. Adequate hydration, by intravenous infusion if necessary.
2. Phototherapy. Skin is exposed to a blue light capable of splitting unconjugated bilirubin into water soluble fragments (Fig. 2).
3. Exchange transfusion. This involves the exchange of twice the baby's estimated blood volume (2 × 80 ml/kg) in 10 to 20 ml aliquots over 1 to 2 hours. This is used only when more simple measures have failed and the level and rate of rise suggest that brain deposition may occur.

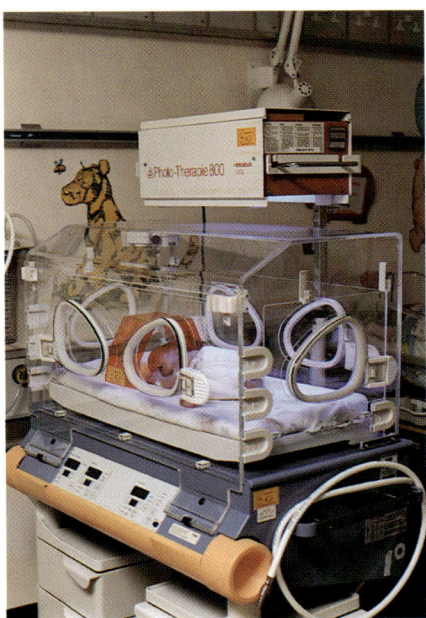

Fig. 2 **Phototherapy.**

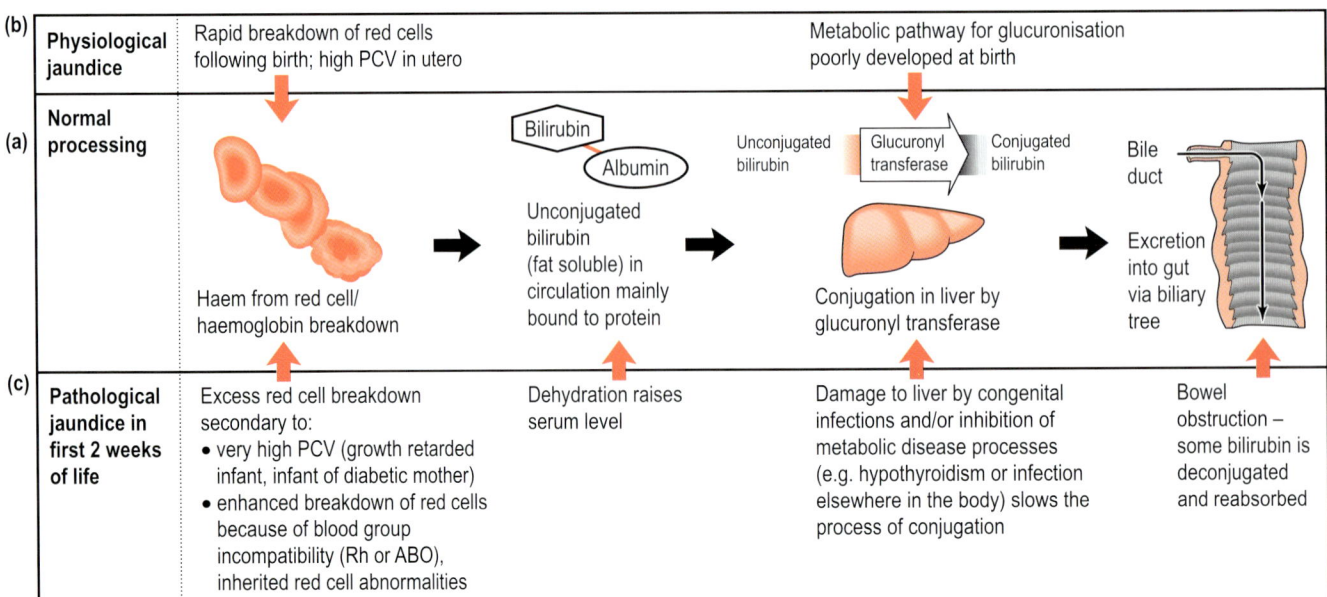

Fig. 1 **Normal processing of bilirubin (a) contrasted with physiological jaundice (b) and pathological jaundice in the first 2 weeks of life (c).**

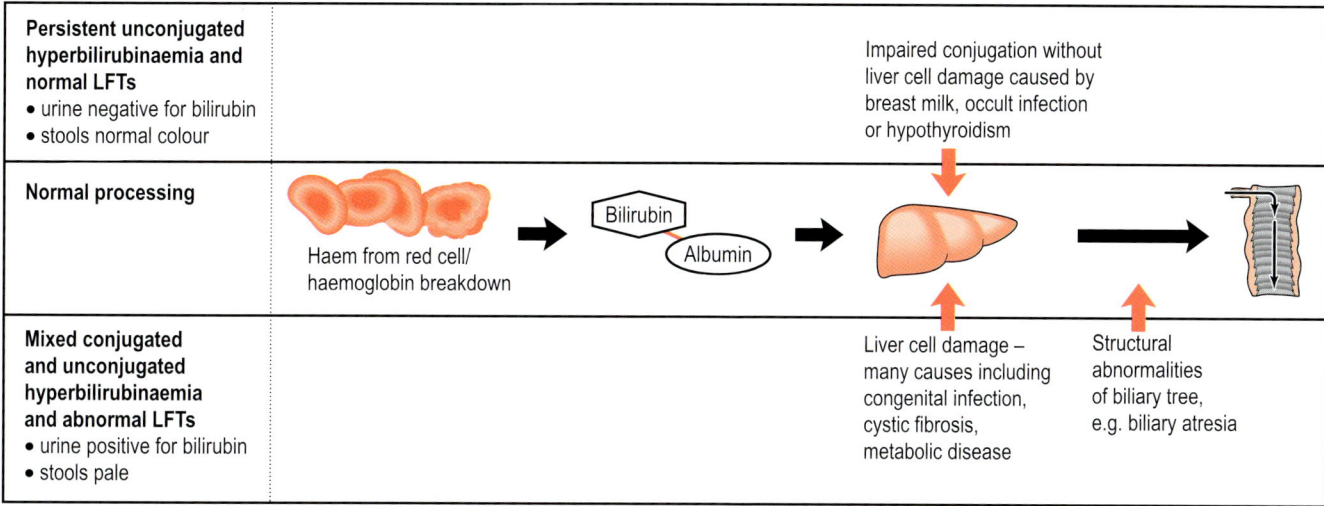

Fig. 3 **Pathological jaundice after the first 2 weeks of life.**

PROLONGED NEONATAL JAUNDICE

The mechanism of physiological neonatal jaundice described above is clearly self-limiting. Where jaundice persists beyond 2 weeks of age an additional diagnosis must be sought. Figure 3 demonstrates that in this situation there are two diagnostic categories.

In the first, the jaundice continues to be predominantly unconjugated and liver function tests are normal. Breast milk jaundice is the most common cause. The factor responsible has not been identified, but the condition is harmless and fades with time.

In the second, the jaundice at 2 weeks is mixed (conjugated and unconjugated) with abnormal liver function tests (i.e. raised cellular enzymes such as aspartate trans-aminase and alanine amino transferase) and the infant is described as having the neonatal hepatitis syndrome. A large number of conditions can produce this picture. One possible diagnosis is biliary atresia. This condition is thought not to be a developmental abnormality but a secondary phenomenon following an early insult to the liver (e.g. an infection). It is amenable to surgery, but in order to have a reasonable chance of success this must be performed before cirrhosis has occurred (i.e. before 6 weeks of age). *Because of this time pressure it is essential that all cases of prolonged jaundice are investigated as a matter of urgency.*

JAUNDICE IN LATER CHILDHOOD

Acute

A large number of viruses infect the liver as part of a generalised infection. Some have a particular propensity for producing an element of acute liver inflammation (hepatitis), e.g. hepatitis A, hepatitis B, and hepatitis C. Others have much less effect on the liver with abnormalities often only detectable on serological testing, e.g. infectious mononucleosis.

Hepatitis A is the most common cause of acute hepatitis and jaundice in the UK. It is spread by the faeco-oral route and is accompanied by flu-like symptoms and anorexia. During the acute phase, urine is typically dark (positive for bilirubin on testing) and the stools pale. It is normally a self-limiting condition.

Hepatitis B and C are both blood spread or transmitted from mother to fetus. They are rare in most Western countries but are relatively common in some parts of Asia. Acute symptoms are similar to those for hepatitis A but liver damage may be much more severe. Both viruses are associated with long-term liver damage which can result in cirrhosis.

CHRONIC LIVER DISEASE

Chronic liver disease in childhood is fortunately rare. The range of causes is shown in

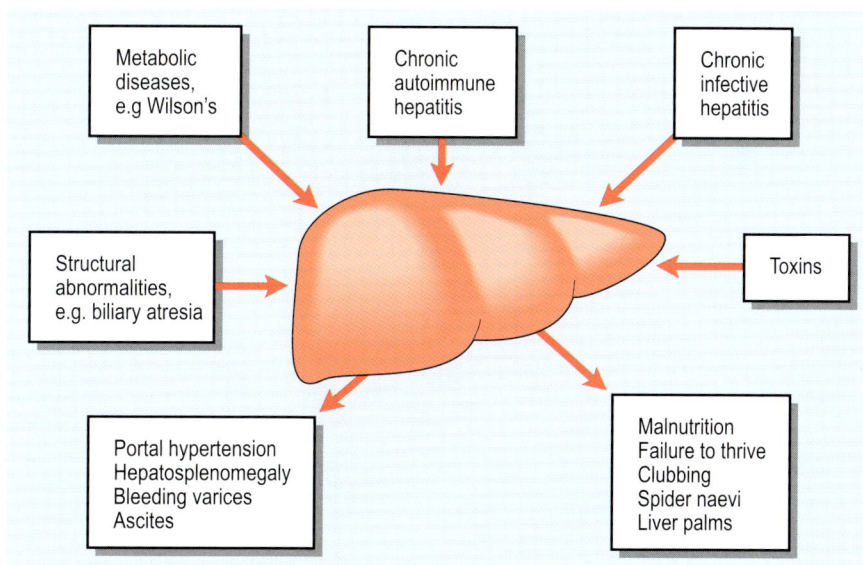

Fig. 4 **Causes and effects of chronic liver disease in children.**

Figure 4. Presentation shows great variation. For some children liver transplantation is beneficial, but conservative management should be pursued for as long as possible.

Jaundice

- Jaundice is not a diagnosis.
- Physiological neonatal jaundice is common and is not a marker of underlying disease.
- Physiological neonatal jaundice never presents before 48 hours of age, peaks around day 4 and is gone by day 14.
- Physiological neonatal jaundice never recurs.
- In later childhood hepatitis A is the most common cause of jaundice.

ABDOMINAL LUMPS

Masses are often felt on examination of the abdomen in infants and children. Many normal structures are palpable (Fig. 1); however, the abdomen is a common site for abnormal swellings (Table 1). These abnormalities may be congenital, the result of obstruction of a viscus or a sign of dysfunction in that organ. The age of the child is important in determining the cause of the abnormality as well as the features of the mass: its mobility, texture, regularity, position in the abdomen or pelvis, whether it is cystic and the presence of other signs such as:

- pain
- fever
- jaundice
- constipation
- vomiting
- haematuria
- dysuria
- systemic symptoms
- bowel obstruction
- ascites
- hypertension
- biochemical and haematological abnormalities.

Careful examination and evaluation of the above features is essential.

NEONATAL MASSES

Some congenital abnormalities may be detected antenatally, e.g. gastroschisis (Fig. 2) and exomphalos (Fig. 3). In gastroschisis there is a defect in the abdominal wall through which the gut protrudes; an exomphalos is an embryological failure of the gut to return to the abdominal cavity and the gut remains outside, in a sac formed by the umbilical cord. Unlike gastroschisis, it is often associated with other congenital abnormalities. Both conditions require urgent surgical correction.

Developmental anomalies such as intestinal duplication cysts and choledochal cysts are identifiable on ultrasound scan before or after delivery. Treatment is by surgical excision. Dysplastic or obstructed kidneys may also be detected antenatally by ultrasound. At

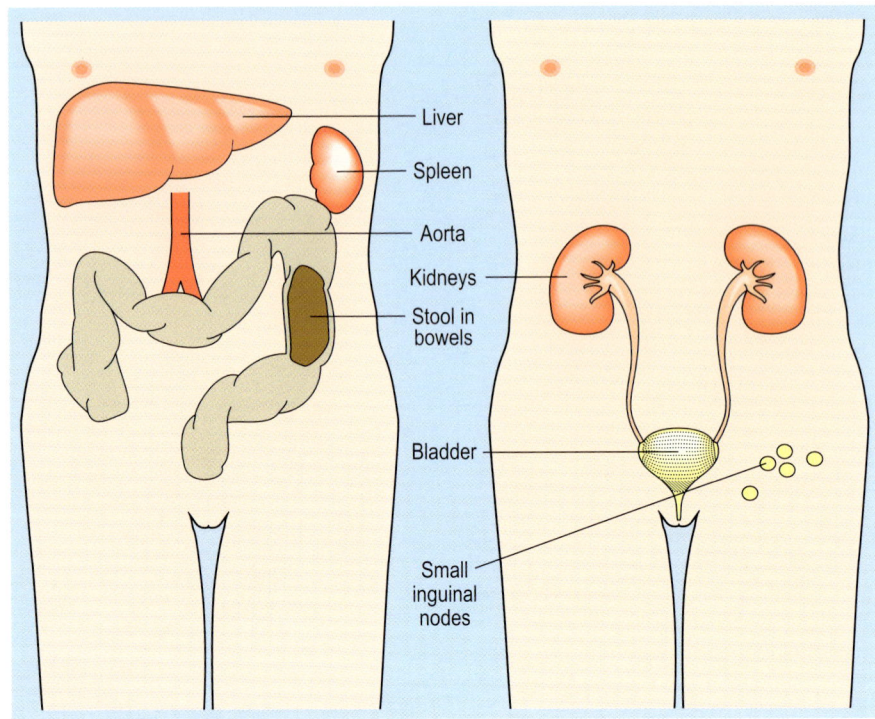

Fig. 1 **Normal structures palpable in the abdomen.**

- Liver
- Spleen
- Aorta
- Kidneys
- Stool in bowels
- Bladder
- Small inguinal nodes

birth, masses will be palpable in the flanks and the abnormal organ can be examined in more detail during postnatal ultrasound scan. Obstructed kidneys due to ureteric narrowing will need surgical drainage. Multicystic, dysplastic kidneys, investigated more accurately by renal DMSA scan, may be managed conservatively as most will involute. Polycystic kidneys need long-term follow-up of renal function and blood pressure. Most pelvic masses, e.g. ovarian cysts, are readily palpable in the neonatal abdomen as the pelvis is small and large masses are displaced into the abdomen.

CHILDREN

The two most common abnormal masses found in childhood are intussusception and an appendix mass.

Intussusception
Intussusception (Fig. 4) may occur throughout childhood; the highest incidence is in the first 2 years of life. Invagination of the bowel occurs into the adjacent distal portion and is associated with pain, rectal bleeding, shock and a palpable sausage-shaped mass in the abdomen. It is spontaneous in most cases but may occur during viral infections because of lymphoid swelling in the abdominal wall, or secondary to lymphomas, polyps, or as a complication of Henoch–Schönlein purpura. After clinical suspicion, diagnosis is made by barium or air enema. This procedure may also produce reduction of the obstruction; alternatively, surgery may be required. If the child is shocked, resuscitation with intravenous fluids and antibiotics is mandatory.

Table 1 **Causes of abdominal lumps**

Congenital	Traumatic	Infective	Neoplastic	Functional	Obstructive
Exomphalos	Haemorrhage into	Appendicitis	Neuroblastoma	Ovarian cyst	Choledochal cyst
Gastroschisis	• liver		Wilms tumour		Renal vein thrombosis
Cystic kidneys	• spleen		Hepatoblastoma		Intussusception
Hydrocele	• kidney		Lymphoma		Pyloric stenosis
Bowel duplication			Testicular tumour		Hernias

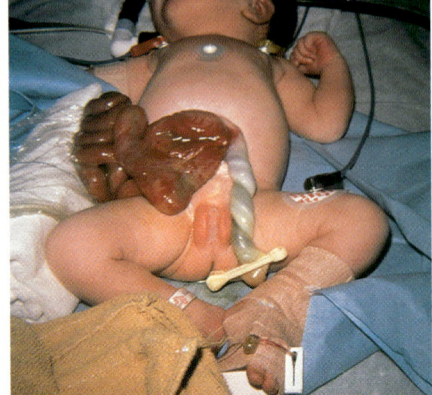

Fig. 2 **Gastroschisis.**

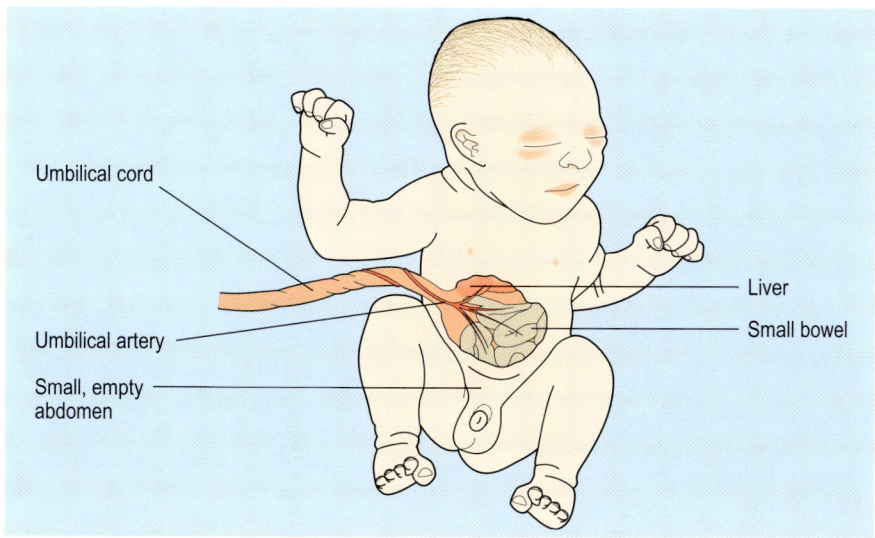

Fig. 3 **Exomphalos.**

Table 2 **Scrotal masses**

Hydrocele
Indirect inguinal hernia
Varicocele
Idiopathic scrotal oedema
Testicular tumour

neonatal period. Many of these resolve spontaneously in the first year of life and can, therefore, be managed conservatively until that time. Hydrocele may present, too, in later childhood, where it is characterised by a painless, usually unilateral, swelling which may vary in size. It transilluminates and has a palpable upper limit.

An indirect inguinal hernia may also cause a painless scrotal swelling but will not transilluminate and the swelling extends to the inguinal canal. Both of these conditions are treated surgically.

Table 3 **Inguinal masses**

Indirect inguinal hernia
Hydrocele
Undescended testis
Lymphadenopathy
Direct inguinal hernia
Femoral hernia

Appendix mass

A fixed mass in the right iliac fossa in association with pain, fever and other signs of infection is typical of an appendix mass. An ultrasound scan is helpful in diagnosis. This intra-abdominal localised infection should be excised surgically.

Pyloric stenosis

Pyloric stenosis occurs in the first few weeks of life, usually in boys. There is a history of increasing vomiting, continuing hunger, eventual dehydration and a metabolic alkalosis. The diagnosis can be made by palpating the hypertrophied pylorus during a feed but is also readily diagnosed by an ultrasound scan. Incision of the circular muscle fibres of the pylorus (Ramstedt's procedure) will relieve the obstruction.

Tumours

Tumours occur both in neonates and in older children. Lymphomas and leukaemia may manifest as hepatosplenomegaly, usually in association with lymphoid enlargement elsewhere, and haematological evidence of these disorders. Intra-abdominal solid tumours are relatively common in early childhood; neuroblastoma, Wilms tumour and hepatoblastoma are all embryonic tumours.

A neuroblastoma most commonly arises from the adrenal gland but may occur anywhere along the sympathetic trunk. Some tumours probably resolve spontaneously without symptoms. Others present with associated weight loss, anaemia, fever and sometimes with evidence of secondary spread. Tumours can be very large and may be palpable across the midline of the abdomen. Diagnosis is made by detecting increased urinary excretion of the catecholamine precursor, vanillylmandelic acid (VMA), bone marrow histology showing

secondary deposits of tumour cells, and/or biopsy of the mass. Therapy involves a combination of surgical resection, radiation and chemotherapy. The outcome depends on the site of the primary tumour, age of the child (infants have a better prognosis; 90% 2-year survival if the tumour is localised) and the degree of secondary spread.

A Wilms tumour may present in a similar way, sometimes with haematuria and hypertension. Wilm's tumour can be associated with congenital abnormalities such as aniridia and hemihypertrophy and is bilateral in 10% of cases. Treatment also involves surgery, chemotherapy and irradiation. If the tumour has not spread, survival is 90% and even if there is secondary spread, survival of at least 50% can be expected.

SCROTAL MASSES

The causes of scrotal swellings are listed in Table 2. A hydrocele is common in the

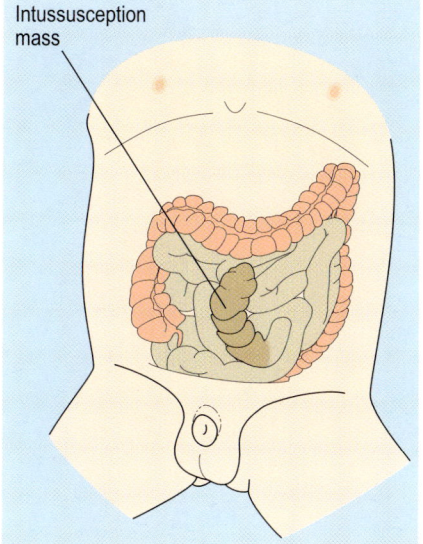

Fig. 4 **Intussusception.**

INGUINAL MASSES (Table 3)

The most common cause of an inguinal lump is an indirect hernia. They are common in preterm infants (5% incidence overall and 30% incidence in those babies under 1000 g at birth), especially in boys. The hernia, which is caused by persistence of the processus vaginalis, may present just as an inguinal lump or may extend into the scrotum. Usually painless unless obstructed, the hernia is often most apparent during crying, coughing or walking. In contrast, an undescended testis will not be felt in the scrotum (which is often underdeveloped on the affected side), but if palpated in the inguinal canal can usually be pulled down into the scrotum. Normal testicular function will not occur unless the undescended testis is placed in the scrotum by 1–2 years of age. Lymph nodes can be identified since they are usually multiple and firm and there may be associated signs of infection or enlargement of glands at other sites in the body.

Abdominal lumps

- Many normal structures may be palpated easily in a child's abdomen.
- Most mobile and cystic masses are benign.
- The abdomen is a relatively common site of childhood tumours.

NON-ABDOMINAL LUMPS

An abnormal mass or lump in a child may be detected by parents or found during a physical examination performed as part of routine surveillance or perhaps in the assessment of a child with symptoms. In early infancy in particular, 'lumps' may be caused by underlying congenital abnormalities. It is important to differentiate such findings from any abnormalities caused during birth. Masses which develop postnatally may be infective, traumatic, neoplastic or functional. Problems causing diffuse swelling are discussed on pages 96–97. Table 1 lists lumps commonly presenting in infancy and childhood.

HEAD AND FACE

Birth injuries to the head and face are common but are usually minor and disappear within days of birth. A caput succedaneum, an oedematous swelling on the back of the head, is due to pressure on the scalp during delivery. It is particularly common during ventouse extraction. A similar swelling may occur in other areas of the body if that is the presenting part. In contrast, a cephalhaematoma involves bleeding under the periosteum of the scalp and, characteristically, the swelling does not cross the margins of the neighbouring suture line and is therefore confined to a single plate of bone. A cephalhaematoma may take weeks to resolve, often producing a hard calcified mass before gradually resorbing into the skull bone. At birth, asymmetry of the head or skull may be noted (plagiocephaly, Fig.

1). Premature fusion of cranial sutures may be responsible for this appearance, but much more commonly it results from a constricted position in utero.

Congenital abnormalities of the central nervous system may be apparent at birth. Generalised swelling of the head, and wide anterior fontanelle, perhaps with associated neurological abnormalities, is characteristic of hydrocephalus. Such an abnormality will require investigation with ultrasound and CT scans, and is usually managed by inserting a shunt between one of the ventricles and the peritoneal cavity. An encephalocoele is a defect occurring in the cranium with an associated swelling containing meninges and sometimes brain tissue. Minor lesions are managed surgically, while large brain-containing defects may not be treatable.

The most serious infection of the face is orbital cellulitis. This may occur at any age. It often presents with rapidly progressive swelling of one periorbital area associated with inflammation, sometimes proptosis, and systemic signs of infection. It may be associated with infection elsewhere, there is often no preceding injury or abnormality. Usually bacterial, it should be treated with systemic antibiotics. Tumours of the eye may rarely present in infancy and childhood. The two most common are a primary tumour of the eyeball, retinoblastoma, (usually hereditary), and secondaries from a neuroblastoma. Both tumours may present with proptosis and an absent red reflex.

NECK

The most common swellings which occur in the neck are due to lymph node enlargement in association with local infection, usually in the mouth or throat. The swellings may be multiple or single and are often tender (Fig. 2). More unusually they may be due to infection of the node itself, e.g. Epstein–Barr virus or mycobacterial infection. Lymphoma or leukaemia may present with similar, but non-tender, enlargement. Response to broad spectrum antibiotics and a normal peripheral white count usually differentiate between infection and neoplasia, although sometimes biopsy of a gland will be necessary.

Infection of the parotid gland with the mumps virus is common in childhood, although it has become less so since the introduction of mumps immunisation (as the MMR).

The sternomastoid muscle may not uncommonly develop a swelling in response to birth trauma. Other causes include upper respiratory infection, local trauma or, rarely, some neurological conditions (Fig. 3). Usually, simple physiotherapy and stretching or neck support in a collar are sufficient treatment.

An abnormality of development of the lymphatic system (lymphangioma or cystic hygroma) or, more rarely, blood vessels (haemangioma) will usually be apparent at birth. These swellings, if large enough, may compromise breathing, or obstruct large blood vessels in the neck and mediastinum.

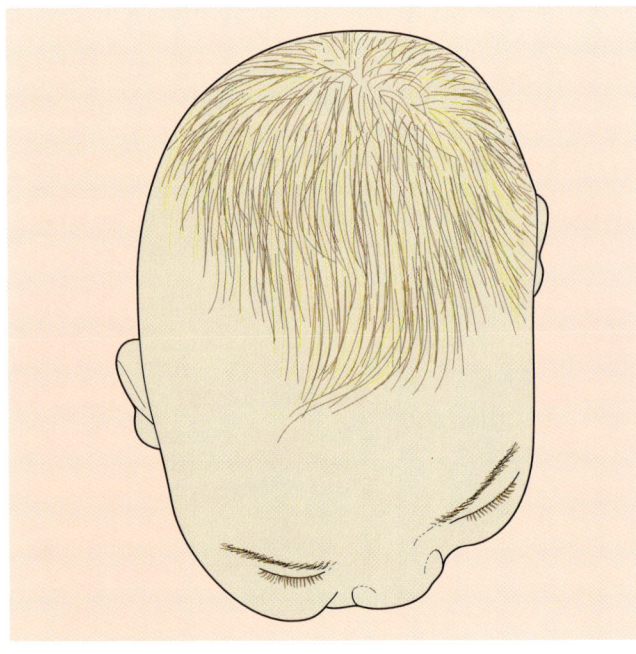

Fig. 1 **Plagiocephaly.**

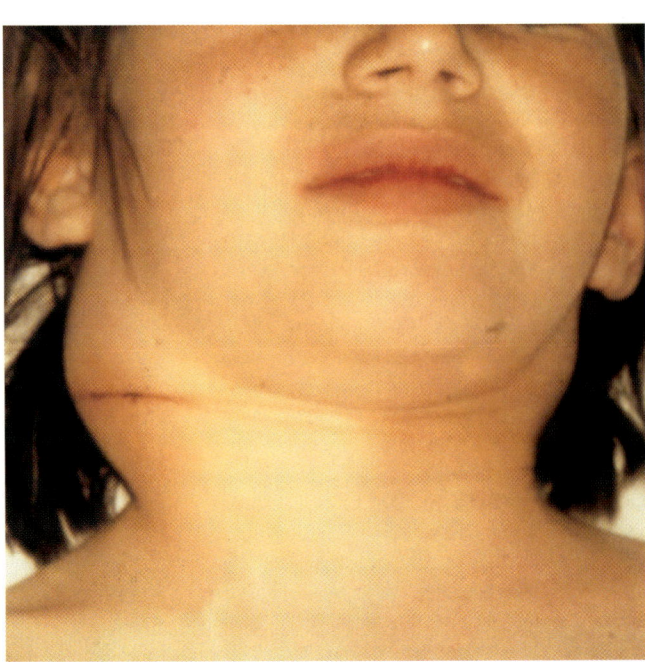

Fig. 2 **Cervical lymphadenopathy.**

Table 1 **Causes of non-abdominal lumps**

Site	Congenital	Birth injury	Infective	Traumatic	Neoplastic	Functional
Head and face	Plagiocephaly Encephalocoele Dermoid Hydrocephalus	Cephalhaematoma Caput succedaneum Skull moulding	Orbital cellulitis Parotitis	Haematomas Skull fractures	Orbital tumours	
Neck	Lymphangioma Bronchial cyst Torticollis Thyroglossal cyst Dermoid cyst		Lymphadenitis		Lymphoma	Goitre
Thorax		Fractured ribs and clavicle	Mastitis			Gynaecomastia
Back	Meningocoele Meningomyelocoele	Fat necrosis				
Limbs	Lymphoedema	Osteomyelitis Septic arthritis		Fractures		
Skin	Haemangiomas Neurofibromas Naevi		Warts Carbuncles			

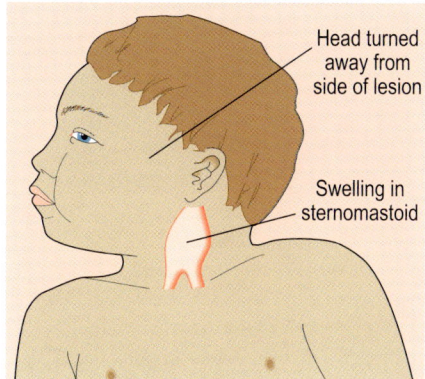

Fig. 3 **Sternomastoid tumour.**

Head turned away from side of lesion

Swelling in sternomastoid

Lymphangiomas often transilluminate. CT scans will indicate the extent of these abnormalities. If small, they can be surgically excised but may be inoperable if diffuse.

Enlargement of the thyroid gland is unusual in children. If associated with other features, investigation for hyperthyroidism is indicated. Asymmetrical enlargement is characteristic of a thyroglossal cyst. Such a swelling often transilluminates and moves on swallowing together with the thyroid gland and will be typically cystic on ultrasound examination. It will require surgical removal.

THORAX

Birth injuries to the thorax are unusual but may involve fractured ribs and clavicles. The resulting callus often causes concern but becomes resorbed into the rib as the child grows. These injuries are managed conservatively. Swelling of breast tissue in both infant boys and girls is common and reflects the effect of maternal hormones. This condition resolves spontaneously. In contrast, infection of breast tissue, usually unilateral and associated with inflammation, systemic signs of sepsis and a raised white cell count will require antibiotics. In pubertal boys, breast tissue may enlarge and become painful under the influence of increasing pituitary hormones. Generally, this will resolve and reassurance is all that is required. However, some boys become particularly embarrassed by this breast tissue and if breast enlargement persists, subareolar removal of breast tissue can be performed.

BACK

A mass on the lower back of an infant may represent a meningocoele or myelomeningocoele and requires careful neurological assessment. A meningocoele does not usually contain nerve elements and most children can be treated with surgical repair of the defect. However, limited neurological damage (e.g. minor degrees of bladder dysfunction) may occur. A myelomeningocoele, which usually contains nerve tissue, depending on the level of the lesion, will have associated limb paralysis, bladder and bowel dysfunction. Ninety percent of cases also have associated hydrocephalus. Surgical correction of these problems is complex and, in view of the variable prognosis, the decision to treat the defect must be made in conjunction with the parents. Most of these neural tube defects can be detected antenatally and termination is offered.

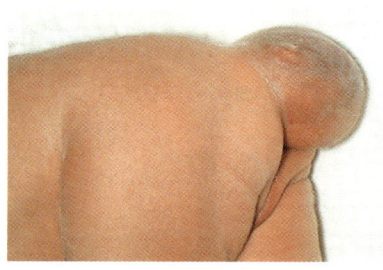

Fig. 4 **Sacro-coccygeal tumour.**

Other back or pelvic swellings include sacro-cocygeal tumour (Fig. 4). These may have malignant elements and therefore need careful assessment.

SKIN

Numerous minor lesions may develop on the skin at any time during childhood. At birth, most naevi and haemangiomas will be noted immediately. Most cavernous haemangiomas typically arise in the period after birth. In general, they will resolve if left alone. Those which compromise vision or the airway may be treated with laser therapy.

Skin infections are common in childhood. Warts can be left to resolve spontaneously, or can be removed surgically, by cryocautery or chemical application. Large bacterial carbuncles may cause systemic symptoms, particularly in young children. They are treated with drainage and/or systemic antibiotics.

Non-abdominal lumps

- Infancy is the most common period for congenital abnormalities to present.
- Birth trauma may commonly produce minor abnormalities which readily resolve spontaneously.
- Although minor conditions may not need treatment, parents find such defects worrying and will need careful explanation and reassurance.
- Conversely, management decisions about serious conditions with variable outcomes must always have parents' involvement.

OLIGURIA

Urine is the end-product of renal excretion. Assessment of aspects of urine output is important not only for disorders of the urinary tract, but can also give valuable information about general disease (Fig. 1),

Urine is produced in utero, and failure of adequate renal function causes oligohydramnios. In renal agenesis, oligohydramnios is profound and results in compression of the fetus, and pulmonary hypoplasia (Potter's syndrome).

At birth, the glomerular filtration rate (GFR) is low (20–30 ml/min/1.73 m^2), and rises in infancy to adult values: 80–120 ml/min/1.73 m^2. However, the full-term neonate, having a high proportion of body weight attributible to fluid, is able to cope with quite wide variations in fluid and electrolyte input, in spite of relative immaturity of tubular and glomerular function.

> Aspects of fluid balance in children should always be discussed in terms of body weight (x/kg) or surface area (x/1.73 m^2).

ASSESSMENT OF URINE OUTPUT

Urine collection is discussed on page 82. The younger the child, the more difficult is accurate direct assessment of urine volume. In general, oliguria is noticed more from decreased frequency of urination than low volumes as such. In hospital, urine bags are useful or nappies can be weighed (wet minus dry). In renal disease, the more important parameter is the relationship between fluid intake and urine output.

ACUTE RENAL INSUFFICIENCY

When established, this usually manifests as oliguria, fluid overload, hypertension and metabolic acidosis, with haematuria and proteinuria. It is caused by any condition that acutely compromises the function of both kidneys.

ACUTE RENAL FAILURE

The causes of acute renal failure are as follows:

- Pre-renal
  — dehydration
  — shock — any cause, e.g. sepsis or blood loss.
- Renal
  — haemolytic-uraemic syndrome
  — acute (glomerulo)nephritis
  — toxic (e.g. drug toxicity).

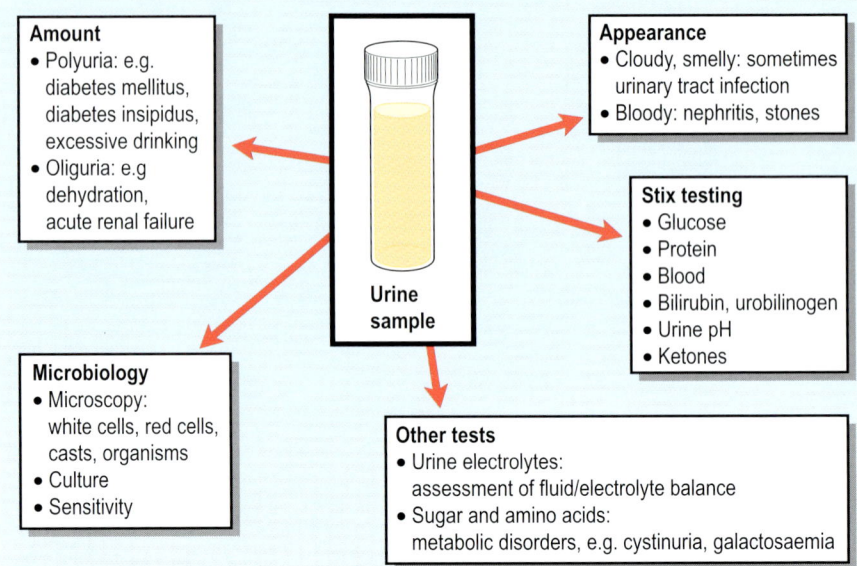

Fig. 1 **Information sources from examination of urine.**

- Post-renal
  — urinary obstruction (e.g. posterior urethral valves).

A common cause of confusion is the relationship of dehydration or hypovolaemia to acute renal insufficiency. If the circulation is insufficient to perfuse organs adequately, the kidneys react with vasoconstriction and conservation of fluid (increased tubular reabsorption). This manifests as oliguria and concentrated urine (high osmolality). However, there is no renal damage at this point, and so no significant proteinuria, haematuria or significant urinary casts. When the insult is severe or prolonged, however, and kidney perfusion sufficiently compromised, there is reversible renal damage (pathologically known as *acute tubular necrosis*, although glomeruli are also affected) and this is manifest by proteinuria (both glomerular and tubular) and haematuria. In the early phase of recovery, dilute urine (concentrating ability affected) is produced.

The most common renal cause of acute renal failure in children in the UK is *haemolytic-uraemic syndrome* (HUS). This combines the onset of acute renal failure with a microangiopathic haemolytic anaemia and thrombocytopenia (Fig. 2). It typically follows an episode of bloody diarrhoea, often shigella dysentery or, most common in the UK, a particular serotype of enteropathogenic *E. coli* (0157/H7). HUS is managed symptomatically and usually resolves spontaneously. Acute peritoneal dialysis is often required.

Nephritis means (non-infective) inflammation of the kidneys. Acute nephritis in childhood most commonly results from an unusual immune response to group A β-haemolytic streptococcal or viral infection elsewhere in the body. Typically, 1–2 weeks after a throat infection, there is acute onset of signs which can include fluid overload

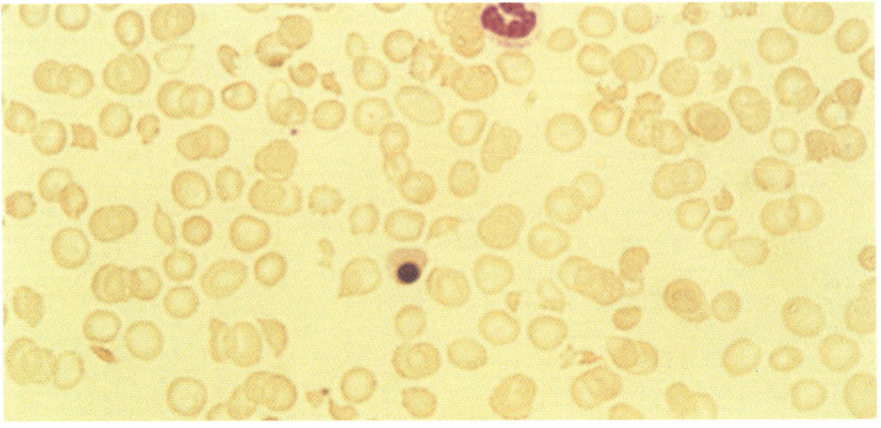

Fig. 2 **Blood film of HUS.**

and hypertension, with haematuria and proteinuria (sometimes gross). Some children are asymptomatic, and in most, the condition is self-limiting. However, in a minority the nephritis is rapidly progressive, with deterioration in renal function. Aggressive management with steroids and cytotoxics can be helpful, but a number progress to chronic renal failure. Worldwide, streptococcal infection (often of the skin) is a potent cause of renal failure and death.

Henoch–Schönlein disease (p. 64) is another cause of acute nephritis.

CHRONIC RENAL FAILURE

This is relatively rare in childhood, and the causes are diverse, including:

- progressive glomerulonephritis (as in severe Henoch–Schönlein disease, or atypical haemolytic-uraemic syndrome)
- renal scarring, as a result of recurrent urinary tract infection, usually due to vesicoureteric reflux (p. 83)
- inherited abnormalities such as the polycystic kidney diseases (Fig. 3), Alport's syndrome, and cystinosis.

It is important to appreciate that once renal function is significantly impaired, there is an element of progression in renal damage leading to further reduction in GFR *whatever the cause of the renal impairment*. So far, there are no treatments that can sufficiently arrest this non-specific deterioration and this is a major area of research. Symptoms do not usually develop until a late stage, but growth, in particular, can be affected earlier. Management is complex and should be supervised in a specialised centre with access to a multidisciplinary team. Aspects of treatment of chronic renal failure are given in Table 1.

When GFR is reduced to <10–20 ml/min/1.73 m^2, end-stage renal failure is reached, and dialysis or transplantation is necessary to preserve life. Renal transplantation is realistic even in infants as small as 10 kg. Below this weight, and at any age while awaiting transplantation, peritoneal dialysis is the preferred method of renal

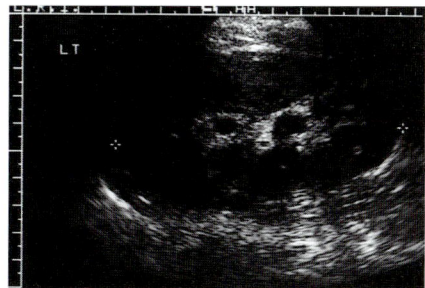

Fig. 3 **Ultrasound scan of a kidney in a child with infantile type polycystic kidney disease.** Note the multiple cysts.

support, allowing children to be at home after suitable parental education.

PROTEINURIA AND HAEMATURIA

Although the combination of proteinuria and haematuria should alert one to the possibility of acute nephritis, there are obviously many other causes of these urinary problems.

For proteinuria, although 'dipstix' are sensitive, morning urine samples for protein/creatinine ratio have replaced 24-hour collections for quantitative assessment, which are usually impractical in young children.

CAUSES OF PROTEINURIA

Transient proteinuria can be caused by any febrile illness or exercise and affects many normal children. The persistent form may be a marker of urinary tract infection. Orthostatic proteinuria (caused by being upright and hence not present in the first morning urine sample) is also relatively common and is easily confused with glomerulonephritis. Nephrotic syndrome is characterised by very heavy proteinuria (pp. 96–97).

CAUSES OF HAEMATURIA

Although the majority of cases of haematuria in childhood are associated with UTIs, blood loss is unlikely to be gross, and usually there are other symptoms in these circumstances.

Haematuria, microscopic or macroscopic, is associated with:

- infection: bacterial, schistosomiasis and tuberculosis (worldwide)
- glomerulonephritis: e.g. Henoch–Schönlein purpura, IgA nephropathy
- stones (urolithiasis) (pp. 82–83)
- trauma
- tumour: Wilms tumour (nephroblastoma) may present with haematuria or more commonly a loin mass in infancy (< 2 years); good prognosis if no blood-borne metastases, e.g. lung or bone
- haematological disorders: e.g. disseminated intravascular coagulation
- iatrogenic: e.g. cyclophosphamide treatment
- recurrent or persistent haematuria: a mixed group, includes benign familial haematuria, IgA nephropathy and Alport's syndrome (hereditary deafness and nephritis, X-linked); if in doubt in these cases a renal biopsy is indicated.

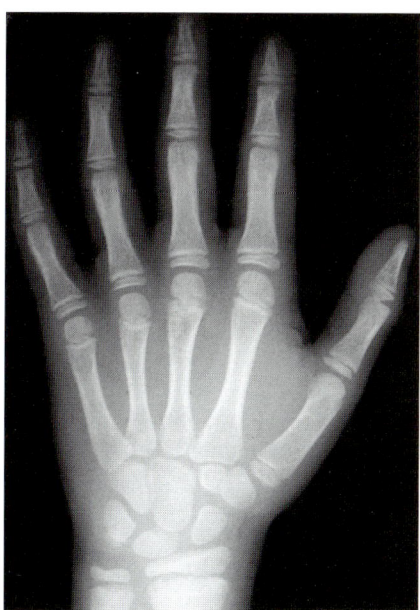

Fig. 4 **Renal osteopathy and rickets in a 7-year-old girl with longstanding chronic renal failure.** Note particularly the resorption of bone on the middle and terminal phalanges.

Table 1 **Effects and treatment of chronic renal failure**

Effect	Cause	Treatment
Growth failure	Poor food intake (poor appetite and nausea)	Dietary assessment and supplementation (calories and vitamins)
	Metabolic acidosis	Sodium bicarbonate
	Anaemia	
	Fluid and electrolyte (particularly sodium) loss	Balance fluid and electrolyte input to output
Renal bone disease (osteodystrophy) (Fig. 4)	Defective vitamin D metabolism	Vitamin D supplements
	Phosphate retention	Dietary phosphate restriction and gut phosphate binders
	Secondary hyperparathyroidism	
Anaemia	Erythropoietin deficiency (formed in the kidneys)	Give erythropoietin injections
	Nutritional	Blood transfusions
Hypertension	Fluid and sodium retention (sometimes)	Correct fluid and electrolyte balance
	Renal damage causing renin release	Antihypertensives

Oliguria

- Haemolytic-uraemic syndrome is the most common renal cause of acute renal failure in children.
- Acute renal failure generally has a good potential for recovery, whereas chronic renal failure tends to be progressive.
- Always ask about urinary stream when assessing potential renal failure; exclude urethral obstruction.

DYSURIA

URINARY SYMPTOMS

Dysuria has come to mean pain on micturition. In later childhood, inflammation of the lower urinary tract usually manifests itself as a 'stinging' or 'burning' sensation on urination, associated with frequency. However, younger children may just refuse to pass urine, or pass very small quantities frequently and seem generally upset. Their toilet habit may be further upset producing wetting problems (p. 30). The most common cause of acute dysuria is urinary tract infection.

URINARY TRACT INFECTION

In pathological terms, this refers to infection anywhere in the renal tract. Symptoms can be very general, particularly in young children, and similarly in sick babies where it is a cause of jaundice. Alteration of pattern of micturition, urinary frequency and 'dysuria' are common in older age groups. Gross haematuria is unusual but smaller amounts of blood in the urine are more common. Urine smell is an unreliable indicator of infection and urine looking 'dark' or 'concentrated' is unhelpful. If the upper tracts are significantly affected, loin pain and high fever with 'rigors' are typical (so-called pyelonephritis). However, it is not helpful in children to talk of 'cystitis', as this term should be reserved for 'insignificant' lower urinary infection as seen in some adults. In children it is better to think of the whole of the urinary tract as being potentially involved in all cases.

URINE COLLECTION

This is one of the most important and difficult aspects of assessment. Several methods of collection are available:

- Older children can cooperate with a midstream urine collection.
- Younger ones can provide a clean catch specimen into a sterile container. The urethral area should be cleaned first with soap and rinsed with water (anterior to posterior). A sterilised plastic potty or large bowl is often useful.
- For babies, urine bags are available (Fig. 1) but can easily be contaminated, particularly with faeces.
- In babies who are acutely unwell, a suprapubic aspirate is valuable, and any bacterial growth is significant if this method is used.
- Catheter specimens are only rarely required.

Dipstix testing of urine for blood and protein, if positive, is suggestive of infection,

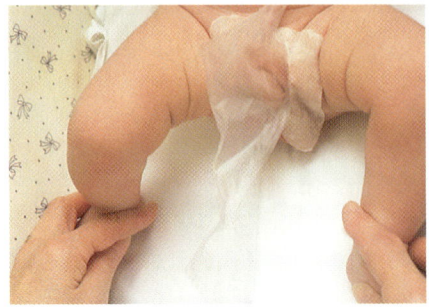

Fig. 1 **Bag for urine collection.** Contamination can be reduced if collected properly.

but not diagnostic, and any febrile illness can cause moderate proteinuria. The nitrite test which relies on the conversion of nitrates to nitrites by bacteria is also useful as a screening test. If infection is present, urine microscopy typically reveals increased numbers of white cells, and organisms can often be seen. However, the laboratory diagnosis of UTI centres on urine culture: more than 10^5 colonies of a pure (i.e. only one species) growth of bacteria (usually Gram-negative) per ml of urine. This is essential for the confident diagnosis of urinary infection.

If symptoms are vague, diagnosis of UTI can be difficult because of problems of collection. Urine cultures often contain 'mixed growths' of organisms, and urine samples should be repeated until they are clear of infection or a pure growth is obtained.

MANAGEMENT OF UTI

Increase fluid intake and give antibiotics. If the child is significantly ill, intravenous antibiotics are indicated. Gentamicin is very effective, but is potentially nephrotoxic (and ototoxic). Otherwise, oral trimethoprim is usually sufficient. Antibiotic sensitivities

will be available the day after culture results; other useful antibacterial agents are nitrofurantoin and cephalosporins, both of which can be given orally. Following a course of antibiotics the young child should remain on a prophylactic dose of an antibiotic, usually trimethoprim, until the urinary tract has been investigated.

COMMON ORGANISMS CAUSING UTIs

- *Escherichia coli* is by far the most common.
- *Proteus* spp. are often associated with stone formation.
- *Klebsiella* spp.
- *Pseudomonas* spp. are usually only found in chronically stagnant urine, e.g. bladder dysfunction.

FURTHER INVESTIGATION OF URINARY TRACT INFECTION

All first cases of UTI in childhood should be investigated further. This is because they are more likely to be associated with urinary tract abnormalities than in adults, and these can result in long-term problems (Fig. 2).

Ultrasound scanning is non-invasive. It gives information about renal size, and whether there is *hydronephrosis*, that is, dilatation of the renal pelvis. This is a non-specific finding and due usually either to vesicoureteric reflux (VUR) or urinary tract obstruction. A micturating cystourethrogram (MCUG) will demonstrate vesicoureteric reflux directly, but is invasive and involves catheterising the child and instilling radio-opaque contrast into the bladder. Vesicoureteric reflux can be mild (Fig. 3) or severe (Fig. 4).

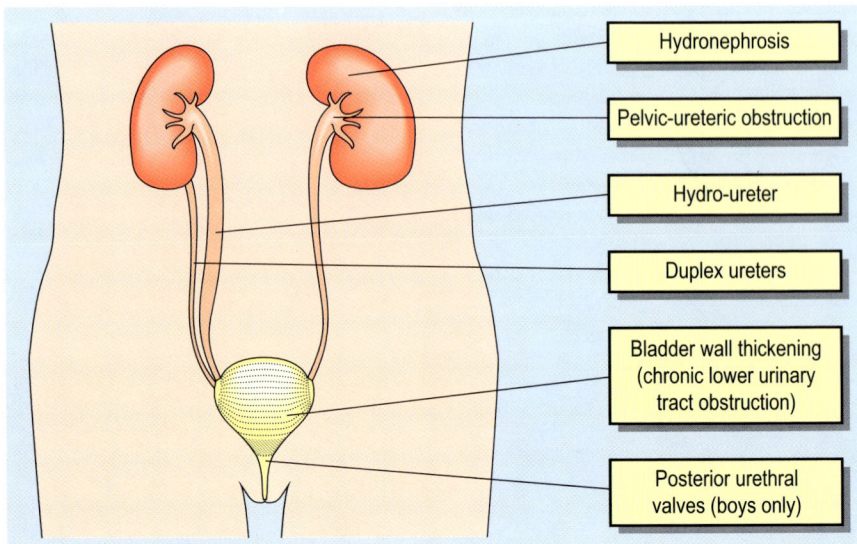

Hydronephrosis

Pelvic-ureteric obstruction

Hydro-ureter

Duplex ureters

Bladder wall thickening (chronic lower urinary tract obstruction)

Posterior urethral valves (boys only)

Fig. 2 **Abnormalities associated with UTIs.**

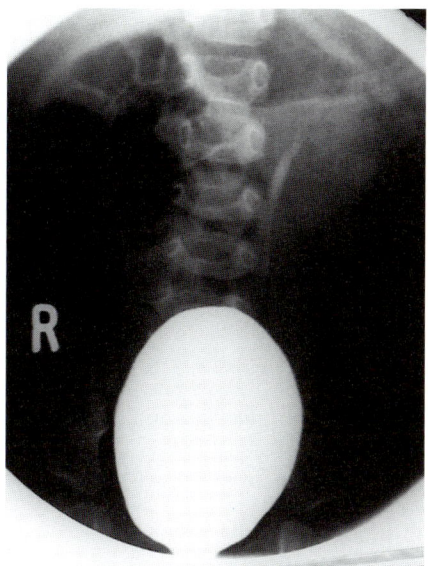

Fig. 3 **Cystourethrogram showing mild unilateral vesicoureteric reflux.**

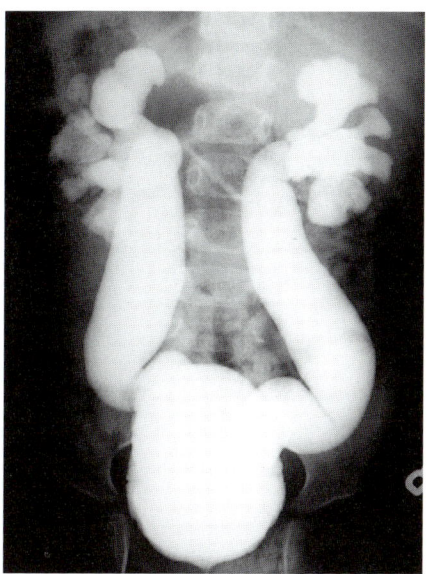

Fig. 4 **Cystourethrogram showing severe bilateral vesicoureteric reflux.**

Counts

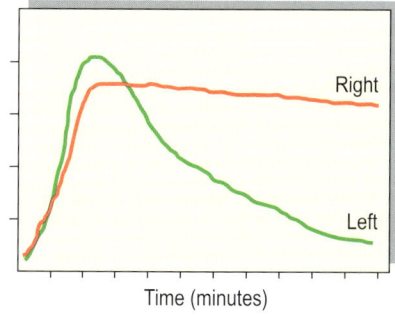

Time (minutes)

Fig. 5 **Dynamic radioisotope scan renal excretion curves showing obstruction to urinary flow on the right side after injection of isotope.**

Recently it has become common to use injected radioisotopic methods to image the urinary tract. DTPA or Mag-3 scans are useful dynamic tests of individual kidney excretion, particularly useful when looking for urinary obstruction (Fig. 5).

The main long-term consequence of urinary tract infection is the formation of renal scars in some children. These predispose to the later development of hypertension, and chronic renal failure if severe and bilateral (Fig. 6). It can be many years before these problems appear. The precise mechanism whereby infection predisposes to later renal damage is not known, but involves interaction between infected urine and back-pressure of urine against renal calyces. The risk is particularly high if vesicoureteric reflux is found—greater in infancy (under 3 years). Therefore, if urinary tract anomalies such as vesicoureteric reflux are found then low dose, long-term antibiotic treatment should be used prophylactically until the child is 3–4 years of age. Obstructive lesions require surgery. DMSA scans (Fig. 7) show renal scars well.

A significant proportion of abnormalities are now found on antenatal ultrasound

scanning. Hydronephrosis can be picked up early in the fetus and specific causes elucidated by later postnatal radiological investigations as above.

Apart from hydronephrosis, other renal abnormalities can be found by antenatal scanning such as infantile polycystic kidney disease, an autosomal recessive condition resulting in large cystic kidneys and liver fibrosis. Adult polycystic kidney disease (autosomal dominant) usually presents later. Multicystic dysplastic kidney is a sporadic condition affecting only one kidney, the abnormal kidney usually involuting spontaneously.

OTHER CAUSES OF DYSURIA

Any febrile illness can be associated with a certain amount of urinary discomfort, but the urine will not be found to be infected on culture. Urinary stones may cause pain, are uncommon in childhood, and usually due to chronically infected, stagnant urine in relation to a urinary tract anomaly. These are normally composed of calcium oxalate/hydroxyapatite and can also be associated with metabolic disorders such as idiopathic

hypercalciuria or hypercalcaemia (rare in childhood). Cystine stones are found in cystinuria, where there is specific failure of tubular reabsorption of the dibasic amino acids cystine, ornithine, arginine and lysine. Uric acid stones are very rare.

Vulvovaginitis is quite common. It usually responds to simple hygiene measures and avoidance of irritants like bubble baths. Balanitis usually occurs with foreskin problems such as phimosis or paraphimosis. One should consider sexual abuse if symptoms are unusual, or there are signs of trauma or bruising.

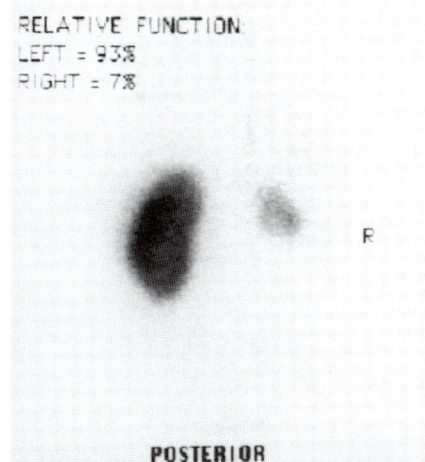

RELATIVE FUNCTION:
LEFT = 93%
RIGHT = 7%

POSTERIOR

Fig. 7 **Static radioisotope scan showing severe scarring of the right kidney.**

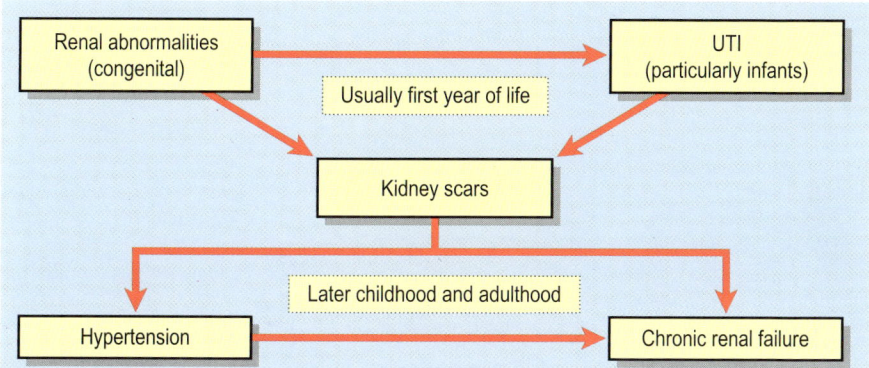

Fig. 6 **Pathogenesis of long-term effects of urinary tract infection.**

| Renal abnormalities (congenital) | → | UTI (particularly infants) |

Usually first year of life

Kidney scars

Later childhood and adulthood

Hypertension → Chronic renal failure

Dysuria

- Urinary tract infection should be confirmed by urine culture.
- Children with UTIs should be investigated to identify urinary tract abnormalities which could predispose to further infection.
- The risk of renal scarring is greatest in infants.
- The consequences of renal scarring may be hypertension and chronic renal failure much later in life.

LOSS OF CONSCIOUSNESS I

PHYSIOLOGY

There is a wide spectrum between the fully conscious and the unconscious. Many acutely ill children will suffer a depressed conscious level as part of their condition. 'Coma' means a state of prolonged unconsciousness and is more unusual.

Maintenance of consciousness depends on the activity of the reticular formation, a collection of neurones spread through the brain stem which acts as an alerting system on the cerebral cortex and the afferent neural pathways. An insult to this structure causes loss of consciousness. The cause may be primary damage to that area, but dysfunction more commonly arises secondary to damage elsewhere in the brain or is due to a systemic disorder.

CAUSES

In only 5% of paediatric cases is consciousness impaired as a result of a primary brain lesion, while 95% result from cerebral depression secondary to a systemic problem.

Primary brain disorder

Primary brain disorders causing unconsciousness include the following:

- vascular, e.g. intracerebral, subdural or extradural haemorrhage
- tumour, benign (e.g. meningioma, craniopharyngioma) and malignant (e.g. astrocytoma, medulloblastoma)
- infection, e.g. meningitis, encephalitis, cerebral abscess
- rapidly expanding hydrocephalus
- trauma, including non-accidental injury.

Adequate perfusion of the brain depends on adequate blood pressure together with a sufficiently low intracranial pressure to allow circulation to take place. In other words cerebral perfusion pressure (CPP) equals mean arterial pressure (MAP) minus intracranial pressure (ICP):

$$CPP = MAP - ICP$$

Anything causing raised ICP therefore reduces CPP and can lead to unconsciousness. This is the mechanism of action of many intracerebral causes of coma. Changes in intracerebral pressure can occur more acutely in children aged over 24 months because the cranial sutures have closed, creating a fixed volume for the brain.

In extreme cases, the ICP may be so great as to push the brain downwards causing the cerebellar tonsils to herniate through the foramen magnum (coning). This has a very grave prognosis. Signs of onset include falling pulse, rising blood pressure, irregular breathing and respiratory arrest.

Secondary to a systemic disorder

A number of conditions can lead to coma since they create an unfavourable environment for normal brain function. Mechanisms include hypoxia, ischaemia, or abnormal biochemical state. These conditions are as follows:

- CVS/respiratory failure
- seizures
- infection — meningitis, septicaemia
- metabolic — hypoglycaemia, hyperglycaemia, hyponatraemia, hypernatraemia, hypocalcaemia and rare inherited disorders of metabolism
- liver failure or renal failure, with consequent rise in toxic metabolites
- toxic ingestion, e.g. drugs, alcohol
- hypothermia.

Many of the above cause cerebral oedema as a secondary effect with a resulting increase in ICP. This contributes to the production of coma.

ACUTE LOSS OF CONSCIOUSNESS

Where loss of consciousness is acute, it represents a medical emergency (Fig. 1). Primary assessment and resuscitation should proceed in parallel. The aim of resuscitation is to minimise any further impairment of brain function, e.g. relieve hypoxia and reduce raised ICP. The assessment serves to identify the immediate resuscitation requirements, and to identify possible causes of the collapse. It is best to have a systematic approach to assessment, as outlined below:

- **Assessment of the airway.** Make sure it is patent and will remain so.
- **Assessment of the child's breathing.** Is the child breathing and is the breathing adequate? Is the child pink? Always give oxygen to a child with a reduced level of consciousness. Bag and mask ventilation or intubation may be necessary.

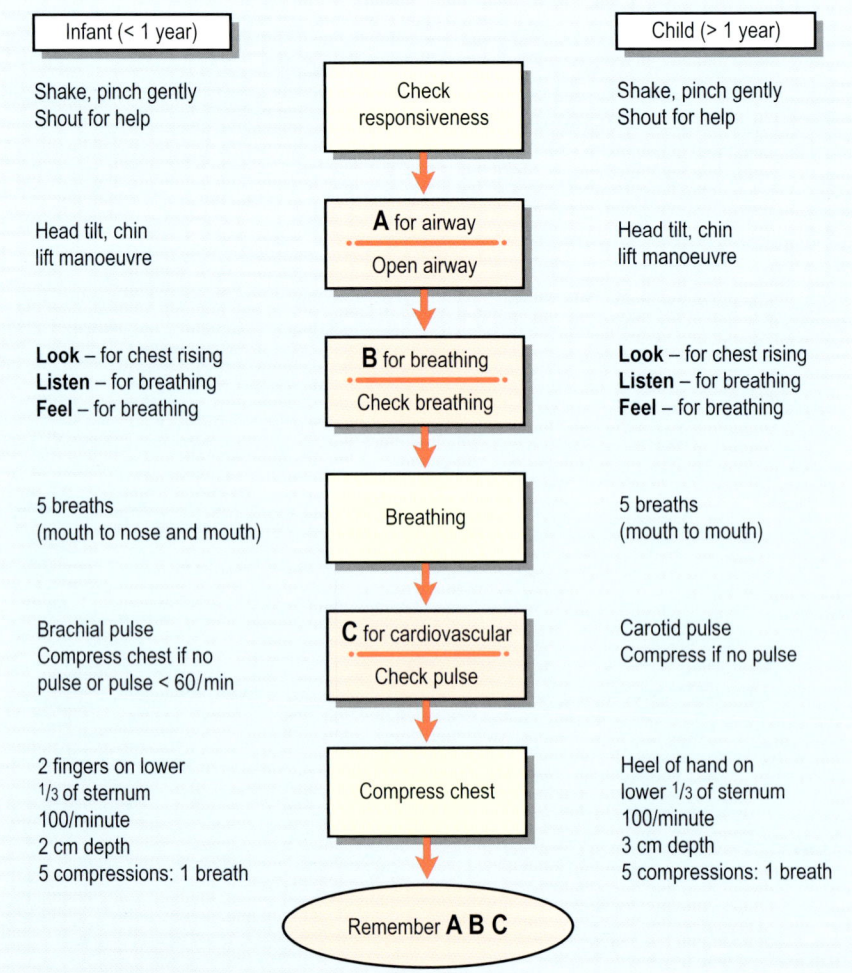

Fig. 1 **Paediatric emergency life support.** Remember **ABC**.

- **Is the circulation adequate?** Monitor pulse rate and volume, blood pressure and capillary refill time. The child should be attached to an ECG monitor, and if the heart rate is less than 80/minute in an infant, or absent in an older child, cardiac massage should be started immediately. Intravenous access (preferably at least two i.v. lines) should be obtained as early as possible. If an i.v. line cannot be sited in the first 90 seconds, intraosseous access should be attempted. If the child is hypotensive or poorly perfused, 20 ml/kg of plasma should be given over 10 minutes (approximately). This may need to be repeated several times.

- **Hypoglycaemia** is an immediately treatable cause of collapse. Blood glucose should be checked immediately after the child arrives in the resuscitation room (Fig. 2). If the blood glucose is less than 3 mmol/l give 10% dextrose 5 ml/kg over 10 minutes, and establish a continuous infusion of maintenance requirements of 10% dextrose.

- **Neurological status** of the child should be assessed. A quick and simple assessment is the 'AVPU' scoring, which puts the child in one of four categories:

  A **A**lert
  V Responds to **V**oice
  P Responds to **P**ain
  U **U**nresponsive.

The 'Glasgow coma score' is more specific, and requires more detailed assessment of the child's neurological status (Tables 1 & 2). The system has clear advantages when it is important to assess progress over time.

- **Pupil size** should always be examined as part of a neurological assessment. Small pupils suggest narcotic or barbiturate exposure, and bilaterally dilated pupils suggest a postictal state.

- Hypertension, bradycardia and irregular respiration presenting together are signs of **'coning'**. Unless the cause is amenable to urgent treatment, death will result.

CLINICAL HISTORY

As part of the initial assessment it is important to establish certain specific points in the history: recent trauma, recent health of the child, seizures, known chronic conditions (e.g. cardiac abnormality) and possibility of poison ingestion.

RAPID GENERAL PHYSICAL EXAMINATION

It is essential to look for clues as to possible causes of collapse. These are summarised in Figure 3.

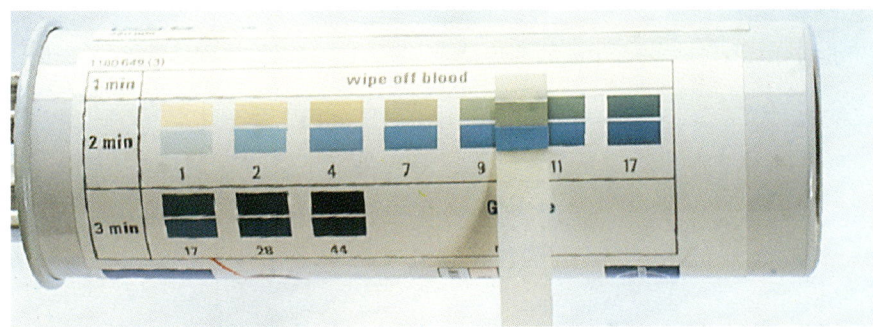

Fig. 2 **Strip used to check blood glucose.**

Table 1 **Children's coma scale (<4 years)**

Score	Eyes	Best motor response	Best verbal response
1	No response	No response	No response
2	React to pain	Abnormal extension to pain	Inconsolable
3	React to speech	Abnormal flexion to pain	Inconsistently consolable
4	Open spontaneously	Withdraws to pain	Consolable crying
5		Localises pain	Smiles and orientates to sound
6		Spontaneous or obeys verbal command	

Table 2 **Glasgow coma scale (4–15 years)**

Score	Eyes	Best motor response	Best verbal response
1	No response	No response	No response
2	Open to pain	Extension	Incomprehensible sounds
3	Open to verbal command	Inappropriate flexion	Inappropriate words
4	Open spontaneously	Flexion with pain	Disorientated and converses
5		Localises pain	Orientated and converses
6		Obeys verbal command	

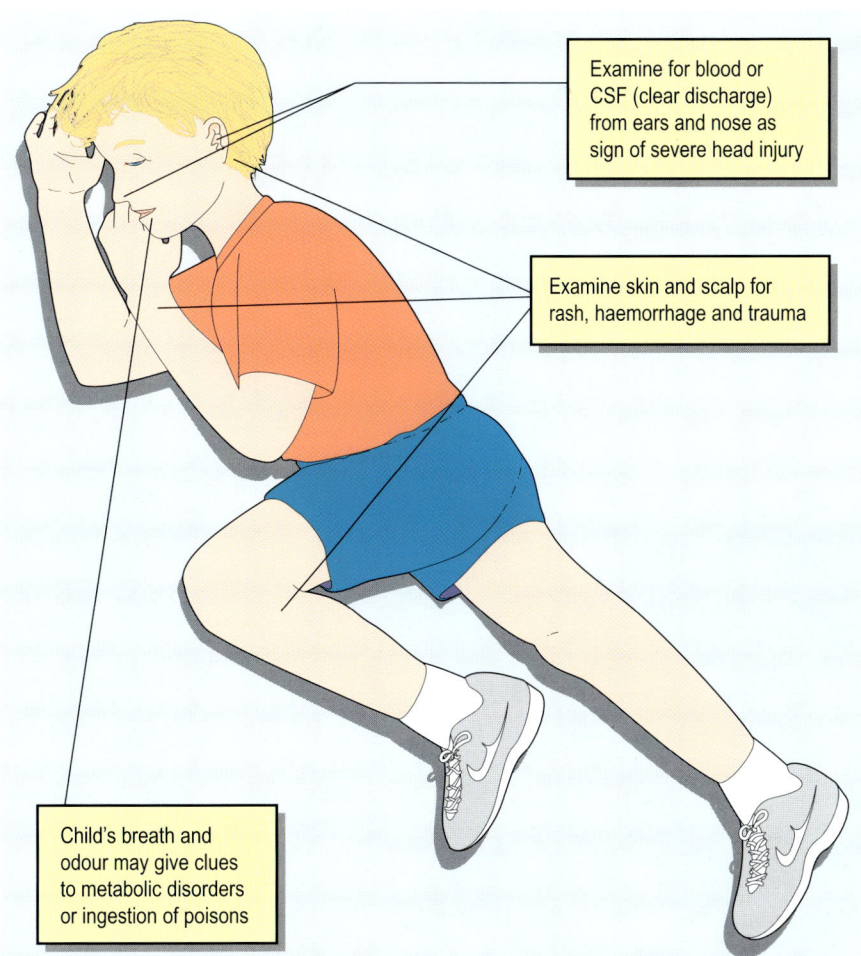

Examine for blood or CSF (clear discharge) from ears and nose as sign of severe head injury

Examine skin and scalp for rash, haemorrhage and trauma

Child's breath and odour may give clues to metabolic disorders or ingestion of poisons

Fig. 3 **Rapid general examination in cases of collapse.**

LOSS OF CONSCIOUSNESS II

REACHING A DIAGNOSIS

Primary brain disorder

Bruising over the head and/or evidence of injury to other parts of the body may make the diagnosis of trauma obvious. However, external signs of trauma are not always apparent in such cases. The fundi should be examined for retinal haemorrhages (Fig. 1), which are a sign of traumatic shaking to the child, often as a result of non-accidental injury. If trauma is the likely diagnosis, then skull X-rays may show a fracture, and a CT or MRI scan may be helpful in revealing intracranial pathology such as a sub-dural haematoma (Fig. 2).

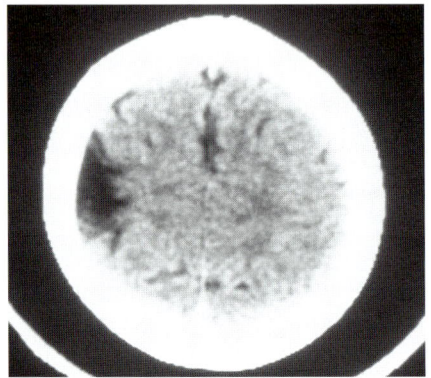

Fig. 2 **CT scan of subdural haematoma compressing adjacent brain tissue.**

A brain tumour typically presents with gradual onset of headaches, worse in the morning and associated with vomiting. Without intervention, this will progress to focal neurological signs such as a squint and more overt signs of raised ICP (e.g. slow pulse and high BP) altered consciousness and papilloedema. Diagnosis is made by CT scan (Fig. 3).

Complications of pre-existing hydrocephalus are suggested by the presence of a

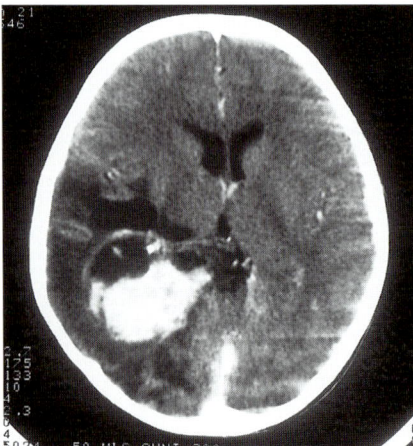

Fig. 3 **CT scan of a brain tumour compressing adjacent brain tissue.**

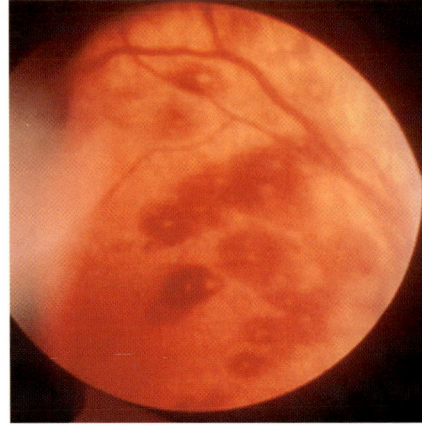

Fig. 1 **Retinal haemorrhages.**

ventriculoperitoneal shunt, easily palpable behind one ear.

Coma due to a systemic disorder

Infection. Infection is the most likely cause of sudden collapse in children, with meningitis (see below) being the most important differential diagnosis. The majority of collapsed children should have a lumbar puncture performed and should be given appropriate broad spectrum intravenous antibiotics very early in the resuscitation. If the lumbar puncture is delayed, for example if raised intracranial pressure cannot be excluded, antibiotics must still be given early, but blood cultures should be taken first.

CVS. A number of cardiac disorders can result in sudden collapse. Mechanisms include arrhythmias, such as supraventricular tachycardia, and acute infundibular spasm in Fallot's tetralogy. All collapsed children should have their ECG monitored on arrival in casualty and throughout their resuscitation. Blood gases may be helpful in reaching a diagnosis; hypoxia and/or acidosis may be present.

Seizure. An unrousable child may have had a fit, due to idiopathic epilepsy, or as part of another disorder, such as an inborn error of metabolism or an infective illness. The history may be helpful in revealing previous fits. Patients who are postictal may have passed urine or bitten their tongue during the episode. Temporary signs following a fit include up-going plantars and dilated pupils. Provided the fit is controlled, consciousness should return over the next few hours.

Metabolic abnormality. Diarrhoea and vomiting can result in hypo- or hypernatraemia, and in consequence fits and coma. The sodium level must be corrected by rehydration with appropriate fluids. Hyperglycaemia, dehydration and acidosis are features of diabetic ketoacidosis and can lead to unconsciousness (see below).

It should be remembered that children with a variety of metabolic disorders may 'decompensate' as a result of intercurrent infection, and must be given antibiotic cover as part of the resuscitation.

Liver or renal failure. Severe abnormalities of liver or renal function cause toxic metabolites to build up in the bloodstream and depress the conscious level. In such cases there is often pre-existing renal or hepatic damage. However, acute failure of either organ can occur. While in renal failure typical serological evidence will be found (i.e. raised creatinine and urea), liver failure may present with hypoglycaemia and raised ammonia with only a modest rise in bilirubin.

Toxic ingestion. A young child may accidentally ingest a toxic substance such as a drug from the parents' bathroom cupboard, or a household material such as bleach. Drug ingestion by teenagers is usually due to a deliberate overdose in a depressed or unhappy child. Only a few of these children will present in a coma. Commonly ingested drugs include paracetamol, aspirin and alcohol. Alcohol or bleach can be smelled on the breath. Blood toxicology helps confirm the diagnosis. Supportive treatment is given, and specific antidotes are used where available, such as acetyl cysteine in paracetamol overdose.

Sudden infant death. An infant presenting with acute collapse may have been at risk of 'sudden infant death'. If successfully resuscitated, the child is said to have had an 'apparent life-threatening event' (ALTE). Such a diagnosis can only be made once all other causes have been excluded.

ONGOING CARE

Those patients that do not make a rapid return to full consciousness require ongoing support in an Intensive Care environment. The following must be kept under regular review:

- general care of the skin, joints, eyes, oral hygiene, fluids and nutrition
- regular clinical monitoring: temperature, pulse, blood pressure, respirations, oxygen saturation, neurological state, and urine output
- regular tests: blood glucose, urea and electrolytes, gases, ICP monitoring if indicated

- specific treatment if underlying cause is known, e.g. antibiotics for meningitis, acyclovir for herpes encephalitis, dialysis for renal failure
- symptomatic treatment where appropriate: treat hypoxia, fits, infection, shock, dehydration, correct metabolic abnormalities and reduce raised intracranial pressure.

OUTCOME

Depends entirely on the cause together with the effectiveness of resuscitation.

MENINGITIS

Although meningitis can result from both bacterial and viral agents, it is unusual for viral meningitis to result in any long-term sequelae or death. In contrast, bacterial meningitis is always life-threatening and carries a high risk of long-term morbidity amongst survivors. Therefore, management guidelines for children presenting with altered consciousness should always include appropriate measures to deal with bacterial meningitis.

Bacterial meningitis is most common amongst young children (i.e. under 5). Presentation amongst this group can be entirely non-specific, perhaps with fever and irritability only. However, many other presentations can occur, e.g. febrile fit, vomiting, lethargy and bulging fontanelle. Therefore, it is important to always consider the diagnosis. In older children the 'classical' symptoms and signs of headache, photophobia, neck stiffness (Fig. 4) and positive Kernig's sign are more likely to be present.

The immunisation programme against *Haemophilus influenzae* type b in the UK has radically altered the pattern of causative organisms seen. Haemophilus, once the commonest pathogen in children under 2, is now rare. Meningococcus is currently the most important organism; infection is typically (but not exclusively) associated with a septicaemia which produces a characteristic haemorrhagic rash (Fig. 5). The rash may develop in minutes and therefore it is important to re-examine any child in whom the diagnosis is suspected. Pneumococcus can also produce meningitis in paediatric patients, but normally in older children.

Management can be summarised as follows:

- Always consider the diagnosis in children presenting with unexplained symptoms.
- Carry out appropriate investigations: full blood count, blood culture, lumbar puncture, serology for bacterial antigens.

- Start antibiotics early: penicillin (covers meningococcus and pneumococcus) and ceftriaxone (covers haemophilus). Do not delay antibiotics in order to complete investigations.
- Consider additional measures where appropriate, e.g. blood pressure support, steroids (to reduce inflammatory damage to the CNS), and anticonvulsants.

DIABETES

Diabetes is one of the commonest serious chronic diseases of childhood (prevalence 1 to 2 per 1000 children). Typical cases in childhood result from damage to the beta cells of the pancreas and, hence, early symptoms represent the effect of lack of insulin (i.e. hyperglycaemia, glycosuria, polyuria, polydipsia, dehydration, weight loss, altered consciousness). Whilst cases may present with marked hyperglycaemia, ketoacidosis and loss of consciousness, children are normally identified at an early stage in their illness and established on therapy. Previously well-controlled diabetics may go markedly out of control over a period of hours in the face of infection. Management of ketoacidosis is summarised in Table 1.

Details of the management of diabetes in childhood are outside the scope of this book; however, basic treatment involves the use of injections of insulin to replace the endogenous supply. The amount of insulin must take account of many factors but, in particular, the child's diet and level of activity must be considered. Any short-term excess of insulin as a result of increased activity and/or reduced carbohydrate intake may result in loss of consciousness through hypoglycaemia. Management of this situation is summarised in Table 2.

Table 1 **Management of diabetic ketoacidosis**

- Resuscitate using ABCD
- Confirm diagnosis immediately using stick test for glucose
- Measure serum glucose, electrolytes, acid–base status, full blood count and perform blood and urine cultures
- Rehydrate. initially use 20 ml per kg of plasma or saline given as bolus. Follow with estimated losses (usually 10 to 15 % body weight) plus maintenance fluids over next 24 hours
- Start insulin as an i.v. infusion (0.1 units/kg/hr)
- Pass a nasogastric tube (paralytic ileus commonly present)
- Monitor electrolytes (especially potassium—replace as necessary) and vital signs

Table 2 **Management of hypoglycaemia**

- Resuscitate using ABCD
- Confirm diagnosis immediately using stick test
- If rousable give oral glucose
- If deeply unconscious give i.v. glucose (5ml/kg 10% glucose)
- If unable to give glucose give i.m. glucagon
- Continue insulin
- Resume oral intake as soon as possible

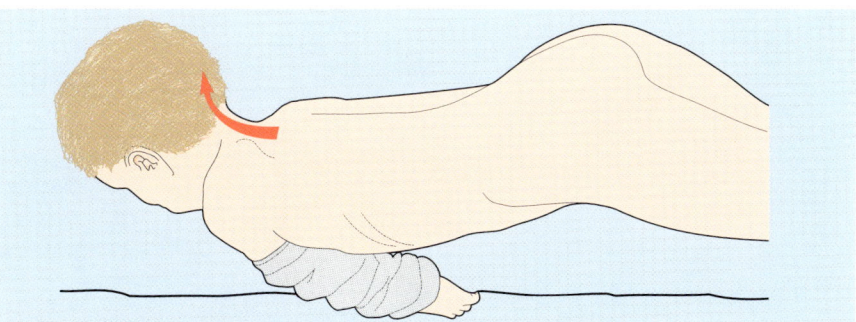

Fig. 4 **Neck retraction in meningitis.**

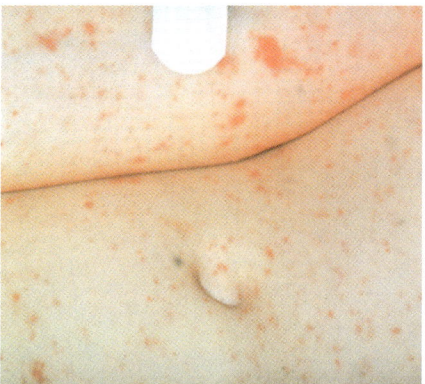

Fig. 5 **Meningococcal rash.**

Loss of consciousness

- Remember ABCD for resuscitation.
- Always do a blood glucose test early in an unconscious patient.
- Babies under 18 months can have meningitis with no neck stiffness and none of the usual symptoms.
- Remember malaria in those who have travelled abroad.
- Fundal haemorrhages are almost always due to non-accidental injury.

HEADACHE

Headache is a common complaint amongst all children with sufficient language development. However, young children (those below 5 years) are poor at localising pain and, therefore, its interpretation as a symptom must be more cautious. Headaches clearly occur in the very young. However, it is possible only to infer the presence of pain from the child's behaviour (e.g. extreme irritability when disturbed or when the head is moved).

Pain in the head can arise from a number of superficial sites (sinuses, external ear, middle ear, teeth and muscle), but there are no pain fibres within the brain, the calvarium or overlying meninges. However, other deep structures are pain sensitive and these include the major blood vessels, the meninges at the base of the skull and the major sensory nerves and nerve roots.

The causes of headache are summarised in Figure 1.

'NON-ORGANIC' HEADACHE

Migraine

Migraine headaches result from vasoconstriction followed by vasodilatation of branches of one carotid artery. The term *migraine* has entered everyday use to mean a severe headache, but it should be reserved for patients whose headaches show evidence of at least some of the following features:

- an aura associated with nausea (with or without vomiting)
- unilateral (although the side affected should vary)
- paroxysmal nature.

The trigger for migraine in an individual is rarely identifiable and many loose associations have been noted. These include:

- certain foods (e.g. cheese, chocolate and fried food)
- allergy
- stress
- obsessional personality.

Although a family history is commonly present, it is important to evaluate each case on its merits and not assume a diagnosis of migraine if the rest of the history is not supportive. In the most severely affected individuals attacks may be accompanied by transient neurological abnormalities such as hemiplegia.

Whilst classical migraine is regularly seen in older children and adolescents, it is comparatively rare in younger children. In this age group attacks may take the form of recurrent abdominal pain often accompanied by vomiting (cyclical vomiting syndrome).

It is unusual to have to resort to specific prophylactic agents in childhood migraine since most patients are satisfactorily controlled by the use of simple analgesics such as paracetamol.

Tension headaches

Simple headaches are of course common in older children, as they are in adults, and may recur from time to time. It is generally felt that they arise from increased muscle tension in the scalp or upper cervical area. However, when assessing a child with this type of problem it is important to consider the following:

- *Duration.* Simple headaches rarely last more than 24 hours.
- *Severity unaffected by simple analgesia.* This would be unusual with this type of headache.
- *Associated symptoms and signs.* Whilst a persistent headache may make the child feel generally unwell, persistent vomiting, fever, neck stiffness, or altered consciousness should not be present.
- *Timing.* Persistent early morning headaches suggest raised intracranial pressure.

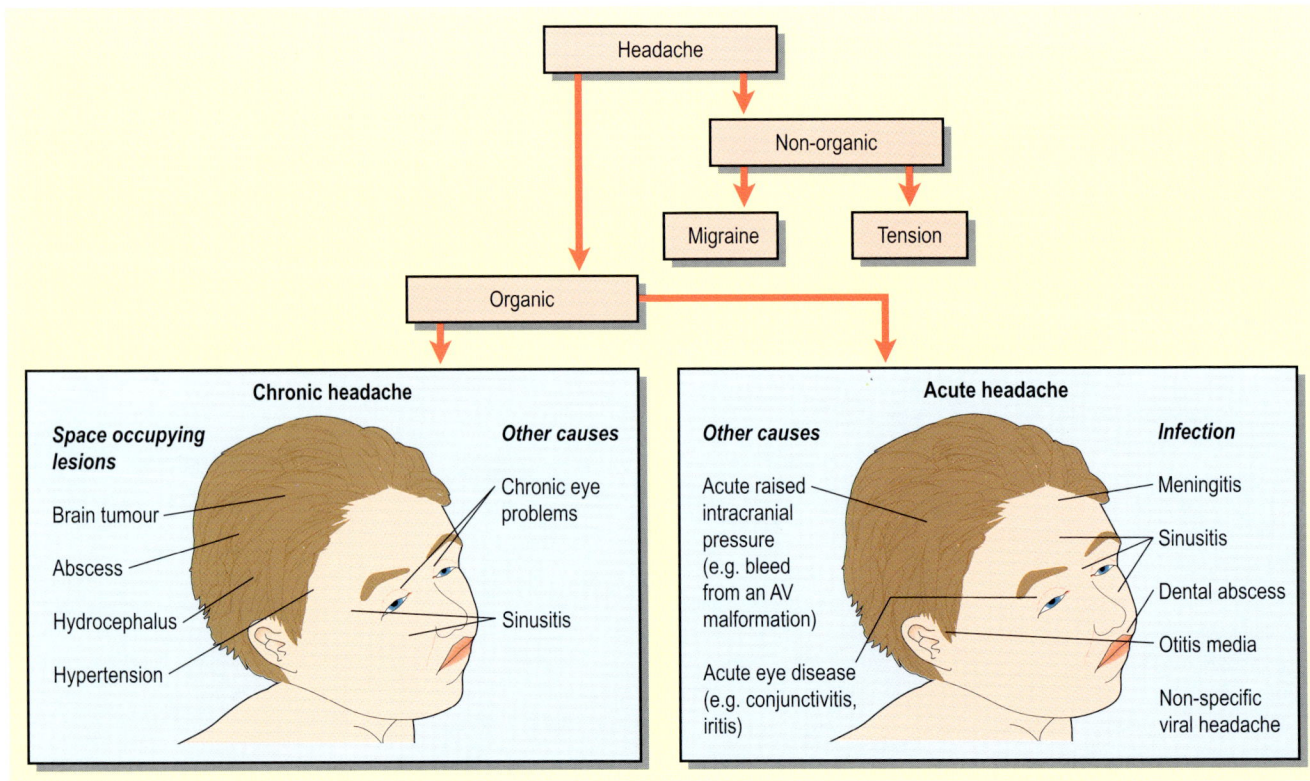

Fig. 1 **The causes of headache.**

ACUTE SECONDARY HEADACHE

Infection

Infection is the most important cause of acute headache in children. It is a feature of many non-specific viral infections but can also arise as a consequence of more localised infection as shown in Figure 1. Some of these, such as dental abscess or otitis media, are fairly readily identified. By contrast, sinusitis is a more difficult diagnosis since, although headaches may be accompanied by nasal congestion, the interpretation of any confirmatory X-rays is hindered by the fact that sinus development is not complete until after puberty.

Clearly, meningitis must always be considered in the differential diagnosis of acute headache. However, during early childhood, other symptoms and signs such as altered consciousness, fever, pallor, vomiting and rash can be equally important in indicating the true diagnosis. Similarly the absence of headache does not exclude meningitis (p. 81).

Non-traumatic intracranial bleeding

This is a rare occurrence in childhood. It is normally a complication of a pre-existing vascular malformation, a tumour, or bleeding disorder (e.g. idiopathic thrombocytopenic purpura). Other signs, such as altered consciousness, are usually also present.

CHRONIC SECONDARY HEADACHE

Space occupying lesions

Although rare in childhood, brain tumours are the second most common form of malignancy. Up to 70% of affected children will present with headache. Two-thirds of CNS tumours in children arise in the posterior fossa where the increased volume rapidly leads to aqueduct compression and secondary hydrocephalus. Pressure headaches of this type are typically a problem during the night or early morning when the child's recumbent posture temporarily adds to the pressure. Such headaches are often accompanied by vomiting and remit during the day. Eventually, if untreated, headache is present both day and night. Although one would anticipate that such headaches would be associated with papilloedema (Fig. 2), this is unreliable, particularly in the early stages.

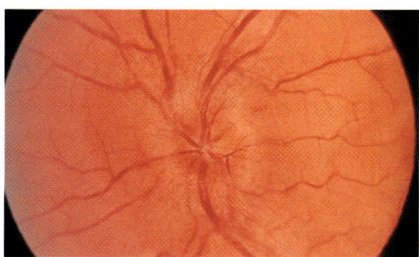

Fig. 2 **Papilloedema.**

Therefore, it is equally important to seek other evidence of posterior fossa 'damage' such as impaired cerebellar function.

Brain tumours in other sites are less predictable in their presentation since the presence of pain will depend on what secondary structures become involved (Fig. 3).

Similarly, headache may or may not be a feature of brain abscess. Such lesions are rare in childhood and normally occur as a secondary consequence of penetrating trauma to the head or local infection, e.g. acute otitis media.

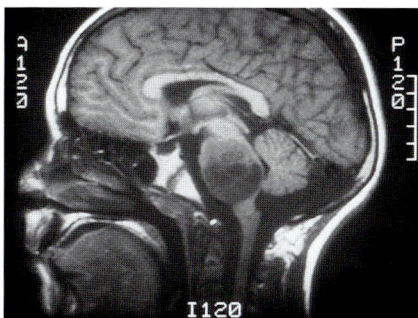

Fig. 3 **Brain stem glioma resulting in moderate hydrocephalus**

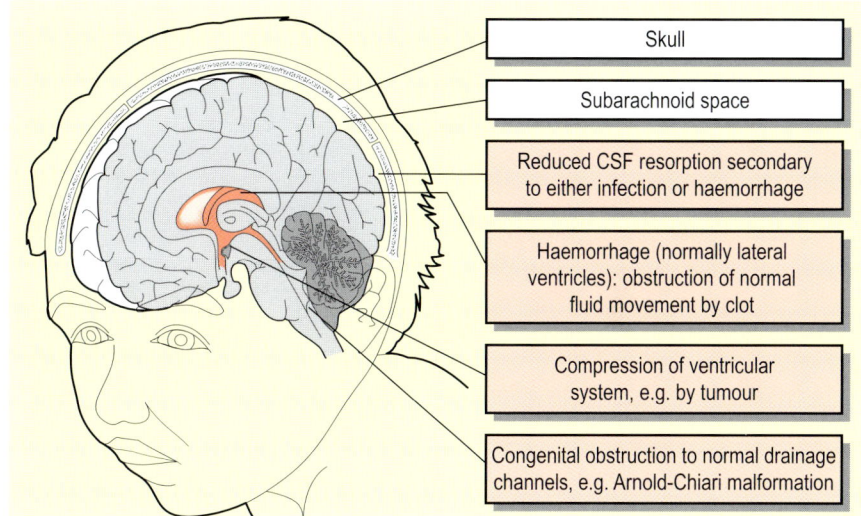

| Skull |
| Subarachnoid space |
| Reduced CSF resorption secondary to either infection or haemorrhage |
| Haemorrhage (normally lateral ventricles): obstruction of normal fluid movement by clot |
| Compression of ventricular system, e.g. by tumour |
| Congenital obstruction to normal drainage channels, e.g. Arnold-Chiari malformation |

Fig. 4 **Mechanisms of hydrocephalus.**

Hypertension

Severe hypertension is rare in childhood. But when present in sufficient severity to cause headache it always requires urgent investigation to exclude renal disease, coarctation of the aorta and phaeochromocytoma. Therefore, it is essential to measure the blood pressure of all children presenting with headache.

It is well known that eye 'problems' can result in headaches and uncorrected refractive errors are the most common example. Therefore, visual acuity should always be assessed and the eyes examined. Headaches caused by simple eye strain should not be accompanied by other neurological symptoms and signs.

Hydrocephalus

Hydrocephalus (Fig. 4) has already been described as a mechanism for headache production in children with posterior fossa tumours. Congenital abnormalities causing hydrocephalus tend to present very early in life with a rapidly enlarging head, not headache. However, children and others who develop hydrocephalus later in life, perhaps following trauma or tumour surgery, require a 'shunt'. This is a tube and valve drainage system which passes from one lateral ventricle to the abdominal

cavity. Such systems are prone to block and allow hydrocephalus to recur with, in consequence, return of the headache.

INVESTIGATION

In cases where the history and examination suggest a clear cause outside the CNS, investigation is clear cut. A cranial CT scan should be performed in those patients in whom the pattern of headache is more ill-defined or where the symptoms are not compatible with non-organic disease.

Headache

- Early morning headache and vomiting always suggest posterior fossa tumour.
- Headache not responding to simple analgesia and/or lasting longer than 24 hours suggests an organic cause.
- Absence of papilloedema does not exclude raised intracranial pressure.
- Blood pressure estimation is an essential element in the assessment of children with headache.

FITS AND FUNNY TURNS

A fit can be defined as 'a paroxysmal, involuntary, excitatory disturbance of brain function'. The terms 'fit', 'convulsion' and 'seizure' are synonymous but the latter two tend to have fewer worrying connotations for the patient and family. Depending on the part of the brain affected, fits may give rise to a huge variety of symptoms including alteration or loss of consciousness, and motor, sensory, behavioural or autonomic abnormalities. Although in many cases the diagnosis is clear cut, in others, particularly in children with behaviour problems, it can be extremely difficult.

Other causes of 'funny turns' (including change or loss of consciousness, loss of colour, abnormal movements and odd sensations) are very common and need to be distinguished from fits. Because they are so variable they may present to the primary care services, Accident and Emergency department or to outpatient clinics. Many will turn out to have a minor self-limiting cause or be a variant of normal behaviour, but there are also important serious diseases that present in this way. It is essential to take a detailed history of the attack from an eye-witness, as the doctor is unlikely to see an attack and the patient may be completely normal by the time of examination. Remember that many parents who see their child collapse think at the time that the child is dying. They may find it very difficult to explain what they have seen because it was so upsetting, although their observations are usually very accurate.

Try to take the witness through a blow-by-blow account of the attack. Some of the appropriate questions and diagnoses are given in Table 1. It is also worth asking how long the attack lasted. This is usually overestimated by parents but one can get some idea by asking what the parent did during the

attack (e.g. pick the child up, attempt resuscitation, telephone an ambulance). The parents' actions may give some help with the difficult but important question of whether the child was unconscious if one asks about his response (or lack of it) to their actions.

In the rest of the history, concentrate on any previous episodes (whether they were the same as or different from the most recent attack), any neonatal problems (which may have caused cerebral damage), birthmarks and abnormalities in development. Recent development of spots or a rash may indicate an infective cause such as meningococcal septicaemia or chicken pox. Because children, are, in general, healthy, any past medical history should be assumed to be significant until proven otherwise.

CHILDREN OVER 1 YEAR

It is easier to make a clinical diagnosis in children presenting with 'funny turns' over 1 year of age and the major differential diagnoses are given in Table 1. Breath-holding attacks tend to occur in younger children (18 months–3 years) and faints in older children (>10 years). Both are common in primary

care. Fits are the most common reason for an acute hospital admission with a 'funny turn' but not every funny turn is a fit.

Fits

The emergency management of a fit is illustrated in Figure 1. A fit is a symptom of brain irritation and in itself rarely causes lasting damage. Classification of fits can be confusing because they can be classified on aetiology (the underlying cause of the fit) or on clinical features of the fit (what sort of fit it is) and the two approaches overlap.

Aetiology of fits

An aetiological paradigm is given in Table 2. Generally this classification is very useful in thinking about a child with an acute illness associated with a fit or after a first fit. The prognosis depends on the underlying cause of the fit.

Simple febrile convulsions are the most common form of convulsion in children. They are most frequently seen in the second year of life and occur in 3% of the population (a third of whom will have a second attack). The criteria for diagnosis are illustrated in Figure 2. These fits are important

Table 1 **Major causes of funny turns in children**

Diagnosis	Factors helpful to making the diagnosis	Useful questions
Fits	Fever Loss of consciousness 1–3/second jerks Postictal	? unwell before attack ? conscious ? postictal
Rigor	Fever No loss of consciousness Exaggerated shivering	? unwell before attack ? conscious
Breath-holding	Antecedent painful or upsetting experience	? events before attack ? events at start of attack
Cardiac arrhythmia	White colour, weak pulse Cardiac history	? look and feel of child
Vaso-vagal (faint)	Emotional upset Postural change	? events before attack ? events at start of attack

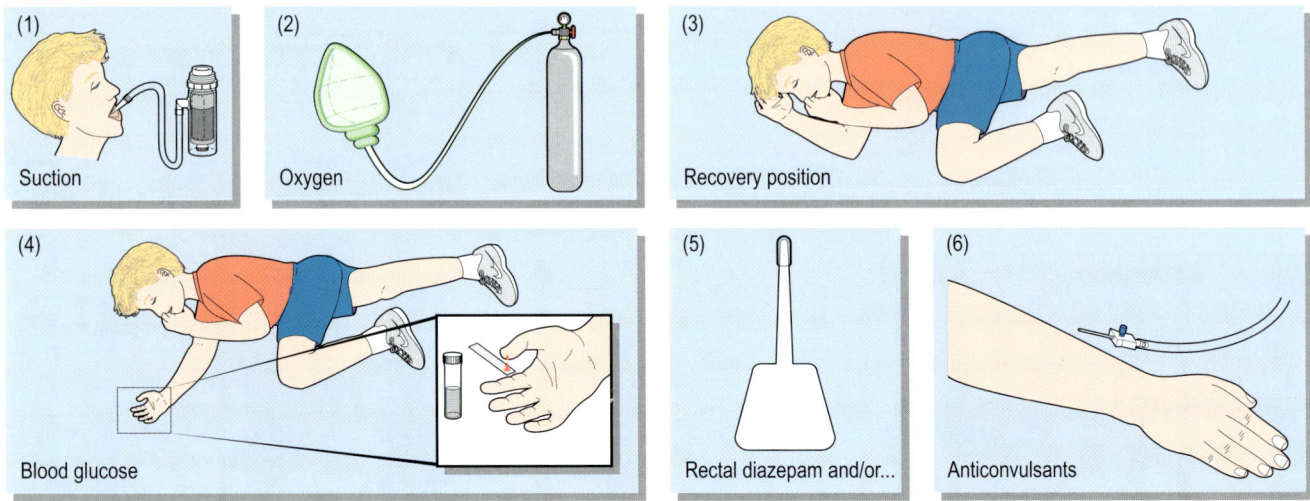

(1) Suction
(2) Oxygen
(3) Recovery position
(4) Blood glucose
(5) Rectal diazepam and/or...
(6) Anticonvulsants

Fig. 1 **Emergency management of a fit.**

because they are common, have a risk of recurrence but, although they cause considerable anxiety, ultimately have a good prognosis. Medication is not usually needed but advice on how to manage fever and further fits is important.

Meningitis rarely presents with fits but is such an important diagnosis that a lumbar puncture should be considered in all children who have a febrile fit, particularly if antibiotics have been given in the previous 2–3 days.

Atypical febrile convulsions (e.g. lasting longer than 20 minutes or with focal features) may need further investigation and treatment as they may be manifestations of underlying epilepsy or other CNS pathology.

Clinical classification of fits

Epilepsy is defined as a tendency to have fits and implies an intrinsic abnormality of the brain, although quite often investigations (EEG, CT or MRI scans) are normal. Epileptic fits are relatively common with a prevalence through the childhood years of about 4 per 1000. In children with established fits, an aetiological diagnosis can be helpful for prognosis but the seizure type is also important.

The most important division of fits is into *partial* (focal) or *generalised* fits. Generalised fits are subdivided into *primary* generalised and *secondary* generalised. The key feature of a generalised fit is loss of consciousness. Different types of generalised or partial fits can be distinguished on clinical features (Table 3).

Advice after fits

As well as treatment of fits with anticonvulsants, which are indicated when the fits are severe or frequent, advice is also important. The first aid management of a fit is to prevent avoidable injury, place the child in the recovery position to reduce the risk of aspiration and call for help. Children with fits should be advised not to cycle on busy roads, not to swim or bath unsupervised, and not to climb to more than 6 feet off the ground. Adults with fits are not eligible for various jobs (e.g. the armed forces and the police) and in the UK cannot have a driving licence if fits have occurred in the previous year and can never hold a PSV or HGV licence.

UNDER 12 MONTHS

In smaller children (particularly under 6 months), the range of possible diagnoses is wider (including inborn errors of metabolism and congenital anomalies) and it is more difficult to differentiate the various causes clinically.

In the neonatal period, both true fits and other funny turns may present with

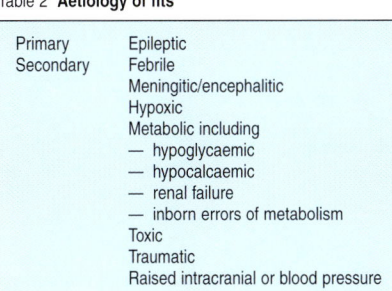

- No history of focal features
- Duration < 20 minutes
- Age 6 months to 6 years
- Previous history of febrile fits may be present
- Source of fever outside the CNS
- Primary generalised convulsion

Full recovery (no residual paralysis)

Fever

Fig. 2 **Criteria for diagnosis of simple febrile convulsions.** Children who breech these criteria are more likely to have suffered an epiletic fit. A positive family history may also be present.

Table 2 **Aetiology of fits**

Primary	Epileptic
Secondary	Febrile
	Meningitic/encephalitic
	Hypoxic
	Metabolic including
	— hypoglycaemic
	— hypocalcaemic
	— renal failure
	— inborn errors of metabolism
	Toxic
	Traumatic
	Raised intracranial or blood pressure

Table 3 **Terms used in epilepsy and apnoea**

Fit, seizure, convulsion	All synonymous
Tonic fit	Stiffening of body associated with apnoea and cyanosis
Clonic fit	Twitching of all or part of the body at about 3/second.
Generalised fit	With loss of consciousness
Primary generalised	No focal features
Secondary generalised	Focal features at beginning or end
Partial/focal fit	Consciousness maintained with fit localised to one part of the brain
Grand mal fit	Generalised tonic then clonic features
Absence fit	Short period of sensory inattention, Loss of consciousness but maintained motor tone
Petit mal fit	Specific primary generalised absence fit with characteristic EEG
Complex partial fit	Focal fit in temporal lobe where consciousness is altered. Semi-purposeful movements may occur
Myoclonic fit	Generalised or isolated muscle twitching which may result in drop attacks in children and infantile spasms in infants
Obstructive apnoea	Cessation of airflow in an infant with continued respiratory effort
Central apnoea	Cessation of airflow in an infant with no respiratory effort

abnormal movements or apnoea. It is normal and quite common for young babies to have single jerks and these can wake them up if they are asleep. More jerky movements suggest fits but these may be very subtle, with lip smacking, cycling movements of the limbs or stiffening of the body rather than the rhythmic jerking seen in later childhood. Where repetitive movements do occur during a fit, they cannot be abolished by holding the arm, unlike simple tremulousness.

The term *apnoea* (i.e. cessation of airflow) is often used to describe funny turns in infants where breathing is affected, but it is a description not a diagnosis. Apnoeic episodes, fits or other funny turns in neonates are a sign that something is not right but are very non-specific. Likely causes of such episodes include asphyxia (which may be obvious from the obstetric history), infection, respiratory disease (including aspiration) and metabolic disturbances. With a positive family history or consanguineous parents, an inborn error of metabolism must be suspected.

In the postneonatal period, fits are less common but apnoeic episodes and choking attacks frequently present to hospital. Upper or lower respiratory tract infections may contribute to these episodes, but in many cases, despite numerous investigations, no obvious cause is found.

Infantile spasms are an important but rare form of convulsion starting in the first year of life. They present with single flexor or extensor spasms (salaam attacks) which may be repeated up to several hundred times a day. In 30% of cases they are

associated with regression of development and a poor neurological prognosis.

Finally, child abuse may present as apnoea or fits. This is very rare, but if there are suspicions in the history and examination, then further investigation may be needed (p. 44).

Fits and funny turns

- A detailed history of the funny turn is crucial to diagnosis.
- Simple febrile convulsions have a good prognosis. Atypical features may need further investigations.
- Meningitis and hypoglycaemia are rare but treatable causes of fits.
- Any funny turn may create enormous anxiety in the family.

PALLOR

Pallor refers to the combination of visible clinical signs resulting directly from anaemia. although many normal children look 'pale' or 'pasty'. Generalised pallor, however, involves the mucous membranes and is recognised in well-vascularised areas such as the conjunctivae, nail-beds and oral mucosa. The thenar eminences are also reliably well vascularised. Even moderate anaemia is difficult to recognise, and if it has developed slowly there may be no noticeable cardiovascular effects even with haemoglobin levels as low as 4 g/dl.

CAUSES OF ANAEMIA

Anaemia is commonly caused by or associated with:

- trace element and vitamin deficiencies: iron, folate and vitamin B_{12}
- haemolysis because of primary red cell abnormalities: hereditary spherocytosis, G6PD deficiency or acquired haemolytic anaemias, e.g. following mycoplasma infection
- deficient production of globin molecules (thalassaemias, e.g. β-thalassaemia); or structural abnormalities of the globin chains (haemoglobinopathies, e.g. sickle cell disease)
- bone marrow problem, e.g. decreased production following marrow aplaisia or infiltration
- blood loss.

CLUES TO DIAGNOSIS

Many types of chronic anaemia are restricted to certain racial groups, for example β-thalassaemia is common in those from the southern Mediterranean and parts of Asia. Inheritance patterns are also useful (hereditary spherocytosis is autosomal dominant; G6PD deficiency is X-linked recessive). The examination (Fig. 1) and the blood count and film (Table 1) are also helpful.

IRON DEFICIENCY ANAEMIA

Iron deficiency is by far the most common cause of anaemia in the UK and worldwide. In some areas of Britain the incidence is as high as 50% of toddlers. It is under-recognised clinically. There is evidence that even mild anaemia (<10.5 g/dl) over a prolonged period can cause a learning deficit. Lack of appetite is usual.

The cause is usually dietary. In all babies there is a normal fall in haemoglobin level after birth to levels below those in adults (Fig. 2). Unmodified cow's milk and breast milk contain very little iron, and so anaemia results after the first 6 months of life when neonatal stores have been depleted, unless a balanced mixed diet has been instituted by this time. Modified cow's milk is fortified with iron, but its absorption is less efficient than from breast milk (containing lactoferrin, an iron binding protein). Only after premature birth (as iron stores are laid down in late pregnancy), or if the mother was severely iron-deficient during pregnancy, will supplements to human milk be needed in early infancy. Worldwide, malabsorption and chronic gastrointestinal bleeding, particularly from hookworm infection, are important causes.

Treatment and prevention involve encouraging a normal healthy diet including fresh vegetables. Short courses of oral iron may be necessary, and often restore appetite.

Megaloblastic anaemia is mainly due to folic acid deficiency, usually secondary to prematurity, infection or malabsorption. There is also greater demand for this vitamin in haemolytic anaemias, and supplements are given if the diet is poor.

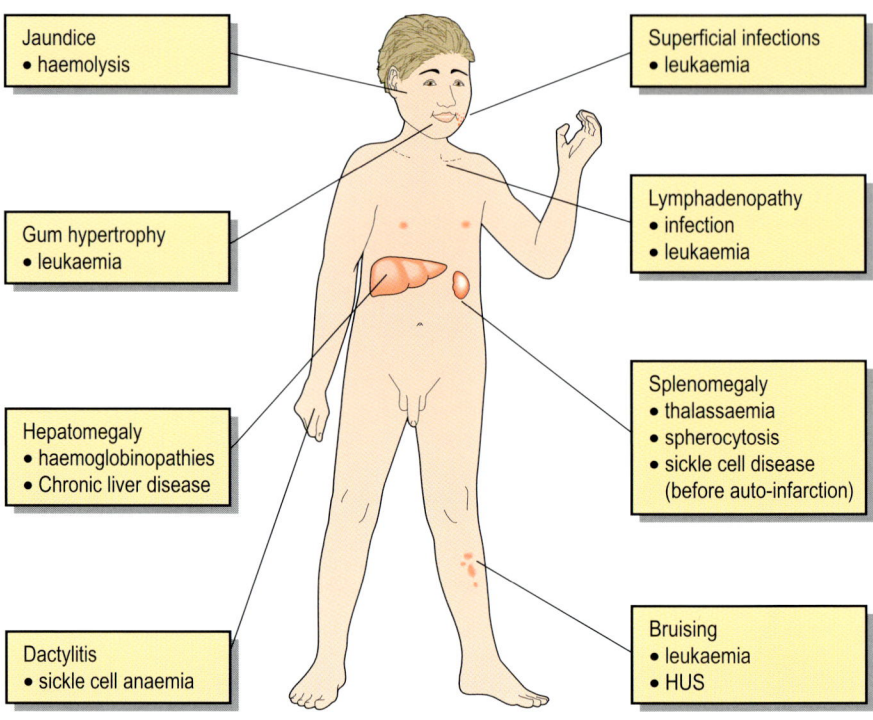

Fig. 1 **Clues to the cause of anaemia from examination.**

Table 1 **Features of the blood film in different forms of anaemia**

	Red cell changes	Other changes
Iron deficiency	Microcytic, hypochromic. anisocytosis (variation in size)	
Folate deficiency	Macrocytic	
Sickle-cell disease	Sickle cells, clumping	
β-thalassaemia major	Microcytic, hypochromic.	
Leukaemia	Lymphoblasts	Thrombocytopenia, neutropenia

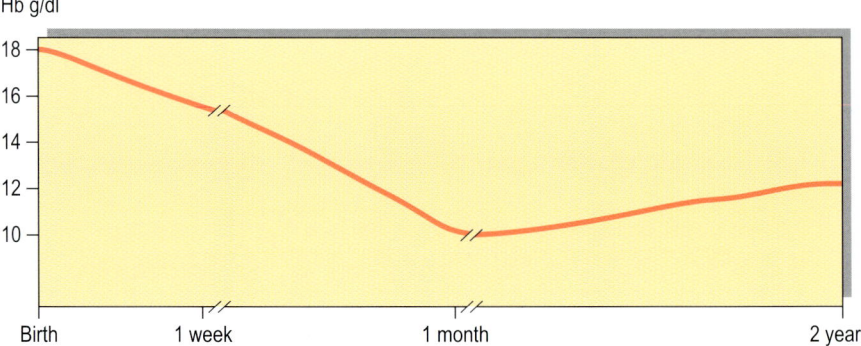

Fig. 2 **Mean haemoglobin concentration in the first 2 years of life.**

THALASSAEMIA

This condition results from genetic defects which diminish production of normal globin molecules (alpha, beta, gamma or delta). There is no actual abnormal haemoglobin produced, but increased proportions of normally vestigial forms to compensate for the lack of available globins (Table 2). In β-thalassaemia major (homozygous disease), the most common severe type, no beta chains are produced.

The clinical features do not start until after the first few months of life because fetal haemoglobins predominate during that time. In the heterozygous form there is a mild anaemia with none of the other clinical problems. The heterozygote state is often mistaken for iron-deficiency anaemia. The 'other' haemoglobins produced in thalassaemia major (Table 2), result in shortened red cell survival. The bone marrow compensates with increased, inefficient, haemoglobin production. Severe anaemia requiring regular blood transfusions results, with splenomegaly. If treatment is inadequate poor and distorted bone growth occurs due to marrow hypertrophy (including frontal 'bossing'). There is chronic iron overload because of the inefficient globin production, and inability to handle the product of frequent blood transfusions.

Regular desferrioxamine is given by intravenous or subcutaneous infusion to chelate the iron and promote excretion. Cellular iron deposition (haemosiderosis) in many organs still occurs with cirrhosis, heart failure and sterility. In the future larger numbers of affected individuals may be able to be cured by bone marrow transplantation.

Table 2 **Haemoglobins in the thalassaemias**

Normal adult haemoglobins	
Hb A	$(2 \times \alpha) + (2 \times \beta)$
Hb A$_2$	$(2 \times \alpha) + (2 \times \delta)$
Normal fetal haemoglobins	
Hb F	$(2 \times \alpha) + (2 \times \gamma)$
Hb Barts	$4 \times \gamma$
Hb H	$4 \times \beta$
Thalassaemias	
α-thalassaemia	Hb A (reduced amounts) and Hb F (and Hb Barts at birth)
β-thalassaemia major	Hb A$_2$ and Hb F
β-thalassaemia minor	Hb A and Hb A$_2$

SICKLE CELL DISEASE

The condition arises from genetic abnormalities which result in the substitution of a single amino acid in the β-globin molecule. In Hb-S, valine replaces glutamine at position 6 of the β-chain. The abnormal haemoglobin is predisposed to distort (sickling) in response to insults such as infection, dehydration and acidosis. This results in intravascular red cell aggregation with thrombosis and obstruction in highly vascular organs such as the spleen and bones. Such events are termed 'crises'

and are often very painful. Small infarcts are particularly frequent in the spleen, leading to auto-splenectomy usually before 5 years of age. Infections are very common, especially after auto-splenectomy.

Treatment of crises depends mostly on prompt recognition of infection and dehydration. Management includes rehydration, pain relief (usually morphine) and antibiotics. Regular blood transfusions are not required and are only used for symptomatic relief, i.e. during a severe episode of sickling (sickle crisis). The abnormal gene is common in Africa, but the heterozygote condition is usually symptom-free and confers decreased risk of cerebral malaria which compensates for the mortality of the homozygous state (an example of balanced polymorphism).

HEREDITARY SPHEROCYTOSIS

This condition is due to an autosomal dominantly inherited intrinsic abnormality of the red cell membrane, and results in an inability to produce the proper biconcave cell shape. Red cells are less viable and liable to be taken up in the spleen. It can cause neonatal jaundice, but often presents later in childhood with anaemia, jaundice and splenomegaly. Splenectomy is greatly beneficial in reducing haemolysis.

GLUCOSE 6 PHOSPHATE DEHYDRO-GENASE (G6PD) DEFICIENCY

Several inherited red cell enzyme deficiencies are known, the most common of which is G6PD deficiency. G6PD is part of the pentose shunt pathway, which produces the co-enzyme needed for the reduction of glutathione. Reduced glutathione protects the red cell from oxidative injury, and its deficiency leads to episodes of acute haemolysis, particularly after exposure to certain drugs (Table 3) or foods. Some people from southern Europe show a particularly severe form of deficiency. All forms show sex-linked inheritance.

ACQUIRED HAEMOLYTIC ANAEMIA

Unlike most inherited haemolytic anaemias, acquired haemolytic anaemias are usually caused by problems outside the red cell (apart from malaria). Auto-immune haemolytic anaemia in children is often due to infection, particularly by mycoplasma.

Table 3 **Some drugs with definite risk of causing haemolysis in G6PD deficiency — dose-related**

Antimalarials:	Primaquine (usually safe in Africans)
Antibiotics:	Sulphonamides, nitrofurantoin
Analgesics:	Aspirin (usually safe in moderate doses)

Haemolytic-uraemic syndrome is described elsewhere (see pp. 76–77).

BONE MARROW DISEASE

Many chronic diseases, particularly infections such as tuberculosis, cause depression of erythropoiesis. The anaemia of chronic renal failure is predominantly due to failure of erythropoietin production in the kidney.

Leukaemia is the most common malignancy in children and 85% of cases are acute lymphoblastic (ALL). The peak incidence in childhood is between 2 and 5 years. The marrow fills with lymphoblasts, and, as a result, presenting signs often include anaemia, bruising (thrombocytopenia) and infection (neutropenia).

Certain factors at diagnosis are important in influencing prognosis:

- age (less than 2 years, or over 10 years of age, generally do worse)
- sex (girls better than boys)
- peripheral lymphoblast count (worse if very high — sometimes over 100 000/mm^3)
- immunogenetic typing of T- and B-lymphocyte surface markers on the malignant cells (those with neither of the above but a 'common' malignant cell antigen have the best prognosis)
- presence of abnormal chromosomes in the malignant cells (carries a worse outlook).

Treatment is standardised in Britain and involves induction, intensification and maintenance cytotoxic regimens, and CNS radiotherapy (cytotoxics are poor at crossing the blood–brain barrier). Cure rate is better than 80% in the favourable prognostic groups. Bone marrow transplants are often done if the child relapses after treatment. Acute myeloid leukaemia (AML) carries a worse prognosis than lymphoblastic leukaemia.

Aplastic anaemia is uncommon. There are inherited (Fanconi's anaemia and *Blackfan–Diamond* syndrome) and acquired forms. The prognosis is worse than for most leukaemias.

Pallor

- Skin pallor does not accurately reflect the haemoglobin level.
- Iron deficiency (dietary) is the commonest cause of anaemia.
- Screening for thalassaemia and sickle cell disease should be performed at birth in at-risk racial groups.
- Leukaemia may present with anaemia.

BRUISING AND BLEEDING

CAUSES OF ABNORMAL BLEEDING

The causes of bleeding can be divided into three broad categories:

- platelet problems
- problems related to abnormalities of one or more of the various clotting factors
- problems related to abnormal blood vessels.

Trauma may exacerbate all of the above problems, but physical child abuse constitutes a special case without other pathology.

Platelet problems

Apart from disorders of platelet function (relatively rare except that caused by aspirin sensitivity), platelet problems relate to thrombocytopenia. Platelet production in the bone marrow, from megakaryocytes, is intimately related to production of red cells and white cells, and diseases affecting the bone marrow (e.g. leukaemias and aplastic anaemias) and cytotoxic drugs regularly cause thrombocytopenia. However, platelet destruction is usually more specific, and idiopathic thrombocytopenic purpura exemplifies this problem in childhood.

Coagulation problems

Coagulation problems are either hereditary or acquired. Although specific inherited defects of all the coagulation factors have been described, they are all very rare except haemophilia A and von Willebrand's disease. Acquired defects are usually caused either by vitamin K deficiency, or severe liver disease leading to failure of cellular synthesis of vitamin K-dependent coagulation factors. Disseminated intravascular coagulation (DIC) occurs when platelets and coagulation factors are abnormally consumed during a severe illness: it is particularly seen in severe infections. More specific coagulopathies are associated with meningococcal septicaemia and haemolytic-uraemic syndrome. Treatment is primarily to treat the underlying disorder, but

fresh frozen plasma and platelet transfusions are often necessary.

Abnormal blood vessels

Blood vessel disorders form a very varied group. Blood vessels are damaged in scurvy and untreated renal failure. Inflammation of blood vessels (vasculitis) causes the bruising in Henoch–Schönlein purpura. Poor quality skin and connective tissue causes excessive bruising in inherited disorders such as Ehlers–Danlos syndrome, an autosomal dominant condition with hyperextensibility of joints, hyper elasticity of skin and poor wound healing. In *hereditary haemorrhagic telangiectasia* (Fig. 1), also autosomal dominant, dilated microvascular swellings appear during childhood, characteristically around the lips, but also on mucosal surfaces. These telangiectases blanch on pressure, unlike bruises, but because they are fragile haemostatic control is poor and mucosal bleeds, especially nose-bleeds, are common.

CLUES TO DIAGNOSIS

Although all causes of bleeding and bruising may show the full range of clinical features, certain manifestations are associated with particular disease categories (Fig. 2).

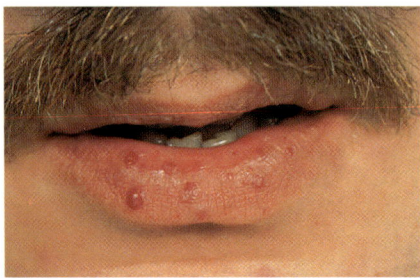

Fig. 1 **Lesions on the father of a child with hereditary haemorrhagic telangiectasia (Weber–Rendu–Osler).**

Table 1 **Terminology**

Bruising	A poorly-defined term, usually applied to any bleeding into tissues and equivalent to purpura
Purpura	Blue-brown discoloration of the skin due to the extravasation of erythrocytes (do not blanch on pressure)
Petechiae	Small, dot-like purpura
Echymoses	More extensive purpura
Telangiectasia	Visible dilatation of dermal arterioles or venules (blanch on pressure)

TESTS IN BLEEDING

Platelets

See Table 2.

Bleeding time

Bleeding time is a measure of the time taken for cessation of capillary bleeding. It is dependent on normal vessel integrity and platelet-thrombus formation. By Ivy's method, a sphygmomanometer cuff is applied to the upper arm and maintained at 40 mmHg. The skin is then punctured by a

Table 2 **Platelet count**

Normal	$150–400 \times 10^9$/litre
<100	Bleeding from operations, trauma
<40	Spontaneous bruising
<10	Serious risk of intracranial bleeding

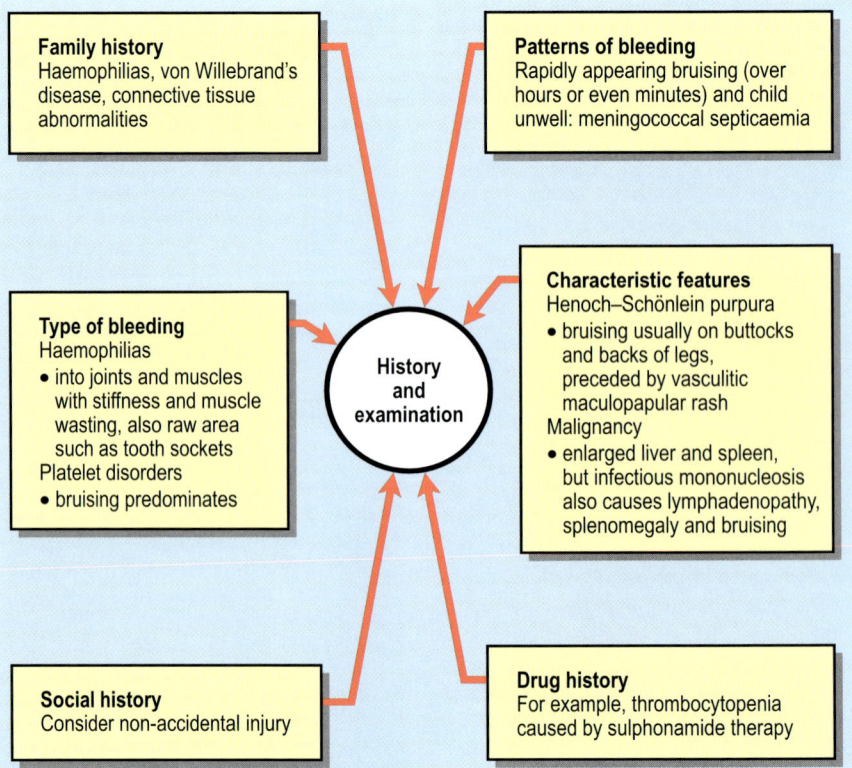

Fig. 2 **Clues to diagnosis in bruising and bleeding.**

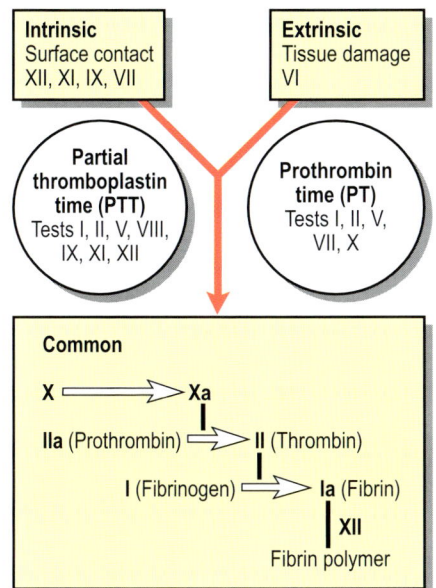

Fig.3 **Simplified coagulation pathway.**

Table 3 **Causes of neonatal bleeding**

Platelet-related abnormalities	Infections: congenital, including toxoplasma, cytomegalovirus, rubella and herpes simplex
	Passive transfer of auto-antibodies in maternal ITP or SLE
	Anti-platelet antibodies from maternal iso-immunisation
	Malignancy: neuroblastoma, leukaemia
	Drugs, including maternal (e.g.thiazides)
Coagulation deficiencies	Coagulation factor deficiency (including haemophilia A)
	Vitamin K deficiency (liver disease, haemorrhagic disease of the newborn)
Mixed	Consumptive coagulopathy: sepsis or birth asphyxia

stilette and blood is wiped away until bleeding stops (normal under 9 min). If prolonged, this usually indicates a defect of platelet number or function.

Coagulation tests
The partial thromboplastin time (PTT) and prothrombin time test the intrinsic and extrinsic pathways, respectively (Fig. 3).

Other tests include thrombin time, fibrinogen concentration and fibrin degradation products (FDPs). These tests evaluate the final common pathway and are particularly valuable in monitoring disseminated intravascular coagulation. In practice it is important to discuss cases of suspected clotting disorders with the laboratory. There are many other tests which further define any deficiencies.

DISEASES
Haemophilia A
A sex-linked recessive disorder, about one-third are new mutations and will have no family history. It is due to synthesis of abnormal factor VIII with limited biological activity. The major problem is bleeding into joints and muscle (Fig. 4). Clinical severity is related to the degree of deficiency of factor VIII:

< 1 %   severe
1–5 %   moderate
5–20% mild.

Diagnosis depends on the demonstration of low levels of factor VIII coagulation activity (VIIIc), despite normal levels of immunogenic factor VIII related antigen (VIII RAG). The factor VIII component concerned with platelet adhesion (VIII von Willebrand factor) is also unaffected. Carrier females can be detected using these assays, and antenatal diagnosis is possible with gene probes.

Treatment is primarily concerned with anticipation of problems and relies on home management with support from the local haemophilia centre. For mild bleeds many patients respond sufficiently to desmopressin (DDAVP), which transiently raises endogenous factor VIII levels. Otherwise, intravenous recombinant factor VIII is given as required, usually at home by the parents. For most bleeds a biologically effective factor VIII concentration of 10–20% is sufficient, but for major surgery up to 50% may be necessary.

Other clotting disorders
Haemophilia B (Christmas disease) is due to factor IX deficiency and is rarer and usually less severe. Von Willebrand's disease is an autosomal dominant disorder involving a failure of synthesis of all moieties of factor VIII leading both to coagulation pathway and platelet function deficiencies. The incidence is difficult to determine as many patients are very mildly affected.

Henoch–Schönlein purpura
This is caused by an immune-mediated hypersensitivity reaction often following an acute infection. This sets up a specific vasculitic response, the resulting rash is characteristic but can be difficult to recognise if mild. Joint and gastrointestinal symptoms are part of the vasculitis. Many patients have mild renal involvement, with haematuria, but only in a small minority does this become a clinical problem with aggressive glomerulonephritis. Treatment is supportive, steroids being reserved for very severe cases.

Idiopathic thrombocytopenic purpura
The thrombocytopenia caused by this disease is associated with immune-mediated platelet destruction. Peak incidence is between 2 and 5 years. It usually presents acutely with superficial bruising when the platelet count falls below 40×10^9/litre. Most patients recover their platelet count spontaneously within a few months, but intracranial bleeding is a hazard. Treatment, if any, is controversial, but in severe cases either steroid or immunoglobulin therapy should be considered. There is no place for routine platelet transfusions, as they are destroyed very quickly by the immune process.

NEONATAL PROBLEMS (Table 3)
Following traumatic delivery, petechiae often appear around the presenting part, and cephalhaematomas can occur (subperiosteal bleeding), particularly following instrumental delivery. Bleeding disorders (congenital and acquired) can present with prolonged bleeding from puncture sites, haematemesis and melaena, or bleeding from mucous membranes including the umbilical cord stump.

Haemorrhagic disease of the newborn is a serious condition caused by vitamin K deficiency. This is now rare as most infants receive prophylactic vitamin K at birth. Breast-fed infants are most at risk since vitamin K content in breast milk is low and breast milk's inherent antibacterial qualities inhibit production by gut bacteria.

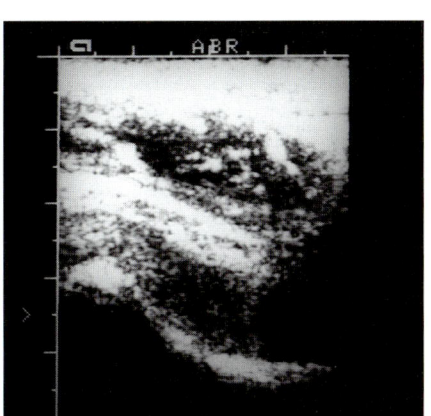

Fig. 4 **Ultrasound scan showing bleeding into the hip joint in a child with haemophilia B.**

Bruising and bleeding

- Characteristic features of bruising and bleeding may give clues to specific diagnoses.
- Some causes of abnormal bruising give rise to no recognisable abnormalities of platelets or coagulation tests, and here the diagnosis is often clinical.
- In thrombocytopenia, or coagulation factor deficiencies, spontaneous bleeding occurs usually only when the deficiency is profound.

SPOTS AND RASHES I

The major function of the skin is as a barrier. As well as the obvious function of preventing access to the body (from chemicals, bacteria, etc.) it also limits loss of fluid in the form of water or serum. If a significant proportion of the skin is disrupted (as in burns for example), large amounts of heat, fluid, electrolytes, proteins and blood cells can be lost.

The skin is also very visible and parents may be concerned that:

- even small lesions may represent underlying serious disease
- there may be social and psychological effects on the child, particularly with facial lesions.

Young children under 5 years tend to be very accepting of their own and other people's physical appearance. However, self-awareness grows during the school years and skin lesions may become a particular problem in adolescence and can be the focus for teasing and bullying. In general, it is not the severity of the lesion that is important in psychological terms but the effect it has on the child's self-image.

To make a diagnosis the important features to define are:

- the type of lesion
- the distribution of lesions
- the time course.

The skin can show manifestations of generalised disease and such a diagnosis may need to be excluded. Obviously there is a spectrum from a 'pure' skin disease (e.g. scabies), through skin diseases which can be associated with a more widespread disease (e.g. psoriasis), to systemic diseases with incidental skin lesions which are nevertheless diagnostically important (e.g. meningococcal septicaemia, SLE).

TYPE OF LESION

Definitions of some of the common skin lesions are given in Figure 1. The distinctions between the types are not always easy and some viruses can produce rashes which are often indeterminate, e.g. coxsackie.

The most important clinical distinction in terms of acute disease is between purpura (which does not blanch) and other red spots (which do). In purpura, the blood vessels have ruptured and the diseases causing this and their investigation is different from primary skin abnormalities.

In addition to lesions within the skin, other lesions from skin-associated tissues may be visible as cysts, lipomas, haemangiomas, etc.

DISTRIBUTION OF LESIONS

Many rashes have a characteristic distribution which helps to identify the process or mechanism responsible for their production. The points to look for are given in Figure 2.

TIME COURSE

The time course of the lesion can be classified as congenital, chronic or acute, although there may be some overlap. The time course of individual lesions within a rash can be a useful guide to pathology. For instance, individual urticarial weals tend to be short-lived (lasting 1–2 hours) but new lesions prolong the total duration of the

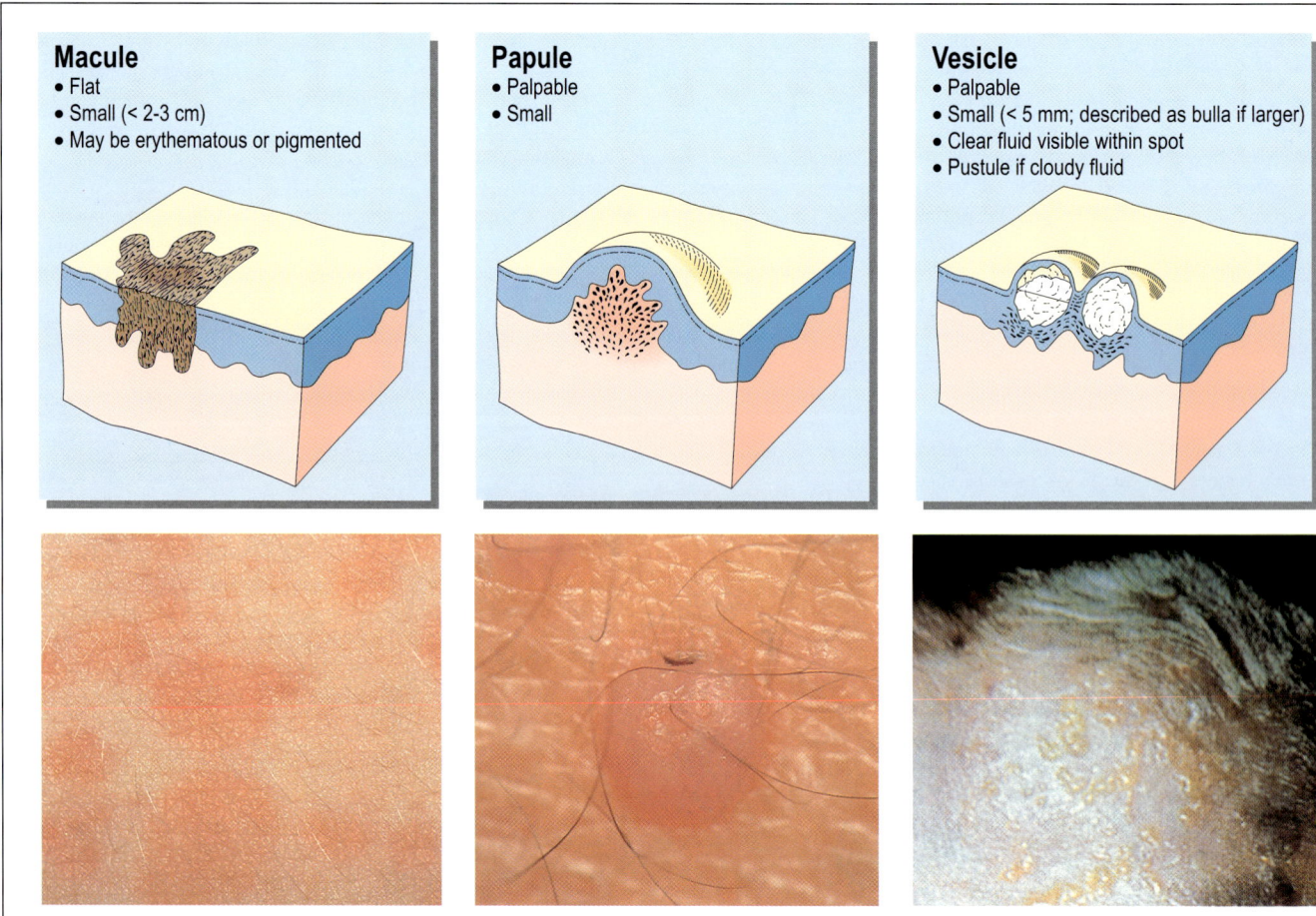

Macule
- Flat
- Small (< 2-3 cm)
- May be erythematous or pigmented

Papule
- Palpable
- Small

Vesicle
- Palpable
- Small (< 5 mm; described as bulla if larger)
- Clear fluid visible within spot
- Pustule if cloudy fluid

Fig. 1 **Some common skin lesions.**

rash. Lesions of chicken pox tend to come in crops with new lesions arriving as the old ones fade.

Congenital

A number of lesions may be present at birth and persist. Some lesions also described as congenital are not, in fact, present at birth but appear soon after (e.g. strawberry naevi and café-au-lait spots). Congenital vascular lesions are quite common. If they are flat with the surface of the skin, they are usually capillary haemangiomata (port wine stain). They do not progress or disappear and can be associated with underlying vascular anomalies. Their cosmetic effect can be improved by laser therapy. Vascular lesions raising the skin level are likely to be cavernous haemangiomata (strawberry naevi) (Fig. 3). These tend to grow rapidly for the first 6–9 months of life and then gradually infarct and regress. By a maximum of 5 years of age they will have disappeared. They cause considerable concern but do not need treatment unless they are obstructing vital organs (airway or eyesight), are large enough to cause haematological problems (heart failure, platelet sequestration), or if they ulcerate and cause recurrent bleeding.

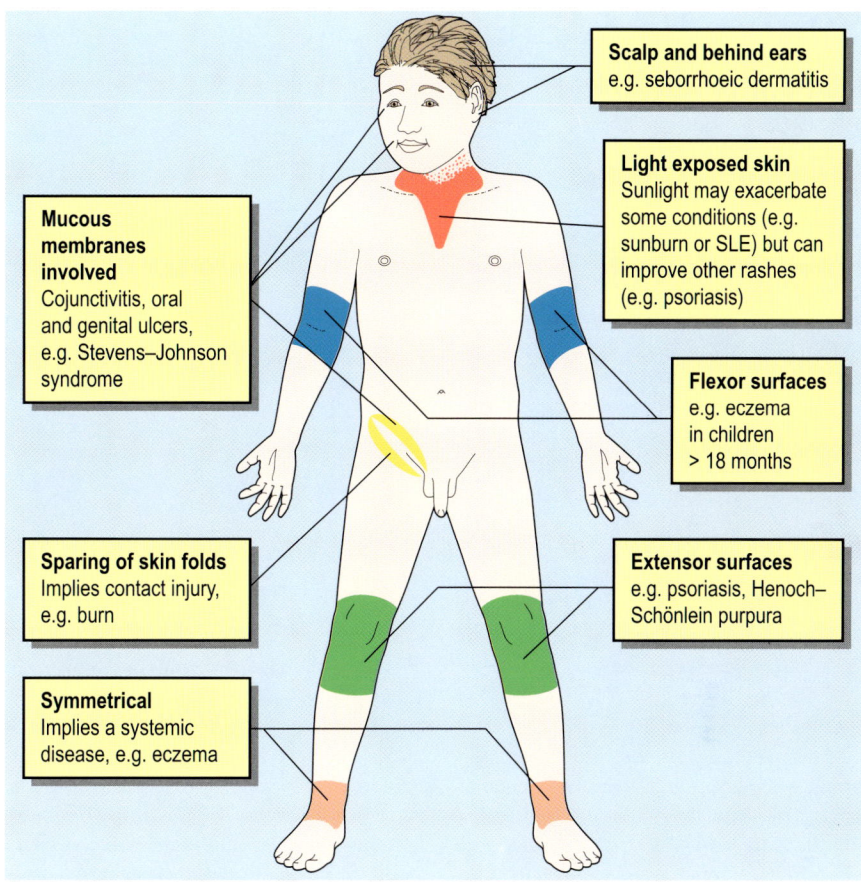

Scalp and behind ears
e.g. seborrhoeic dermatitis

Light exposed skin
Sunlight may exacerbate some conditions (e.g. sunburn or SLE) but can improve other rashes (e.g. psoriasis)

Flexor surfaces
e.g. eczema in children > 18 months

Extensor surfaces
e.g. psoriasis, Henoch–Schönlein purpura

Mucous membranes involved
Cojunctivitis, oral and genital ulcers, e.g. Stevens–Johnson syndrome

Sparing of skin folds
Implies contact injury, e.g. burn

Symmetrical
Implies a systemic disease, e.g. eczema

Fig. 2 **Characteristics of lesion distribution.**

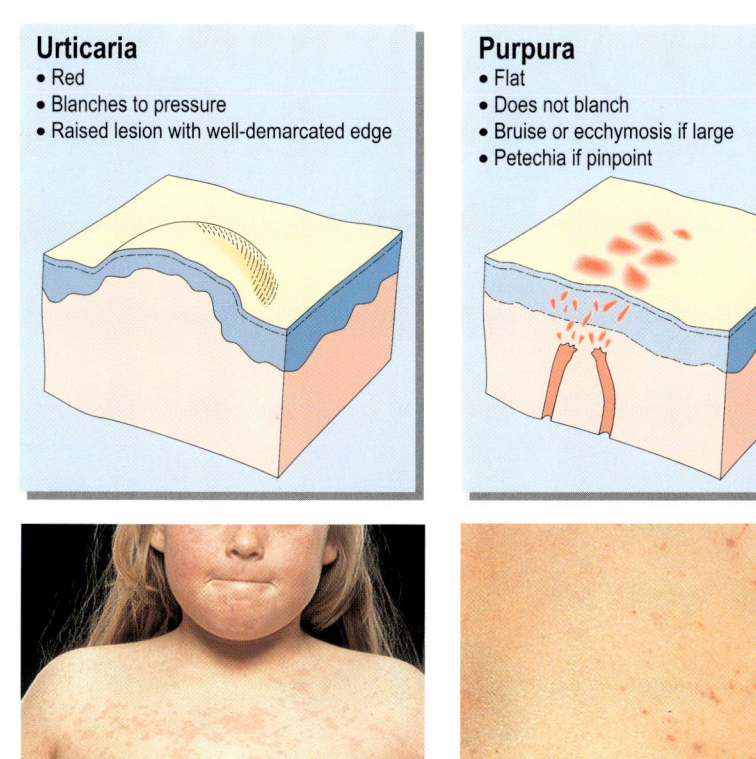

Urticaria
- Red
- Blanches to pressure
- Raised lesion with well-demarcated edge

Purpura
- Flat
- Does not blanch
- Bruise or ecchymosis if large
- Petechia if pinpoint

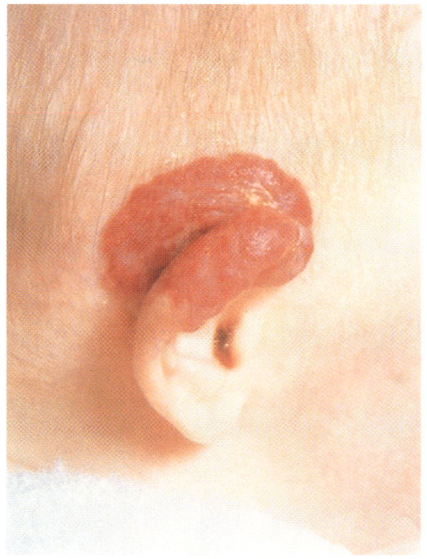

Fig. 3 **Strawberry naevus.**

Spots and rashes I
- Psychological factors are important in chronic skin disease.
- Purpura must be differentiated from other rashes.
- Skin lesions may be a marker for systemic disease.

SPOTS AND RASHES II

CHRONIC

Nappy rash

Nappy rash is easy to diagnose as it has a characteristic distribution, often with sparing of the skin folds. There is no single cause (Fig. 1), but irritation of the skin from infrequent nappy changes appears to be an important factor. Candidal infection is often present (this is normally acquired via the GI tract and oral candidiasis should be excluded by inspecting the mouth). Elements of treatment are given in Table 1.

Table 1 **Treatment of nappy rash**

1	Prevent skin becoming wet by exposure to air and use of barrier creams
2	Topical anticandida treatment
+/– 3	Oral anticandida treatment (if present in mouth)
+/– 4	Steroid cream for inflammation

Eczema

Eczema (Fig. 2) is the most common chronic skin eruption, with a prevalence of about 10% through childhood. It presents with an itchy vesicular, usually symmetrical, rash. In infants it tends to be on the face and trunk whereas in older children it tends to localise to the flexures (wrists, elbows, knees and ankles). Infantile eczema does not necessarily progress into later childhood and 90% of childhood eczema resolves by 15 years of age, although later relapse does occur. The vesicles may not be seen but scratch marks are typically present and, in chronic lesions, thickening of the skin (lichenification). Fissures may also be present. Genetic predisposition to atopy is a factor in the disease (in two-thirds of patients there is a family history of atopic disease) but enviromental exposure to allergens is also necessary. The interplay of these two factors and the reason for the increasing rates of childhood eczema in the developed world are a matter of intense research.

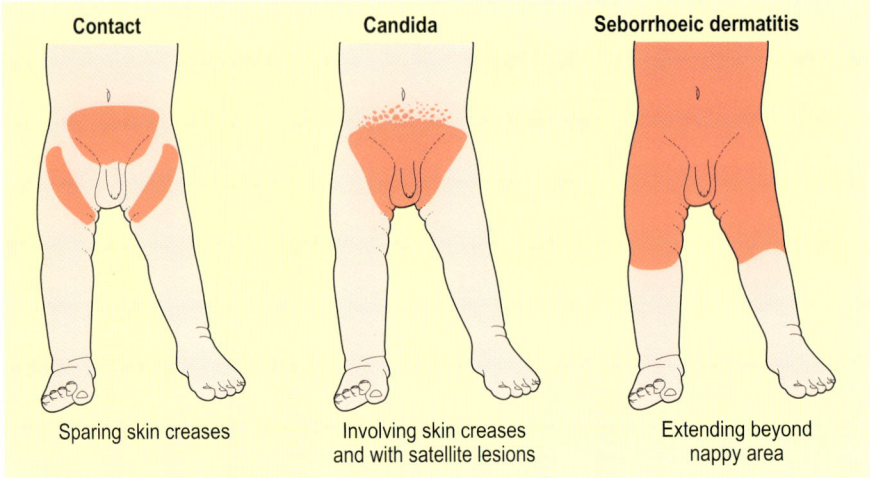

Fig. 1 **Different patterns of nappy rash.**

Contact — Sparing skin creases

Candida — Involving skin creases and with satellite lesions

Seborrhoeic dermatitis — Extending beyond nappy area

The principles of treatment are given in Table 2. Because eczema is a chronic visible condition which is not curable, it is a fertile ground for alternative therapies. Some of these may have a place in treatment but most are of no proven benefit. Some alternative practitioners recommend stopping conventional treatment, so it is worthwhile exploring the family's views and whether other advice and treatment is being given. Complications of eczema are mainly infective, iatrogenic effects of treatment or secondary psychological effects. The infective complications are caused partly by disruption of the natural barrier of the skin and partly by the intrinsic T-cell dysfunction that is probably the primary lesion in eczema. Topical steroids may also play a minor role in enhancing the risk of infection.

Warts

Warts (Fig. 3), verrucas and molluscum contagiosum (Fig. 4) are extremely common local viral skin infections. Eventually the host defences will eliminate the disease, but individual lesions can be treated (usually by freezing with liquid nitrogen).

Table 2 **Principles of eczema treatment**

Aim	Methods
Preserve the suppleness and oils in the skin	Emulsifiers applied to skin Emulsifiers added to baths Avoid soaps and detergents
Avoid obvious precipitants	Use non-biological washing powder Double rinse clothes when washing Natural fibre clothes to reduce sweating Consider house-dust mite control, dietary manipulations
Reduce scratching	Occlusive dressings at night Antihistamines
Anti-inflammatory	Steroid creams Evening primrose oil

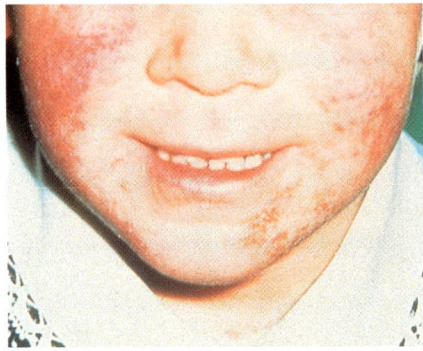

Fig. 2 **Eczema.** The skin is generally dry with inflammation particularly on the cheeks. The vesicles in eczema are often not visible but scratch marks are common.

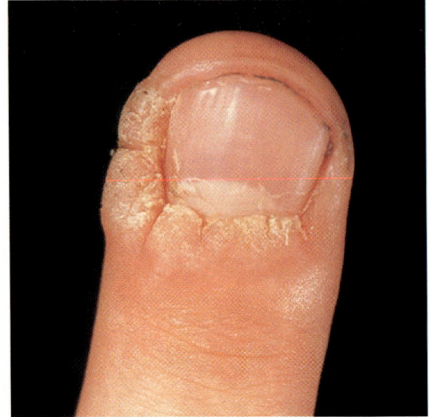 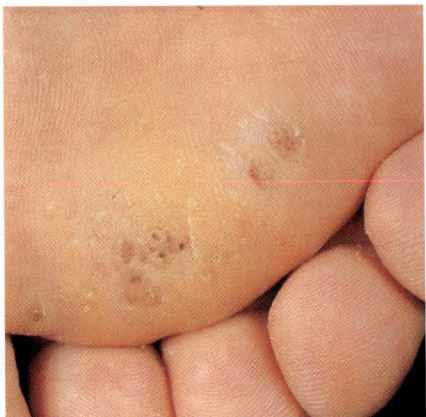

Fig. 3 **Viral warts.** Periungal warts (left); plantar warts (right).

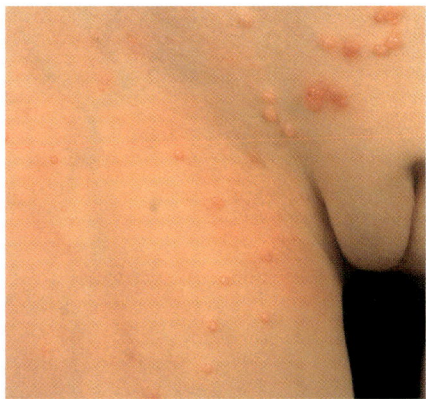

Fig. 4 **Molluscum contagiosum.** Viral infection like warts, recognised by umbilicated lesions.

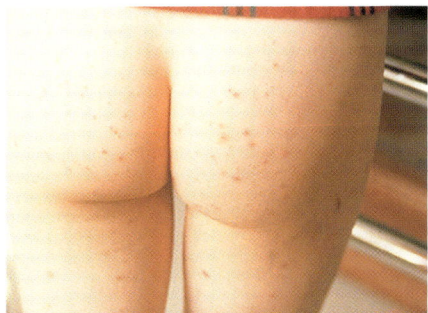

Fig. 5 **Henoch–Schönlein purpura.** The rash is purpuric with urticarial features over extensor surfaces.

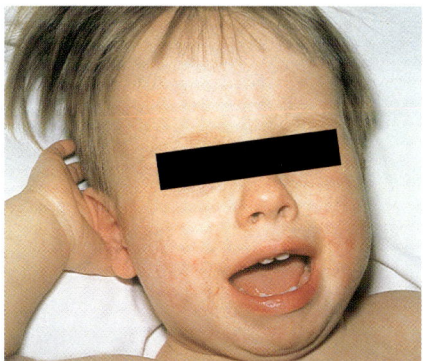

Fig. 6 **Measles.** Blotchy macular rash.

Acne

Acne is almost universal in teenagers and is secondary to an increase in sebum secretion in the hair follicles and the resulting colonisation by bacteria. In severe cases, treatment can be given to reduce the bacterial proliferation topically or orally. As acne results from hormonal stimulation of the skin, it may also be a complication of abnormalities of steroid and sex hormone production in younger children.

ACUTE

With an acute rash it is vital to assess whether the child is systemically unwell. Insect bites, urticaria, and many causes of purpura (Fig. 5) (pp. 90–94) can occur in otherwise well children. Non-specific rashes are quite common as part of a viral infection and often appear as the fever settles and the child is improving. A purpuric rash in a febrile child should be considered to be meningococcal septicaemia until proven otherwise. A number of exanthemata with important complications are shown in Table 3. Immunisation history is important as vaccination virtually excludes that particular disease as a cause of the rash. As a result of good uptake of immunisation in developed countries, clinical experience of these diseases has decreased and in the general population the term 'measles' or 'German measles' tends to be applied to any maculopapular rash associated with fever.

Other rashes may occur as a result of generalised infection, drug reactions or systemic conditions (Figs. 8 & 9).

Newborn infants commonly display transient erythema which is not significant (Fig. 10).

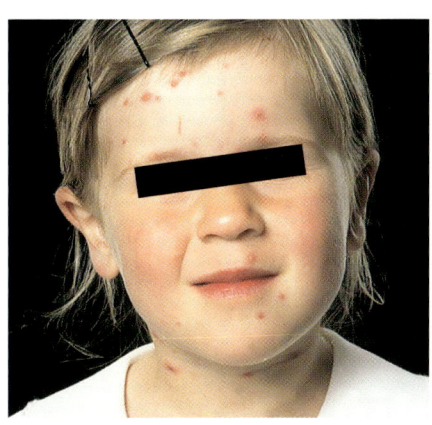

Fig. 7 **Chicken pox.** The central vesicles are starting to scab over.

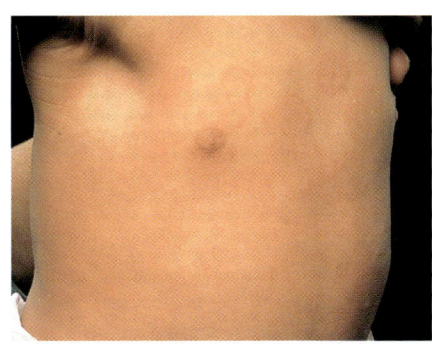

Fig. 9 **Erythema multiforme.** Common causes are viral infections and drug reactions.

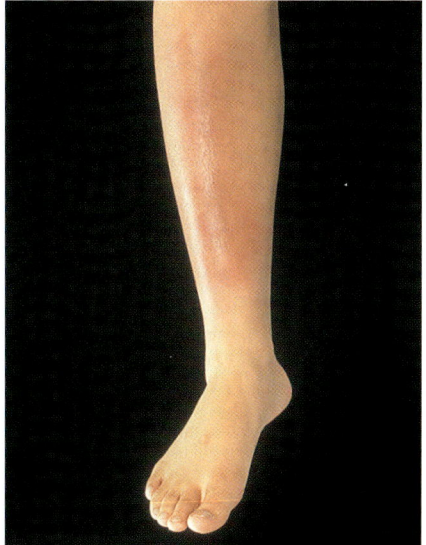

Fig. 8 **Erythema nodosum.** The main causes are post-infection (streptococcal, TB), drug reactions and inflammatory bowel disease.

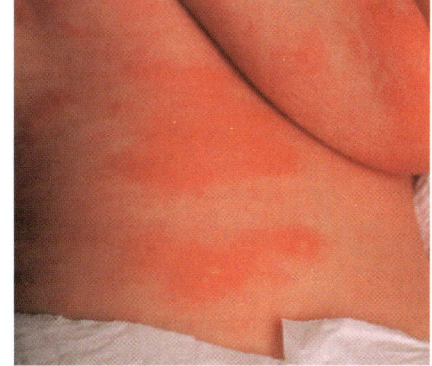

Fig. 10 **Erythema toxicum neonatorum.** A common transitory rash in the first few days of life.

Table 3 **Exanthemata and their complications**

Disease	Incubation period (days)	Clinical	Complications
Measles (Fig. 6)	7–10	Maculopapular rash spreading from behind ears Lymphadenopathy Conjunctivitis Koplik's spots	Pneumonia Otitis media Encephalitis (acute or late) Death (even in normal children)
Chicken pox (Fig. 7)	14–21	Pustules Central distribution Crops of lesions	Cerebellar encephalitis Death in immunocompromised Teratogenic risk
Rubella	7–10	Maculopapular rash spreading from behind ears Occipital lymphadenopathy	Teratogenic risk

Spots and rashes II

- Treatment of nappy rash is exposure, barrier creams and anticandidal therapy.
- Treatment of eczema is with emulsifiers and topical steroids.
- Alternative therapies are often tried on children with eczema.

SWELLING

Visible swelling in a child may result from:

- an increase in tissue fluid (oedema)
- the distortion of normal morphology resulting from enlargement of underlying viscera.

Oedema occurs when the normal mechanisms that control the distribution of fluid at tissue level have been disrupted. Increased venous pressure, reduced plasma oncotic pressure and increased vascular permeability may all result in oedema which characteristically pits when pressed. The mechanisms may be generalised (e.g. resulting from a loss of albumin) or localised (e.g. when local trauma leads to inflammation and increases vascular permeability). Obstruction to lymphatic channels also produces oedema. However, this type of oedema is typically associated with a secondary increase in connective tissue and does not pit on pressure.

It is important to note that congenital forms of oedema can also arise from each of the mechanisms identified above.

Swelling that results from the enlargement of an organ should be readily identified since in general such swelling will be firm and related to the anatomy of the particular structure. Diffuse abdominal swelling in the young child is perhaps the exception. Other hard swellings are discussed on pages 72–75.

ACQUIRED GENERALISED OEDEMA

The main conditions producing generalised oedema are those that lower serum albumen (and hence oncotic pressure) and those that increase venous pressure.

Those that *lower serum albumin* include:

- *Renal disease* resulting in heavy proteinuria (nephrotic syndrome).
- *Hepatic disease* of sufficient severity to impair albumin production. This is rare in children but is seen in liver failure when portal hypertension may also be involved in the pathogenesis.
- *Gastrointestinal disease* of sufficient severity to cause protein loss into the bowel lumen as a result of altered permeability of the gut mucosa — protein losing enteropathy. This may occur in coeliac disease, Crohn's disease, ulcerative colitis, cystic fibrosis or intestinal lymphangiectasia.
- *Malnutrition* with poor protein intake resulting in hypoproteinaemia, e.g. kwashiorkor (Fig. 1).

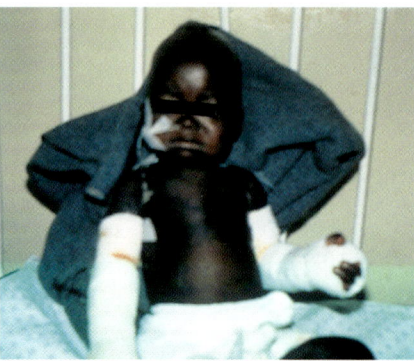

Fig. 1 **Kwashiorkor causing oedema.**

Those that *increase venous pressure* include:

- *Cardiac failure*. All causes of pump failure can produce increased tissue fluid. The distribution of the oedema will depend on the nature of any underlying pathology and whether one or both ventricles fail.
- *Fluid imbalance*. During intravenous fluid therapy, gross fluid overload can occur if mistakes are made in calculation or administration. This situation is normally recognised by a physiological deterioration in the patient, e.g. tachycardia. However, peripheral oedema may result where the overload is less acute and if oncotic pressure is also relatively low (e.g. the premature neonate).

Nephrotic syndrome

The most common cause of generalised oedema in children in the Western world is nephrotic syndrome (NS). 85% of cases of nephrotic syndrome in Caucasian children are called 'minimal change' type. The detailed aetiology is unknown, but it is thought to be related to the host's immune reaction to an intercurrent infection. The term 'minimal change' comes from the light microscopy appearances of the glomeruli. Electron microscopy shows fusion of the epithelial foot processes. Children with minimal change NS have a good prognosis — 90% respond to corticosteroid therapy within 8 weeks.

During the acute phase there is massive proteinuria (0.05–0.1 g/kg/24 h) which results in hypoalbuminaemia (<26 g/l) and generalised oedema. The incidence is 2 per 100 000 Caucasian children and most frequently occurs between the ages of 1–5 years (M:F, 2.5:1). The clinical presentation is with periorbital and dependent oedema and ascites (Fig. 2). Additional symptoms are common and include lethargy, irritability, gastrointestinal upset and abdominal pain. Complications are hypovolaemia with

circulatory collapse (this may result from injudicious use of loop diuretics) and infections (primary pneumococcal peritonitis is a particular risk whilst oedema is gross).

In those children that do not respond to steroids, other pathological conditions that cause nephrotic syndrome must be considered. These include focal segmental glomerulosclerosis and membrano-proliferative glomerulonephritis. These are more likely to be associated with haematuria and hypertension and do not carry such a good prognosis.

Management (Fig. 3). Diuretics are rarely used in the management of NS. Salt-poor albumin infusions will be necessary to correct hypovolaemia in some children. In the oedematous phase, prophylactic penicillin should be given and some check should be kept on fluid intake if this is excessive. Corticosteroid treatment should be started when the diagnosis of NS is confirmed.

ACQUIRED LOCALISED OEDEMA

Infection is the most common cause of acquired localised oedema. Oedema results from the associated inflammatory response. In these circumstances swelling is accompanied by other symptoms (e.g. pain and loss of function) which indicate the diagnosis. Common examples include:

- conjunctivitis (swelling of conjunctive and periorbital tissues)
- sinusitis (swelling over affected sinus +/– cellulitis)
- parotitis (pain and swelling localised to parotid — may be viral or bacterial, the latter tending to be recurrent)
- arthritis (swelling of affected joint accompanied by pain and loss of function).

Angiodema (acute allergic oedema) can produce localised oedema of any distribution. However, it is normally accompanied by other evidence of allergy, e.g. itchy skin weals.

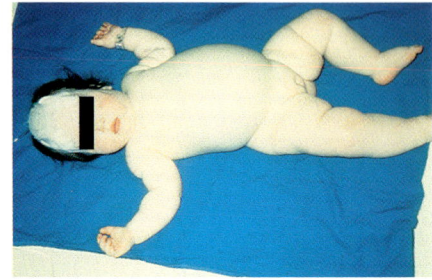

Fig. 2 **Child with nephrotic syndrome.**

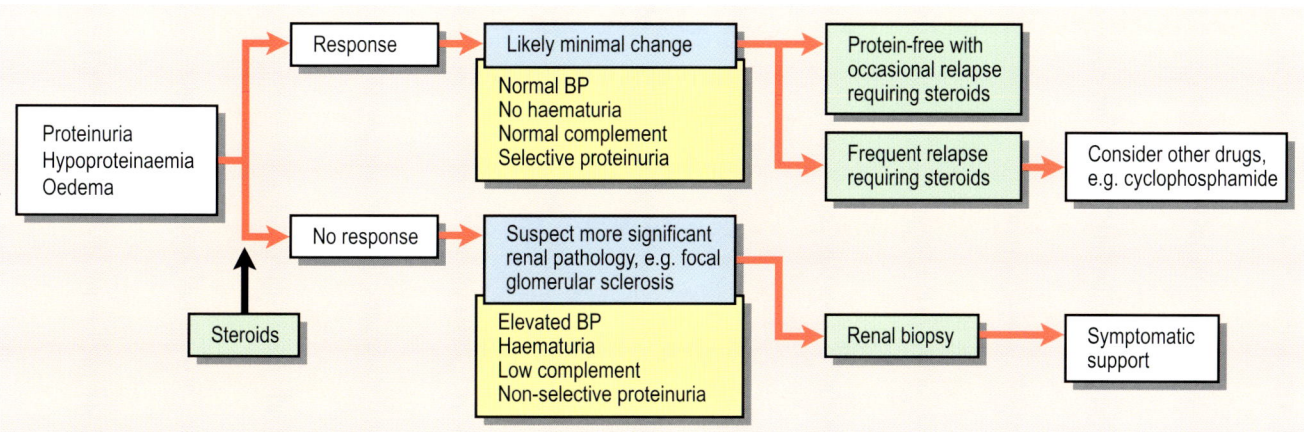

Fig. 3 **Management of childhood nephrotic syndrome.**

Obstruction of venous or lymphatic channels by either malignant or benign tissue enlargement may also lead to localised oedema. Again, other symptoms and signs are normally present.

CONGENITAL OEDEMA

Generalised oedema at birth is rare. Affected babies are called 'hydropic'. In only 50% will a cause be able to be identified and the overall mortality is very high.

Turner's syndrome (XO karyotype) is associated with localised lymphoedema present at birth (also detectable in utero). The swelling is normally peripheral and is particularly seen in the feet. This syndrome has important long-term sequelae (Fig. 4) and therefore, if lymphoedema is present, Turner's syndrome must be considered (see p. 107).

ABDOMINAL SWELLING

Babies and young children often have rather protruberant abdomens. This is caused by a relative lack of abdominal musculature and (in toddlers) a relatively lordotic posture. Any increase in abdominal contents, including gas, therefore, results in distension. In young children presenting with acute abdominal swelling, simple explanations (e.g. an excessive intake of fizzy drinks or simple constipation) must be excluded first. In those where this is not the cause, intestinal obstruction must be considered. Additional symptoms supporting such a diagnosis include abdominal pain, vomiting (especially if bile-stained), failure to pass wind or faeces rectally.

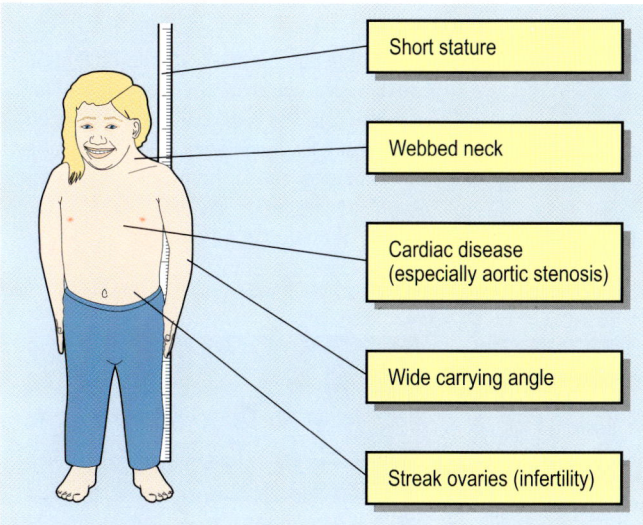

Fig. 4 **Features of Turner's syndrome.**

Causes of intestinal obstruction vary with age. In the *neonatal period*, causes include:

- gut atresia (present from birth)
- inperforate anus (present at birth but may be missed if fistulous connection allows limited passage of meconium)
- volvulus (associated with malrotation of the gut — may not present until later childhood)
- paralytic ileus (may arise secondary to any systemic illness, e.g. respiratory distress syndrome)
- Hirschsprung's disease (if severe may cause acute obstruction — see page 32.
- meconium ileus (occurs in 10% of infants with cystic fibrosis — it may be possible to wash the bowel clear)
- necrotising enterocolitis (gut infection secondary to vascular insufficiency of the gut — can cause perforation — predominantly a disease of premature infants).

Childhood causes of intestinal obstruction:

- volvulus (associated with malrotation of the gut)
- paralytic ileus (associated with systemic illness or abdominal pathology, appendicitis must be considered)
- obstructed hernia (herniae are relatively common in infants born prematurely).

Abdominal swelling may occur over a more prolonged period. Under these circumstances the presence of a mass should be considered (pp. 72–73). Alternatively, the presence of a relative increase in the amount of intestinal gas in association with particularly poor musculature may produce this picture. This latter situation may arise in untreated coeliac disease or cystic fibrosis.

Acute swelling in the scrotum, if it is associated with pain, must be regarded as torsion of the testis until proved otherwise. It can occur at any time and confirmation of the diagosis is urgent in order that surgery can be carried out before necrosis occurs. Other causes of acute swelling in the scrotum are hernia, hydrocele, epididymo-orchitis or trauma (p. 73).

Swelling

- Oedema is a marker of underlying disease.
- Nephrotic syndrome is the most important cause of generalised swelling.
- Nephrotic syndrome in childhood generally has a good prognosis.
- Abdominal swelling and bile-stained vomiting is always significant.

IMPAIRED MOVEMENT: MUSCULOSKELETAL

During normal development children progress from being incapable of locomotion to being fully competent at both walking and running. This process results from a combination of learned behaviour and neuronal maturation. There is great natural variation, so that whilst it is the norm for children to be able to walk independently around 1 year of age, some infants will have developed this skill at 8 months whilst others will not achieve it until after their second birthday.

Many factors affect the time at which a child walks, including the child's personality, the amount of stimulation given, the space available at home and the child's size. In addition, some children progress to walking via a stage in which they move by shuffling on their bottoms. Such children usually do not walk until around 18 months to 2 years of age. However, it is important to remember that late walking can be a marker of a more serious problem (e.g. muscular dystrophy), especially where other aspects of development are also not progressing normally. For example, very poor vision or mental retardation may both affect how quickly a child walks as well as other aspects of development.

It is important when assessing a child's gait to consider how long he/she has been walking. It is quite usual for children who have only recently acquired walking to adopt a broad-based unsteady gait, at times going on to tip-toe. However, they should progress steadily from this situation to a more mature pattern of walking and later running.

Figure 1 indicates those systems which if damaged in some way can be expected to affect locomotion. On pages 100–101, attention is paid to the effects of CNS and muscle problems. Clearly, where that type of impairment exists it is likely that gait will be affected. However, although some reference will be made to neuromuscular problems, this section will centre on problems of the skeletal system.

CHRONIC PROBLEMS AFFECTING LOCOMOTION

Table 1 summarises the effects of CNS and primary muscle disease.

The two most important structural problems to be considered are rickets and congenital dislocation of the hip (CDH).

RICKETS

This condition results from a lack of vitamin D and leads to poor bone mineralisation. Because the bones are soft, bowing of the legs occurs. The ends of long bones also become splayed and tender (Fig. 2). Most commonly the condition is a consequence of an inadequate diet. Those at particular risk include some racial groups whose diet is restricted for religious reasons and whose pigment limits the ability of sunlight to produce vitamin D in the skin.

Rickets may also complicate other conditions, e.g. malabsorption or severe renal disease.

CONGENITAL DISLOCATION OF THE HIP (CDH)

At the time of birth the hip joints (both ball and socket) are largely cartilaginous. In order that the hip develops normally, the ball must lie within the socket. If not, the acetabulum becomes shallow and the femoral head malformed. Should this be allowed to occur when the child attempts to stand and walk, the femoral head on the affected side is displaced superiorly. This effectively shortens the leg and the child limps. Every newborn baby is examined for CDH in an attempt to avoid these long-term problems. A number of risk factors for the condition have been identified including breech delivery, family history and female sex.

There are two degrees of severity in CDH. In the most serious form the affected hip is completely dislocated at birth. During examination (using the position shown in Fig. 3), as the hips are abducted, the femoral head is brought back into the acetabulum and this can be felt (often described as a clunk — Ortolani's test). Less severely affected hips lie within the acetabulum but can be dislocated when stressed. Such a problem can also be identified by using the manoeuvre described above but at the midpoint of abduction pushing backwards to displace the femoral head (if this is possible). Again, on completing abduction the femoral head comes back into the acetabulum but the sensation is less marked (often described as a click — Barlow's test). Ultrasound allows confirmation and in future may become the standard screening test for congenital dislocation of the hip in all children.

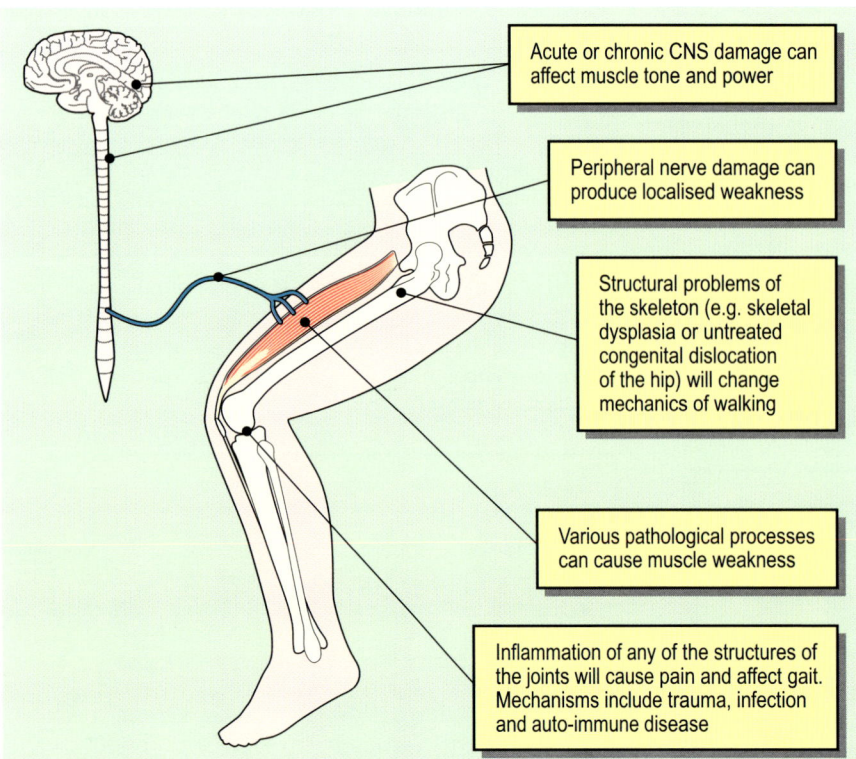

Acute or chronic CNS damage can affect muscle tone and power

Peripheral nerve damage can produce localised weakness

Structural problems of the skeleton (e.g. skeletal dysplasia or untreated congenital dislocation of the hip) will change mechanics of walking

Various pathological processes can cause muscle weakness

Inflammation of any of the structures of the joints will cause pain and affect gait. Mechanisms include trauma, infection and auto-immune disease

Fig. 1 **Mechanisms of damage which can affect locomotion.**

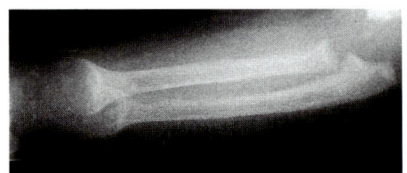

Fig. 2 **Rickets seen on X-ray.** Note poorly calcified distal radius and ulnar with widening of metaphyses.

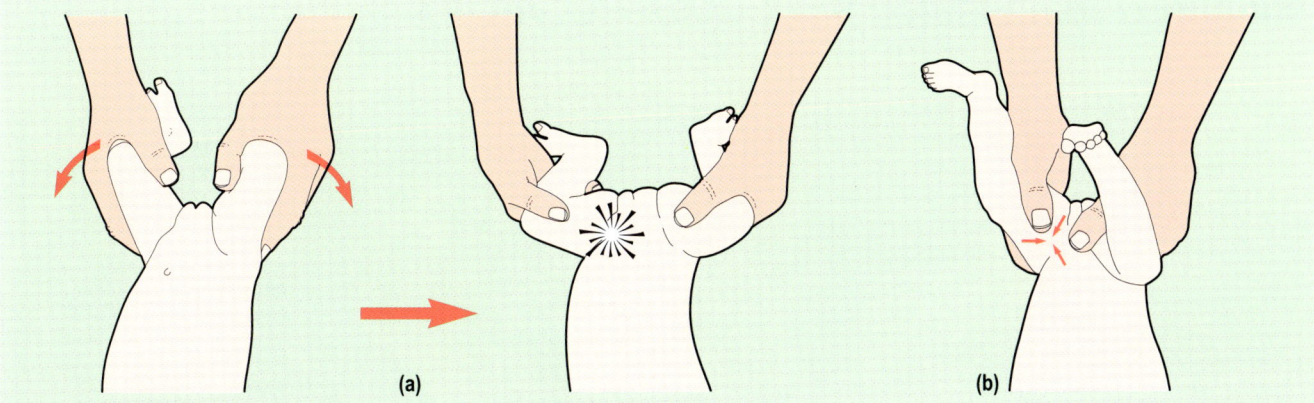

Fig. 3 **The Ortolani (a) and Barlow (b) tests (left hip).**

Treatment consists of splinting to hold the joint in correct alignment during early growth, or where this fails, surgery.

ACUTE PROBLEMS AFFECTING LOCOMOTION

Acute neuromuscular diseases may present with altered gait. These are largely dealt with on pages 100–101. The major skeletal problems are described below.

TRAUMA

Fractures will clearly affect mobility. A careful assessment must be made to consider the possibility of child abuse, especially where the history is unclear or if the child is very young. Indeed, there may be no history: the child may simply present with a limp, and a fracture diagnosed on X-ray. It is important to realise that small children just starting to walk rarely suffer fractures as a result of a fall. Radiology may be particularly helpful since non-accidental injuries caused by pulling a leg (or arm) typically result in spiral fractures or fractures through the epiphysial plate.

ATRAUMATIC SKELETAL PROBLEMS

Transient synovitis of the hip (irritable hip) is the most common cause of a limp in children. The aetiology is unclear but the condition frequently follows a viral infection, suggesting that it is related to the immune response. Although the hip is commonly affected, it can occur in any joint. Typically there is no history of injury and no systemic upset. The condition resolves with rest.

Perthes disease

This condition is caused by spontaneous avascular necrosis of the femoral head. It is most common in boys aged 4–8 years. The presentation may be with pain or with a painless limp. Healing occurs with time but during this period (up to 4 years) the affected hip joint must be protected, normally with the use of a brace.

Slipped upper femoral epiphysis

During the pubertal growth spurt both sexes are vulnerable to a shearing separation of this epiphysis. Obese children with delayed sexual development seem particularly at risk. Presentation may be with pain (in the hip or knee) or with a limp. Treatment is by urgent surgical fixation.

INFECTION

Both osteomyelitis and septic arthritis may present in young children simply with a limp of acute onset. Older children will clearly report pain made worse by movement. The presence of some recent penetrating injury (however minor), fever, local inflammation, reduced movement and swelling all support the diagnosis. It is essential that infections of this type are diagnosed and treated aggressively since:

- septicaemia may follow
- permanent damage to a joint or reduced bone growth may result.

Plain X-rays are rarely helpful in the early stages. White blood cell count, C-reactive protein, blood cultures, isotope bone scan and examination of aspirate from the site are the most important investigations to be considered. Staphylococci and streptococci are the most common pathogens. Treatment is with antibiotics and surgery to remove any dead tissue.

Non-infective arthritis

A number of diseases may present in childhood with arthritis. These can, in some cases, be confined to one or two joints and present with a limp. This is discussed more fully on pages 102–103.

Table 1 **Chronic neuromuscular disease and gait**

Diagnosis	Pathology	Effect on gait
Cerebral palsy*	Unilateral damage to pyramidal system	Spastic hemiplegia * increased tone with foot in extension * arm immobile and flexed * walking may be delayed
	Extensive bilateral damage to pyramidal system	Spastic quadraplegia * as above but bilateral * children may not walk independently
	Localised bilateral damage to pyramidal system	Diplegia * increased tone especially marked in legs * Achilles tendon will be tight (as above) * legs are also adducted (tend to 'scissor') * walking may be delayed
	Cerebellar damage	Broad-based staggering gait Walking may be delayed
	Basal ganglia damage	Involuntary movements make gait very unsteady Walking may be delayed
Muscular dystrophy	Generalised muscle damage	Delayed walking Increasing weakness
* Damage to central control; severity varies as does distribution		

> **Impaired movement: musculoskeletal**
>
> - All newborn infants must be examined for congenital dislocation of the hip.
> - Sepsis must always be excluded in children who present with an acutely inflamed joint.
> - An unexplained limp of acute onset may be the result of child abuse.

IMPAIRED MOVEMENT: NEUROMUSCULAR

All movements are the result of a complex interplay of the central nervous and musculoskeletal systems. In this section consideration will be given to those conditions which can disrupt the functional components of this process. Figure 1 indicates the broad patterns of damage that can occur.

UPPER MOTOR NEURONE LESIONS

Congenital

This clinical situation is largely covered by the general descriptive term *cerebral palsy*. A wide variety of mechanisms may operate to damage the developing motor system (Fig. 2), but in approximately 50% of affected children no cause can be found. The origin of neuronal damage, when identified, most commonly relates to the perinatal period. However, increasing circumstantial evidence supports the concept of a prenatal origin for many of the cases that are currently unexplained.

It is clear that following a generalised insult to the CNS the consequent lesion is unlikely to be confined simply to the motor system. As a result, children with cerebral palsy often have associated problems. These include mental retardation, epilepsy and damage to the special senses.

The pattern of motor deficit reflects the distribution of CNS damage (Fig. 3). The extent of neuronal damage may show great variation between individuals. For example, injury to the right internal capsule may be so severe as to cause a dense left hemiplegia, or in another individual so minor as to produce neurological deficit that can only be detected by the most careful testing.

Although the CNS injury may be complete at or soon after birth (i.e. the insult is non-progressive), the extent of the resulting damage may take time to become apparent. For example, it may be obvious at birth that a child has a dense hemiplegia, whilst in another, less severely affected child it may take some weeks or months before anyone notices that one hand is used less competently than expected. Similarly, the manifestations of the damage may change as the child develops. In both the above cases the affected limbs may initially be hypotonic but with time show steadily increasing tone.

Subacute lesions

A number of rare conditions exist which result in progressive CNS damage. Mechanisms include toxic damage (e.g. untreated phenylketonuria), storage disorders (e.g. Tay–Sachs' disease in which

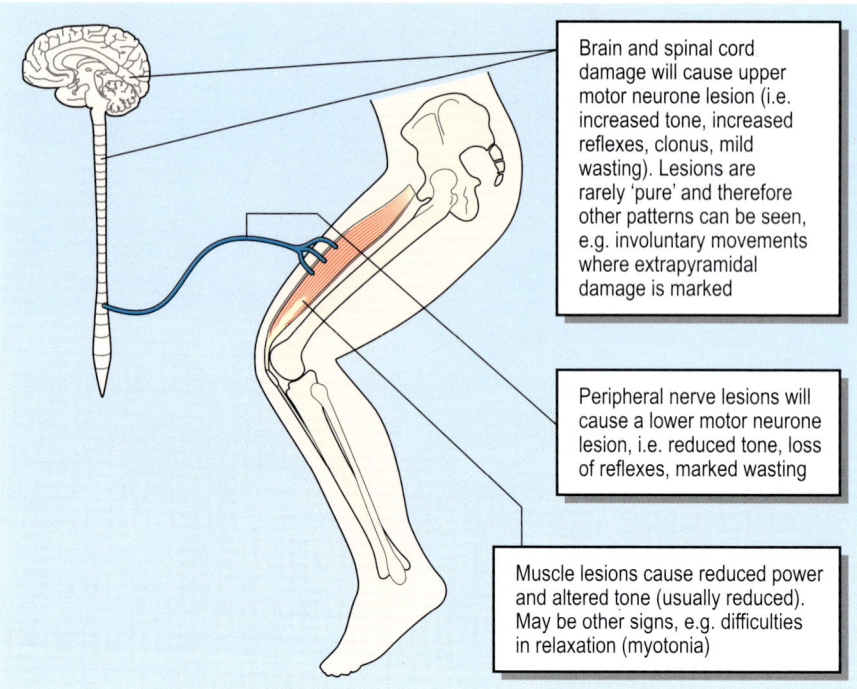

Fig. 1 **Patterns of CNS and muscle damage that can lead to impaired movement.**

ganglioside GM2 accumulates in grey matter) and other metabolic disorders (e.g. Leigh's disease). These conditions produce degenerative changes in the brain and, unlike cerebral palsy, increasing motor and other neurological deficits.

New problems with movement may also be encountered in children who develop tumours. However, other symptoms (e.g. headache and vomiting) often dominate.

Acute lesions

Sudden loss of function may occur in transverse myelitis. In this condition, acute demyelination of the cord is produced as a post-infectious phenomenon. Normally there is accompanying sensory loss.

LOWER MOTOR NEURONE LESIONS

Congenital

Approximately 1 in 20 000 infants are born with Werdnig–Hoffman disease and present with an early onset flaccid paralysis. This is a recessive disorder that leads to progressive degeneration of anterior horn cells and death by 18 months of age. In this condition (as in most diseases which damage anterior horn cells), fasciculation is common and may help make the diagnosis: it is seen most clearly in the tongue and hands. Despite the neurological problems, affected babies typically stay responsive and alert. A variant of this condition (Kugelberg–Welander syndrome) occurs in later childhood.

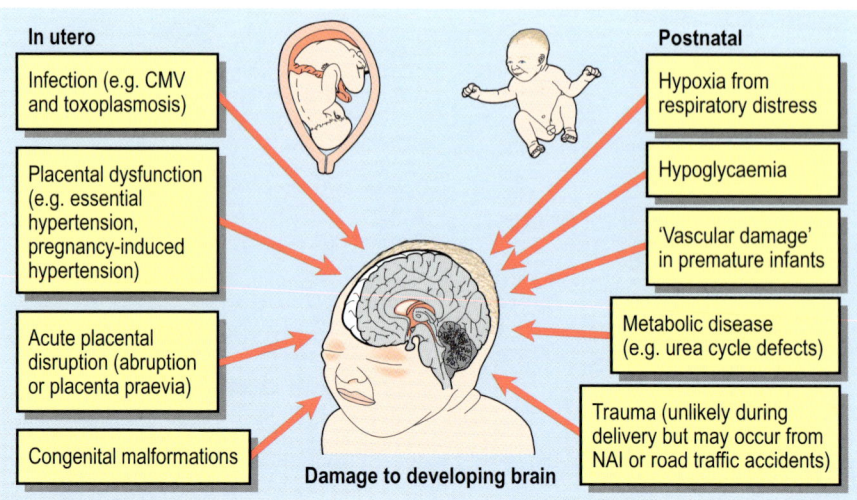

Fig. 2 **Origins of cerebral palsy.**

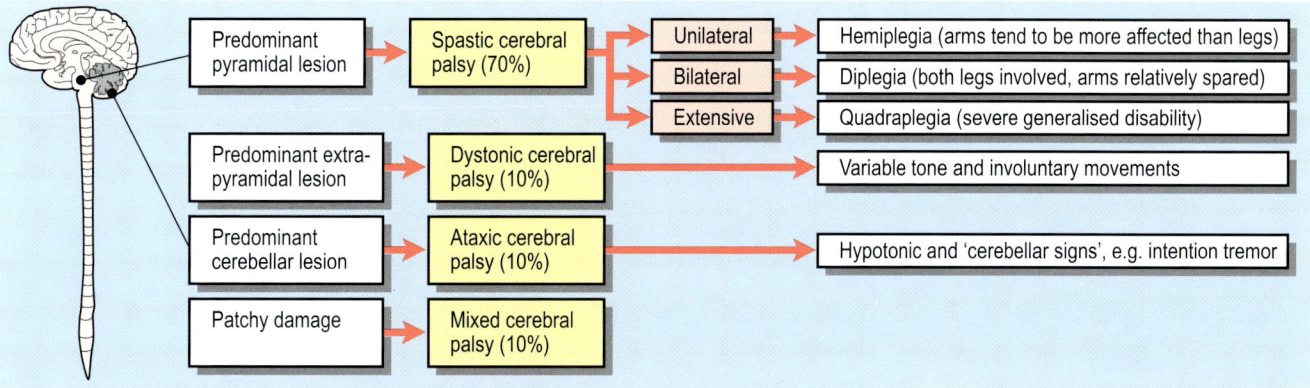

Fig. 3 **Patterns of motor deficits reflecting distribution of CNS damage.**

Acute lesions

'Infective' polyneuropathy or Guillain–Barré syndrome is a condition that follows an acute viral infection. It predominantly affects peripheral nerves and nerve roots. Lumbar puncture typically shows increased protein but few cells. The disease produces a flaccid paralysis which progresses over a number of days before stabilising. A slow recovery phase then follows. During the height of the illness, intensive care including ventilation may be necessary.

Historically, poliomyelitis has been the most important cause of acquired paralysis and in the Third World remains so today. Infection can take the form of a flu-like illness alone, lead to a meningitic picture (with symptoms of headache, photophobia and neck stiffness), or produce acute paralysis. In this latter situation active destruction of anterior horn cells occurs and fasciculation is prominent. Recovery is variable and in an epidemic, unless long-term ventilation is available, deaths will result from respiratory failure.

MUSCLE DISEASE

A number of congenital muscular dystrophies exist (dystrophy implies abnormal muscle structure and function) but all are rare and in general their effect on muscle power is not marked. Later in childhood dermatomyositis, an autoimmune disease, can result in primary muscular inflammation and weakness whilst other diseases may produce secondary muscle impairment (e.g. thyrotoxicosis, malignancy). All of these situations are uncommon.

However, a number of inherited forms of muscle disease exist which lead to increasing muscle dysfunction (muscular dystrophies). They are characterised by weakness that does not conform to the distribution of a nerve or group of nerves. Of these the most important is Duchenne dystrophy.

Duchenne dystropy

This is an X-linked recessive disorder which affects approximately 1 in 7000 liveborn boys. Even in the first few days after birth, muscle damage can be detected by the presence of excessive amounts of the muscle enzyme creatine phosphokinase (CPK) in the blood. Symptoms and signs do not usually emerge until 1–2 years and can include delayed walking (i.e. beyond 18 months), toe walking and difficulty in standing up. Rising from the floor can be so difficult that an affected child will often use his hands to 'walk up his body' (Fig. 4). This is the basis of Gower's sign. The condition is progressive with children being wheelchair bound by approximately 11 years. Death, from myocardial failure, is to be expected any time from the late teens to the early twenties. The site of the gene for Duchenne muscular dystrophy has now been identified on the X chromosome and the normal product of the gene 'dystrophin' has been manufactured. As yet, human therapy with this substance has not been established.

INVESTIGATION

Differentiating between muscle disease and disorders of peripheral nerves can be difficult on clinical grounds. The most helpful investigations in this situation include:

- nerve conduction velocities
- electromyograms
- peripheral nerve biopsy
- muscle biopsy.

FLOPPY BABY SYNDROME

Normal tone results from inputs that arise from several central nervous and peripheral neuromuscular structures, as well as the presence of normal connective tissue. Children who display marked hypotonia immediately after birth are often described as 'floppy'. Many of the neuromuscular disorders described above can produce this pattern but a number of other conditions must be considered. These include syndromes for which hypotonia is a specific feature (e.g. Prader–Willi syndrome — hypotonia and excessive appetite) and in addition those syndromes associated with mental retardation (e.g. Down's syndrome). Benign congenital hypotonia refers to those children who are profoundly hypotonic but who have normal muscle strength and no underlying medical condition.

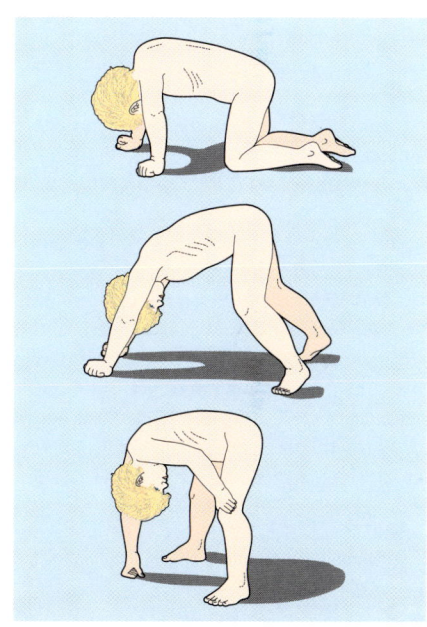

Fig. 4 **Gower's sign in Duchenne dystrophy.**

Impaired movement: neuromuscular

- Cerebral palsy is the most important cause of neuromuscular dysfunction in childhood.
- In approximately 50% of cases the cause of cerebral palsy cannot be identified.
- When assessing a child with cerebral palsy, evidence of neurological damage outside the motor system should be sought.
- Boys who are not walking by 18 months of age should be screened for Duchenne muscular dystrophy.

PAINFUL JOINTS AND BONES

In children it is often very difficult to localise pain, and any clinical assessment of joint problems must consider the surrounding bones and soft tissues. Inflammation in or around a joint is the usual cause of pain. It may result from trauma, infection or an immune response to internal or external stimuli. The signs of joint inflammation are pain, swelling, heat and/or disability.

THE PAINFUL JOINT

Acute infection

Acutely, injury is the most common cause. However, injuries are very common in children, and there is often a history of trauma even if the problem is not causally related.

Septic arthritis, although uncommon, is the most important cause of a painful joint of acute onset. If not diagnosed early, irreversible joint damage can result. *Staphylococcus aureus* is the main organism involved, often by haematogenous spread from a distant focus, perhaps a minor skin wound. Large joints are usually affected. Antibiotic treatment needs to be given for several weeks to ensure penetration and eradication of infection.

The distinction between osteomyelitis and septic arthritis is often blurred, with a similar presentation and management. The metaphyses of long bones are most commonly affected. Spread of infection across the growth plate into the joint is uncommon, but the two (osteomyelitis and osteoarthritis) can coexist, particularly at the proximal radius and proximal femur because the metaphysis is intracapsular (Fig. 1). In infants, vascular connections between the epiphyses and metaphyses still exist, making spread more common.

Less acute presentation

Insidious onset of swelling or pain around a joint may indicate chronic infection. Tuberculosis of bone is rare in the UK but a common cause of morbidity worldwide. Infection of vertebrae leads to kyphoscoliosis, and if the spinal cord is involved, paraplegia. Bone cysts and tumours usually present with pain and tenderness, or 'pathological' fracture. The majority are benign, often with typical X-ray features (Fig. 2). Two primary malignant bone tumours are relatively common: osteogenic sarcoma, affecting people between 10 and 25 years, and Ewing's sarcoma, arising from cells of mesenchymal origin, usually in younger children.

Other diseases

Haemarthroses are common in haemophilia and must be treated aggressively with factor VIII infusions because recurrent episodes are destructive leading to deformity. In sickle cell disease, painful crises often involve bones and joints (p. 89).

Multiple joints

Septic arthritis can affect more than one joint, but usually this indicates a more generalised disorder. Viral infection frequently causes 'arthralgia', but an actual reactive arthritis, probably resulting from immune complex deposition, is also quite common, particularly with rubella (Table 1). Henoch–Schönlein disease (p. 64) also commonly causes troublesome joint problems. Rheumatic fever is very uncommon in the UK but still common worldwide. Following an acute β-haemolytic streptococcal infection, either in the throat or the skin, the child develops a polyarthritis, fever, and often an acute carditis. Although the acute cardiac inflammation settles, permanent valvular damage may result from endocarditis, presenting clinically sometimes several decades later.

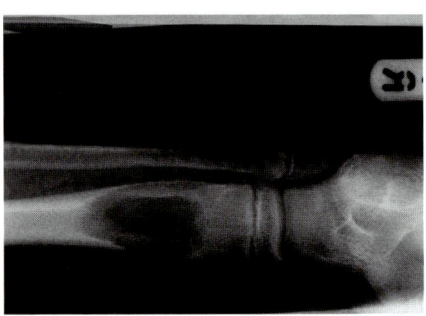

Fig. 2 **Bone cyst in the tibia which could cause a pathological fracture or local pain.**

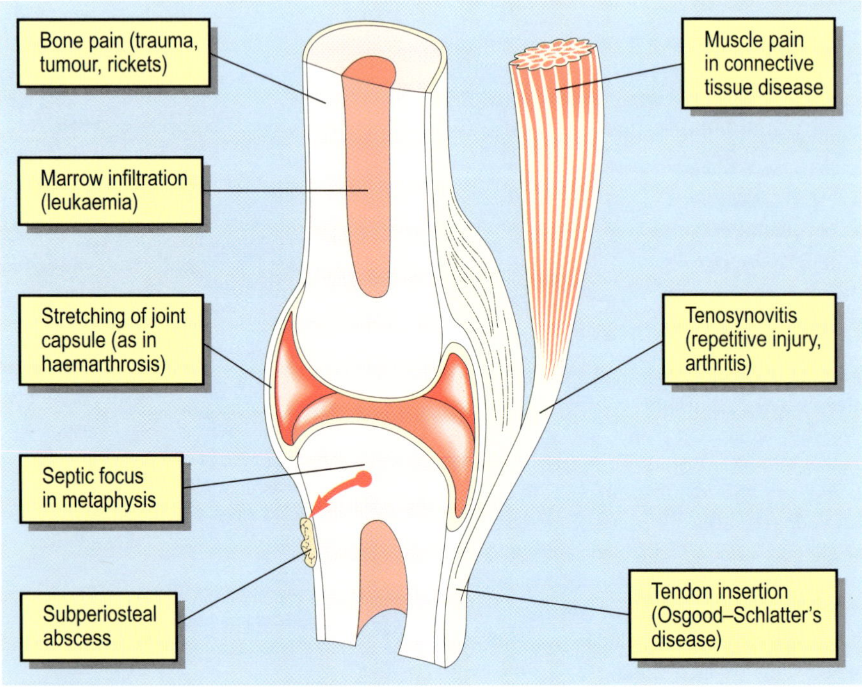

JUVENILE CHRONIC ARTHRITIS (JCA)

This is defined as joint inflammation persisting in a child for more than 6 weeks in the absence of another specific cause. The definition is important because it is entirely a clinical diagnosis, and a diagnosis of exclusion of other relevant possibilities such as the above. The pathogenesis of the synovitis is not well understood, but the immune system is thought to play a central role. Three clinical subtypes have been defined (Table 2) mainly for prognostic purposes.

The pauci-articular type tends to affect older girls (sex ratio more than 10:1), and is commonly associated with an anterior uveitis (iridocyclitis) (Fig. 3). This can be asymptomatic until a late stage, and needs careful ophthalmic examination (with a slit-lamp) in order that it is recognised. In poly-articular disease the eyes are less often involved, but the presentation with arthritis, rather than systemic symptoms, is otherwise similar.

Fig. 1 **Some sites of pain around joints.**

- Bone pain (trauma, tumour, rickets)
- Marrow infiltration (leukaemia)
- Stretching of joint capsule (as in haemarthrosis)
- Septic focus in metaphysis
- Subperiosteal abscess
- Muscle pain in connective tissue disease
- Tenosynovitis (repetitive injury, arthritis)
- Tendon insertion (Osgood–Schlatter's disease)

Table 1 **Some viral infections associated with arthritis**

Rubella and rubella vaccination	Parvovirus
Infectious hepatitis	Adenovirus
Mumps	HIV
Glandular fever	Chicken pox

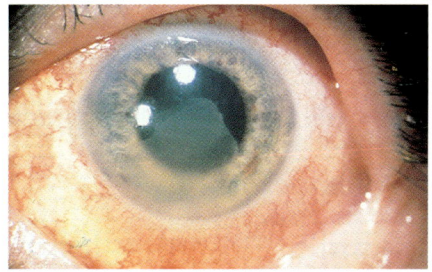

Fig. 3 **Severe acute anterior uveitis as associated with chronic arthritis.** Long-term eye damage is often worse when the presentation is more insidious.

By contrast, in systemic onset disease (also called Still's disease) the child is often much younger and the joint problems are usually initially only minor. There is more generalised illness, with fever. Initial features also usually include many of the following:

- widespread rash
- lymphadenopathy
- hepatomegaly
- splenomegaly
- anaemia
- pericarditis.

Distinction from leukaemia is sometimes difficult. In most cases of JCA, active disease continues for months or years, but eventually remits spontaneously. Management is primarily concerned with preserving joint mobility during and after periods of active inflammation. Physiotherapy and, in particular, hydrotherapy are very helpful. Occupational therapists are involved, especially if there are problems with the hands or feet. Anti-inflammatory drugs, and intra-articular steroid injections, help improve mobility. Methotrexate may help the disease more specifically (Fig. 4).

Other diagnostic labels are used in this condition and commonly lead to confusion. In the USA the same disease is called juvenile rheumatoid arthritis, and older texts use 'Still's disease' in this sense.

KNEE SYMPTOMS

The knee is the most complex joint in the body. It is perhaps surprising that in childhood, even in this joint, permanent traumatic injury is rare. However, particularly in adolescence, certain specific conditions

Table 2 **Types of juvenile chronic arthritis**

	Pauci-articular	Poly-articular	Systemic onset
Number of joints affected	1–4	5+	Several and symmetrical, but not usually a major feature
Age	Older	Older	Younger
Sex ratio	Girls ++	Girls ++	Equal
Iridocyclitis	Common	Unusual	Unusual
Anti-nuclear antibody titre	If positive: eyes even more commonly affected	Usually negative	Usually negative

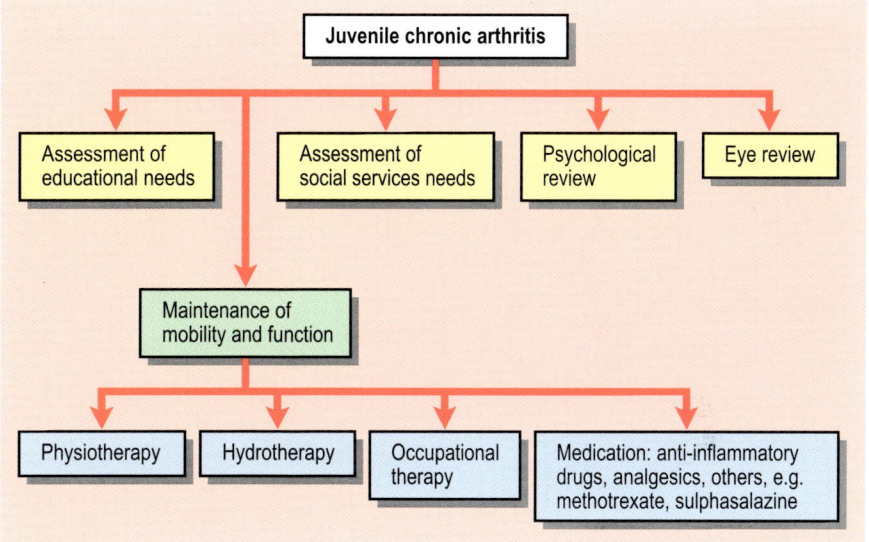

Fig. 4 **Aspects of management of JCA.**

occur which may be said to be 'overuse' syndromes. These were previously seen mostly in athletic young adults, but with greater emphasis on athletic activities at all ages, these have become more common in younger people. Chondromalacia patellae arises because of stresses on the patella resulting from the pull of the quadriceps muscle, and is common in teenage girls particularly. In Osgood–Schlatter's disease, there is pain, and often swelling over the tibial tubercle after exercise. This is more common in boys (Table 3). In both cases, treatment involves avoiding activity that brings on the pain, and encouraging exercise to strengthen the muscle groups around the joint.

SPINAL SYMPTOMS

Chronic back pain is uncommon in children. Causes include:

- *Osteochondritis:* Schuermann's disease in adolescent males — cause unknown.

- *Malignancy:* intrinsic (very rare) or extrinsic (neuroblastoma, lymphoma, Ewing tumour).
- *Infection:* tuberculosis.
- *Arthritis:* ankylosing spondylitis usually after 15 years of age.
- *Scoliosis:* may be postural or structural. Whereas a postural curve will correct with adjustment of posture, a structural curve is accompanied by vertebral rotation. Secondary structural scoliosis can be caused by many of the above conditions, and also by neuromuscular imbalance as in cerebral palsy or muscular dystrophies. Most cases of primary (idiopathic) structural scoliosis are seen in adolescent girls. Treatment is by surgical correction.

Painful joints and bones

- Septic arthritis can cause irreversible joint damage.
- Most cases of childhood arthritis remit spontaneously.
- Always consider the eyes in childhood arthritis.
- Physiotherapy is the mainstay of treatment of childhood chronic joint problems.

Table 3 **Features of three overuse syndromes**

	Chondromalacia patellae	Osgood–Schlatter's disease	Hyperextensibility
Sex ratio	Girls > boys	Boys > girls	Girls > boys
Age at onset	Adolescents and young adults	Adolescents	School age
Symptoms	Knee pain on exertion. Need to sit with straight legs (pain on prolonged flexion)	Pain over tibial tubercle exacerbated by exercise	Pain after exercise, especially knees, elbows, hands and ankles
Signs	Patellar tenderness on compression Quadriceps weakness	Tenderness and swelling at insertion of patellar tendon	Pain worse at night

FEVER

DEFINITION

Fever means an elevated body temperature. Normal temperature varies depending on the site at which the temperature is being measured. A child can be flushed, hot to touch and sweating without having a fever, for example after exertion or when well-wrapped in bed. Environmental factors such as over-wrapping rarely cause true fever in children, but may do in infants. A fever often impairs thermal homeostasis and as a result a person may feel hot or cold whilst febrile. Similarly, a 'rigor' occurs when the fever is so high it results in inappropriate violent shivering, often with chattering of the teeth.

MEASURING THE TEMPERATURE

The best method in older children is to use a thermometer in the mouth; the rectum or axilla are preferred in infants. It must be held carefully in place for at least 1 minute in order to obtain an accurate record. A normal temperature is not above 37°C in the axilla, 37.2°C in the mouth or 37.5°C rectally. A 'fever strip' can be used on the forehead by parents at home, but this is not as accurate as a thermometer and must be done very carefully to obtain a good result.

A fever may be *acute* or *chronic* (Fig. 1).

ACUTE FEBRILE ILLNESS

Many very serious conditions such as meningitis, pyelonephritis and appendicitis often appear trivial at the onset of the illness, sometimes with fever as the only sign. It can be difficult to tell the difference between a harmless, viral illness and one which is about to develop into a serious, life-threatening infection. It is important to search for a focus of infection (Table 1). A careful search will reveal a focus in many cases. Reassessment over time is valuable to identify a developing significant illness.

If there is no focus to suggest an aetiology, further action is guided by:

- the height of the fever
- the age of the child
- the degree of 'illness' apparent in the child.

For example, if the child has a temperature of 38°C to 39°C and looks well, only anti-pyretic measures are required, e.g. give paracetamol, strip off warm clothes and perhaps use a fan. (It is important to remember not to chill the child, as shivering may increase the temperature.)

If there is a temperature of 38°C to 39°C in a child who looks ill, keep under review and consider tests and treatment as suggested below for a higher fever.

If there is a temperature above 39°C, 10% of these children will have bacteraemia which may proceed to serious infection such as meningitis. Therefore, unless a viral cause is obvious, these children merit investigation and treatment.

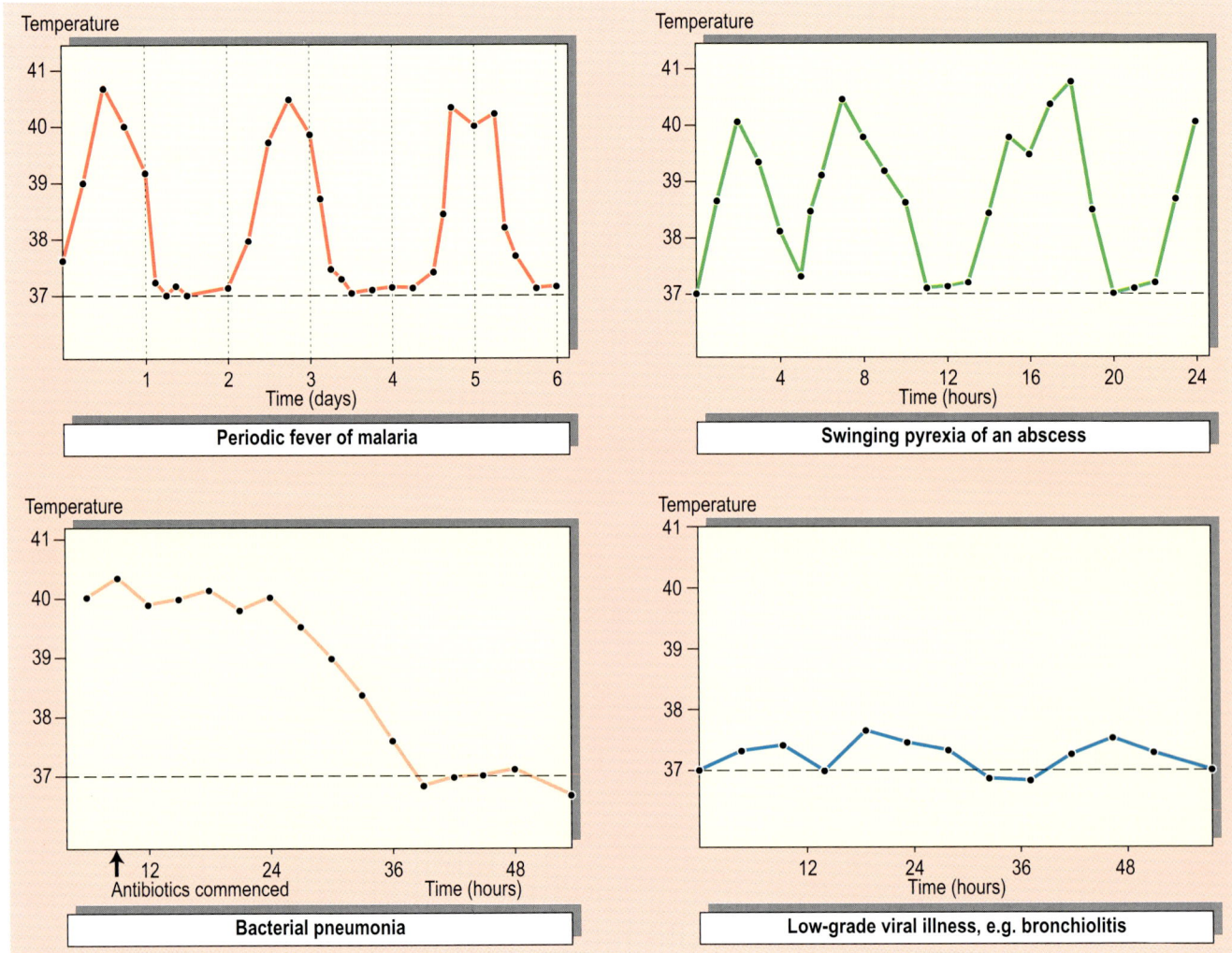

Fig. 1 **Temperature in four common types of febrile illness.**

Management is also influenced by the age of the child. For example, at 0–3 months of age, bacteraemia associated with high fever is common, therefore full investigation should be undertaken, and antibiotics started until a diagnosis is clear. Beyond 3 months of age it is easier to assess children and a more conservative approach may suffice.

Investigations

Minimum investigations should include:

- urine culture
- blood count with differential white cell count
- blood culture.

Lumbar puncture is indicated in all very young infants and older children with signs of meningitis. Chest X-rays will be necessary if clinical signs indicate pneumonia may be present.

Treatment

If the child looks well, wait for the results of tests and treat accordingly. If the child looks ill, commence empirical, broad-spectrum, intravenous antibiotics while waiting for test results.

CHRONIC FEVER — PYREXIA OF UNKNOWN ORIGIN (PUO)

A PUO is a fever which has persisted for 2 weeks and for which there is no obvious cause. There are several possible aetiologies.

Infectious disease

Possible infectious causes of fever include:

- malaria (travel abroad)
- salmonella (travel abroad, abdominal pain, known contact)
- tuberculosis (contact, ethnic origin)
- AIDS (failure to thrive, persistent diarrhoea, recurrent infection, mother in high risk group).

Non-infectious inflammation

Rheumatoid disease and connective tissue disease can produce low-grade fever over a long time. It is important to look for the presence of other related symptoms and signs such as swollen, painful joints, rashes and an enlarged spleen.

Features of Kawasaki disease include high fever of acute onset, enlarged lymph nodes, rash, inflamed mucosa, conjunctivitis and swelling or peeling of hands and feet.

Malignancy

Neuroblastoma is a tumour which normally arises from the adrenal gland. It commonly presents as a mass and is identified on palpation or on ultrasound of the abdomen. It

Table 1 **Some common causes of fever**

Disease	Possible symptoms	Possible signs	Organism	Tests	Treatment
Pneumonia	Cough Sputum Breathing probs	↑Respiratory rate Toxic child Focal signs	Pneumococcus H. influenzae Mycoplasma	Sputum, blood culture, CXR	Antibiotics Physiotherapy
Otitis media	Earache	Red, bulging drum	50% viral 50% bacterial	None	Paracetamol +/- antibiotic
Tonsillitis	Sore throat	Follicular tonsillitis Inflamed throat	80% viral 20% Streptococcus	Throat swab	Paracetamol +/- antibiotic
Appendicitis	Abdo. pain Vomiting	RIF tenderness	—	FBC, urine for bacteriology	Appendicectomy
UTI	Dysuria Haematuria Loin pain	Loin tenderness	Gram-negative organisms	Urine for bacteriology, FBC	Antibiotics
Peritonitis	Severe abdominal pain	Guarding		FBC, blood culture	Laparotomy
Gastroenteritis	Diarrhoea Vomiting	Dehydration	E. Coli Shigella Salmonella Campylobacter Rotavirus 70%	Stool culture and virology	Rehydration: oral or intravenous
Meningitis	Headache Vomiting Photophobia	Neck stiffness Kernig's	Meningococcus Pneumococcus H. influenzae	Blood culture, LP	i.v. antibiotics in high doses
Skin sepsis	Localised swelling and pain	Cellulitis Infected eczema abscesses	Streptococcus Staphylococcus	Swabs, blood culture	Penicillin Flucloxacillin
Childhood exanthema		Typical rash	Measles, rubella parvovirus, chicken pox (Fig. 2)	Viral titres, EM of fluid from lesion	Anti-pyretic measures

can cause a high, 'swinging' pyrexia in a very ill child. Leukaemia is the most common malignancy in childhood. Bacterial infections are often active at presentation and result in high fever.

Factitious

Children may use a temperature to avoid school or as a means of seeking attention for a variety of psychological reasons. A factitious fever may also be produced by a mother with a psychological disturbance who wishes the child to appear ill (Munchausen syndrome by proxy).

INVESTIGATING A PUO

Tests as for acute infection may be appropriate but additional investigations on a case by case basis may include the following.

Acute phase reactants. These are proteins or cells which increase at the time of infection or inflammation, e.g. the white blood count shows raised granulocytes in bacterial infection. The ESR, C-reactive protein (CRP) and plasma viscosity are elevated in most infections and non-infectious inflammation. These tests are non-specific, and do not give a diagnosis.

X-rays, ultrasound or isotope scans. These may help with the diagnosis of septic arthritis, osteomyelitis or malignancy.

Other tests include: Mantoux or Heaf test for TB, immunological tests including autoantibodies for connective tissue disorders, Widal test for typhoid, HIV antibody test and blood film for malaria parasites.

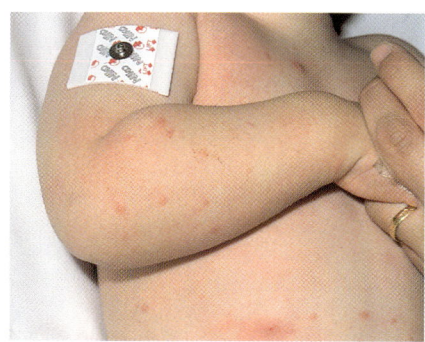

Fig. 2 **Chicken pox is a potential cause of fever in children.**

Fever

- In practice only a few tests are usually necessary to diagnose a febrile illness.
- Look for the purpuric rash of meningococcus in all febrile children.
- In suspected meningitis, give antibiotics *as an emergency before* an LP.
- LP can be dangerous in severe shock or with raised intracranial pressure.
- In chronic pyrexia, do the investigations in a logical order.

SEXUAL DIFFERENTIATION I

The sex (male or female) of a normal adult depends on three factors: the genetic constitution (the genotype XX in females, XY in males), the external appearance of the genitalia (the phenotype), and for each individual the identification of their sexual role (the gender). If there is any imbalance of these three factors, abnormal sexual development can occur. In paediatric practice the problems relate to abnormalities of either the external genitalia or of the genetic constitution. These disorders are usually either noticed at birth, when the sexual phenotype is uncertain, or around puberty, when there is an abnormal pattern of sexual maturation.

NORMAL SEXUAL DEVELOPMENT

Sexual differentiation

The basic pattern of sexual development is always female; this is only overridden by the presence of a Y chromosome carrying a gene which encodes the testes determining factor (TDF), a DNA binding protein which stimulates the undifferentiated gonad to develop into a testis. In turn, Müllerian inhibiting factor (MIF) is secreted by Sertoli cells which inhibits the differentiation of the Müllerian ducts into a uterus and fallopian tubes whilst Leydig cells secrete testosterone which maintains the Wolffian duct and the development of the internal male genitalia. Testosterone that is secreted into the circulation is converted to dihydrotestosterone (DHT) which virilises the basic female pattern of external genitalia. When there is no TDF (usually because the Y chromosome is absent), the undifferentiated gonad becomes an ovary and the Müllerian duct differentiates into female internal genitalia and the external genitalia remain female. Most of this process occurs in the first 12 weeks of a pregnancy.

Puberty

Puberty is the period when sexual maturation occurs. Tanner in 1962 divided it into five stages. The first endocrinological event in puberty is increased gonadotrophin secretion secondary to increased pulsatile secretion of GRH. The LH and FSH from the anterior pituitary stimulate sex hormone production from the gonad. The age of onset of puberty can be influenced by both socioeconomic and racial factors. In the UK the mean age of onset for girls is 11.4 years and in boys 12 years. The first sign of puberty in a girl is breast development, together with an increased growth velocity which reaches a peak when the breasts are

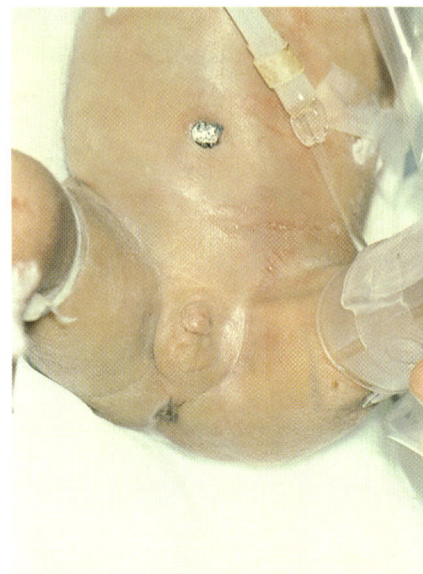

Fig. 1 **Ambiguous genitalia.**

Tanner stage 2–3. Menarche occurs late in puberty when breast development is around stage 4. In boys the first sign of puberty is testicular enlargement (i.e. larger than 4 ml) and this is usually associated with a slight growth deceleration. When the testes have reached volumes of 10 ml the growth spurt starts. Disturbances in the normal process of maturation result in precocious or delayed sexual development.

AMBIGUOUS GENITALIA

When a baby is born with ambiguous genitalia whose sex is uncertain (Fig. 1), the management of that baby is a medical and social emergency. Although an appropriate gender will be established, and the parents should be told that their child has a sex, it may take time to determine this. The baby's birth should not be registered (because the sex of the child on the register cannot be changed subsequently). The parents may wish to give the baby a name appropriate to either sex (e.g. Chris or Jo). Cases of ambiguous genitalia are either masculinised genetic females (female pseudohermaphrodites) or incompletely masculinised genetic males (male pseudohermaphrodites) (Table 1).

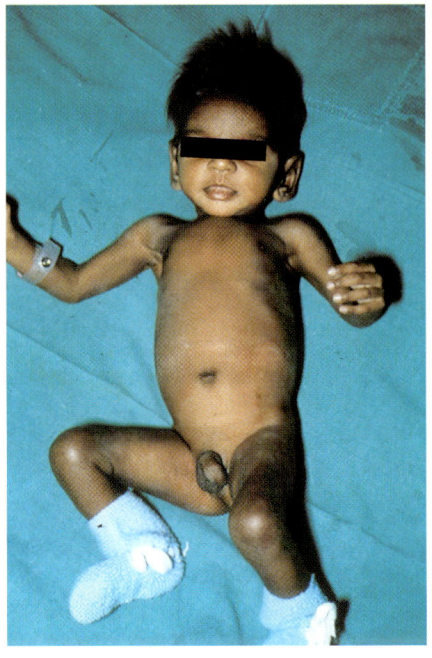

Fig. 2 **Virilised male due to congenital adrenal hyperplasia.**

Differential diagnosis of ambiguous genitalia

Female pseudohermaphrodite

The most common cause of this by far is congenital adrenal hyperplasia (CAH). In this condition there is an inherited metabolic block in the synthesis of cortisol from cholesterol. 95% of cases of CAH are due to 21 hydroxylose deficiency. The cortisol precursor is 17 hydroxy progesterone (17 OHP) which is hugely raised in the plasma. This is converted to androstenedione and then to testosterone which causes virilisation of the external genitalia. The cortisol deficiency causes an increased production of ACTH by the pituitary from negative feedback. This causes adrenal hyperplasia which results in continued excessive production of androgens.

When an affected female is born, because of the excessive androgen production, there is a variable degree of virilisation — enlarged clitoris, labial fusion. Affected males, despite high levels of testosterone, may have anatomically normal genitalia at birth, although there may

Table 1 **Clinical differences between a male and female pseudohermaphrodite**

	Female pseudohermaphrodite	Male pseudohermaphrodite
Genitalia	Clitoromegaly/penis with hypospadias	Variable phallic development
Labia	Variable fusion	Variable labial scrotal fold fusion
Gonads	Not palpable	Gonads in inguinal regions
Internal genitalia	Vagina, cervix and uterus present	Orifice in perineum opening into urogenital sinus or blind-ending vagina
Chromosome karyotype	46 XX	46 XXY

be a greater degree of pigmentation (Fig. 2). Many children with this condition also lack mineralocorticoids and in the second week of life become severely salt depleted and collapse with vomiting, dehydration and hyponatraemia, a medical emergency that needs prompt diagnosis and treatment. All forms of CAH are inherited in an autosomal recessive manner and occur equally in both sexes. Affected girls and salt-losing boys with CAH present in the first weeks of life; non-salt-losing boys are often not diagnosed until they present with advanced growth and premature sexual development from the excess amounts of androgens. The condition is diagnosed by determining the chromosome karyotype and measuring the raised plasma 17 OHP and ACTH levels together with the plasma sodium and potassium. Management of CAH consists of initial resuscitation and correction of the salt deficit if present, followed by mineralocorticoid treatment and corticosteroid replacement therapy (Table 2). The correct sexual identity has to be established, and the long-term management planned with the parents.

Table 2 **Emergency management of salt losing state in congenital adrenal hyperplasia**

- Resuscitate with i.v. albumin, normal saline
- Correct hypoglycaemia
- Treat with corticosteroids and mineralocorticoids

Male pseudohermaphrodite

This relatively rare state occurs when an individual has testicular tissue and a karyotype which usually contains a Y chromosome but has been incompletely virilised. There are numerous causes of this condition and a wide range of genital anomalies:

- Gonadal dysgenesis: this group includes true hermaphrodites, i.e. individuals with testicular and ovarian tissue. There is always a high risk of gonadal malignancy in these cases.
- Production of abnormal testosterone levels, e.g. from hormone secreting tumours.
- Normal testosterone production with abnormal response.
- Biosynthetic defects such as gonadotrophin (LH and FSH) deficiency, e.g. Kallman's syndrome.

In these cases, as well as establishing a definitive diagnosis, great skill is needed to determine which sex the child should be reared as. If it is unlikely that surgery will be able to create a boy who can stand up to pass urine and, as an adult, a male able to achieve and enjoy normal 'male' sexual function, then it may be much more appropriate and ultimately more fulfilling for that child to be raised as a female. Such a decision is only taken after informed discussions between the parents and an experienced team of paediatric urologists, paediatric endocrinologists and in some situations geneticists and psychologists.

TESTICULAR FEMINISATION SYNDROME (COMPLETE ANDROGEN INSENSITIVITY)

This is a rare X-linked condition where there is a metabolic block in the activation of androgens in the tissues. An affected individual has female looking external genitalia, but is a genetic male with testes. Presentation is usually in late childhood or young adult life and can be with an inguinal hernia which is found to contain a gonad (a testis) at surgery. Otherwise, the testes may be palpable in the labia majora. Ideally, those testes should be left *in situ* so that any testosterone and oestrogen production can help to effect a satisfactory puberty. They need to be removed after puberty because there is increased chance of malignant change after the age of 30. These individuals are always brought up as girls. Imaging of their pelvis shows they have a blind ending vagina but no fallopian ducts or uterus. They virtually always require oestrogen replacement therapy.

SEX CHROMOSOME ANOMALIES

These anomalies usually result from non-disjunction of sex chromosomes during metagenesis in one or other parent.

Klinefelter syndrome

Karyotype 47 XXY. This is a relatively common condition which occurs in approximately 1 in 500 males. Most cases are detected in late childhood, the testes are small and there are associated long limbs. Spermatogenesis is impaired and there is usually associated infertility.

Turner's syndrome

Karyotype 45 XO. This condition occurs in approximately 1 in 2500 female fetuses. It can be diagnosed at birth if the characteristic lymphoedema of the feet and hands is noticed and a chromosomal analysis is undertaken. Other clinical features which become more obvious as the child gets older include a short, wide, webbed neck, a broad chest with widely spaced nipples, an increased carrying angle at the elbow (cubitus valgus), and short stature (see p. 97). There can be associated cardiac anomalies such as coarctation of the aorta. The uterus and vagina may be small and the gonads are rudimentary streaks. Secondary sexual characteristics usually do not appear. Hormone therapy is given for breast development and to induce menstruation. Most cases of Turner's syndrome are infertile. The characteristic short stature is currently treated with growth hormone at a young age in order to maximise height.

UNDESCENDED TESTIS

The testis descends from the urogenital ridge to the scrotum in two phases. The first transabdominal migration is dependent on MIF whereas the second stage of inguino-scrotal descent is dependent on androgens. The processus vaginalis (a peritoneal extension) elongates into the gubernaculum which migrates into the scrotum. Between weeks 26 and 28 of gestation the testis descends through the processus vaginalis into the inguinal canal and reaches the scrotum by 35 to 40 weeks. An undescended testis is one that does not sit in the scrotum and cannot be manipulated into the scrotal sac. The other sites for a testis are: intra-abdominal, intracanalicular (within the inguinal canal), in the superficial inguinal pouch, or it can lie outside the normal line of descent of the testis (an ectopic testis which is rare). An undescended testis has to be differentiated from a retractile testis (very common) which is a testis that has descended but because of an active cremasteric reflex stimulated by cold, anxiety or local stimulation retracts out of the scrotum. Undescended testes are common in infants of less than 32 weeks' gestation. The majority of these descend by term. If a testis has not descended by 3 months post-term, it will stay undescended until it is treated. A complication of an undescended testis is an inguinal hernia. The undescended testis delays the closure of the processus vaginalis by holding it open which may cause bowel to herniate through and cause a symptomatic indirect inguinal hernia. These herniae are at high risk of strangulating and always need prompt surgical repair together with orchidopexy if necessary. The best age for an uncomplicated orchidopexy is 9 to 12 months.

ABNORMAL PUBERTY

Puberty can be abnormal either because it occurs too early (precocious puberty) or too late (delayed puberty). Normal pubertal development is a steady, harmonious process. If there is a divergence away from this progression, i.e. loss of consonance, that is also an abnormal puberty.

Early puberty

There are two conditions of early puberty — isolated premature thelarche and precocious puberty.

Isolated premature thelarche is a common, harmless, self-limiting condition comprising unilateral or bilateral breast

SEXUAL DIFFERENTIATION II

development. It usually occurs in the first 2 years of life and is thought perhaps to relate to oestrogen in the mother's milk, the episodic formation of ovarian cysts producing oestrogen, or increased sensitivity of the breast tissue to oestradiol stimulation. In a typical case there is unilateral breast development which waxes and wanes every 4 to 6 weeks. There are no other signs of puberty, no pubic or axillary hair, growth velocity is normal and there is no evidence of advanced bone age. The management is first to diagnose and then to reassure.

Precocious puberty (Fig. 3) is due to either central (gonadotrophin dependent) precocious puberty, i.e. activation of the whole hypothalamic-pituitary-gonadal axis where a normal pattern of puberty occurs early, or pseudopuberty, where there is the development of early disorganised puberty resulting from sex steroid production independent of the axis arising from, for example, the adrenal glands or gonads. Puberty is considered precocious if it occurs in girls younger than 8 years and boys younger than 9 years (Table 3).

The McCune–Albright syndrome, almost always seen in females, is rare. These girls have hyperpigmented patches, bone lesions with X-ray changes of polyostotic fibrous dysplasia and multiple endocrinopathies which often present with precocious puberty.

The management of both central precocious puberty and precocious pseudopuberty is directed toward treating the underlying cause. In central precocious puberty, if no cause is found, many factors have to be determined before deciding whether or not to suppress gonadotrophin secretion, e.g. age of child, rate of progression and social state. Currently, the management is with GnRH analogues, which are specific and effective in switching off central precocious puberty by blocking the action of naturally occurring GnRH from the hypothalamus. Treatment is stopped when the time is appropriate for puberty to progress.

Delayed puberty

In girls, delayed puberty is an onset of puberty later than 14 years and in boys later than 14.5 years. The most common cause of delayed puberty is constitutional delay of growth in puberty, when pubertal development and growth occur at the edge of the normal range. The problem is more pronounced in boys who have their growth spurt relatively late on in puberty so when puberty is delayed there are concerns about short stature. These boys require reassurance that they will attain a satisfactory final height. Chronic disease, such as coeliac disease, asthma, inflammatory bowel disease and juvenile rheumatoid arthritis are often associated with delayed puberty. The main distinction to make in delayed puberty is between constitutional delay (above) and hypogonadotrophic hypogonadism, i.e. deficiency of gonadotrophin releasing hormone which can present as either failure to enter puberty, failure to progress in puberty for a period of 18 months or more, or failure to attain normal reproductive function (Table 4).

Table 3 Causes of pathological precocious puberty

Central precocious puberty	95% of these cases occur in girls in whom the majority are idiopathic. In males 50% of cases are due to CNS tumours and 50% are idiopathic: • idiopathic • CNS lesions (e.g. trauma, tumours, raised intracranial pressure) • neurofibromatosis • gonadotrophin producing tumours
Pseudopuberty	In males and females congenital adrenal hyperplasia is the most common cause: • adrenal: congenital adrenal hypoplasia, adrenocorticoid tumours, Cushing's syndrome • gonadal: ovarian tumours, testicular tumours • ingestion of sex steroid (accident or child abuse) • primary hypothyroidism
McCune–Albright syndrome	A gonadotrophin independent precocious puberty

Table 4 Causes of delayed puberty

General	Constitutional delay Malnutrition Chronic diseases, e.g. diabetes mellitus, cystic fibrosis, renal failure, coeliac disease
Hypothalamic	Intensive sports training Anorexia nervosa Hypogonadotrophic hypogonadism Kallmann syndrome } Rare Cranial irradiation
Pituitary	Complete/partial hypopituitarism Tumours, e.g. craniopharyngioma Langerhans cell histiocytosis } Rare Cranial surgery/irradiation
Gonadal	Turner's syndrome Down's syndrome Chemotherapy — rare

Treatment of delayed puberty includes treating any systemic disease appropriately.
Endocrine therapies can be used to closely mimic the physiological hormone levels found in normal puberty so that puberty can progress. In boys testosterone preparations are used and in girls ethinyloestradiol is used to induce puberty.

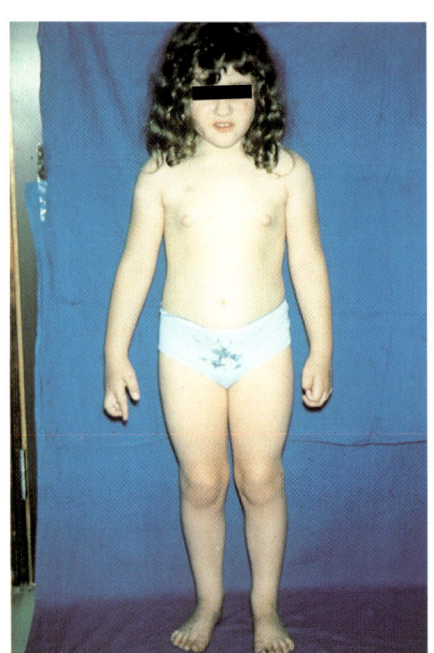

Fig. 3 **Precocious puberty.**

Sexual differentiation

- In cases of intersex, decisions regarding allocation of gender should not be rushed.
- Both early and delayed puberty can cause great distress.
- Puberty should follow a normal physiological progression.
- Undescended testes are at increased risk of torsion and malignant change.

PAEDIATRICS IN THE DEVELOPING WORLD

THE MALNOURISHED CHILD

INTRODUCTION

Protein energy malnutrition (PEM) results when the body's need for protein, energy fuels or both cannot be satisfied by the diet. The origin of PEM can be primary (when it is the result of inadequate food intake) or secondary (when it is the result of other disease that prevents adequate nutrition). The conditions likely to have a role in the production of secondary PEM are covered elsewhere in the book. The causes of primary PEM are shown in Figure 1. All age groups can be affected, but the condition is seen most frequently among infants, especially premature and LBW children. Chronic intake of insufficient food can result in marasmus, which is the most common form of severe PEM before one year of age. The oedematous form of the disease (kwashiorkor) is more frequent after 18 months of age and typically occur in children who are fed diets consisting of starchy gruel, diluted cereal-based beverages and vegetable foods.

PATHOPHYSIOLOGY AND ADAPTIVE RESPONSES

The full picture of PEM develops gradually over many days or months. This process allows a series of metabolic and behavioural adjustments that result in decreased nutrient demands and a nutritional equilibrium compatible with a lower level of cellular nutrient availability. Typical changes include:

1. Decreased interactions with the physical and social environment.

2. Alterations in protein metabolism:
   - decreased protein synthesis in viscera and muscles
   - increase in muscle protein catabolism to increase amino acid availability for essential protein production
   - recycling of amino acids and a reduction in urea synthesis
   - adaptive changes at the intracellular level in relation to energy and protein metabolism.
   - the rate of albumin breakdown decreases
   - shift of albumin from the extravascular to the intravascular pool.

   When adaptive mechanisms fail, the concentration of serum proteins decreases, especially albumin. The reduction in intravascular oncotic pressure and outflow of water into the extravascular space contributes to the development of oedema in kwashiorkor.

3. A variety of endocrine changes which contribute to:
   - increased glycolysis, lipolysis and amino acid mobilisation
   - decreased storage of glycogen, fats and protein
   - decreased energy expenditure.

4. Changes to cardiovascular and renal function:
   - decreased cardiac work and functional reserve
   - preservation of central circulation at the expense of peripheral circulation (leading to postural hypotension and eventually peripheral circulatory failure)
   - renal perfusion decreases but water clearance and the ability to concentrate and acidify urine appear unimpaired.

5. Changes to the immune system:
   - marked depletion of lymphocytes from the thymus and atrophy of the gland
   - altered complement function, and opsonic function of the serum
   - impaired phagocytosis, chemotaxis, and intracellular killing
   - circulating levels of B cells and immunoglobulins are maintained
   - there is an increased susceptibility to infection.

6. Changes in gastrointestinal function:
   - reduction in gastric, pancreatic and bile products as well as brush border enzyme activity
   - impaired intestinal absorption of lipids and disaccharide and a

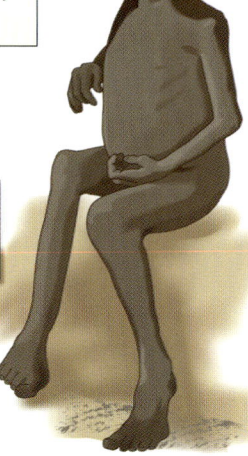

Biological factors
- maternal malnutrition prior to and/or during pregnancy
- infectious diseases, e.g. diarrheal diseases, measles, by producing anorexia and a catabolic state
- poor diet, e.g. use of over diluted milk formula or bulky vegetable foods that have low nutrient densities

Environmental factors
- climatic conditions/natural disasters
- man-made catastrophes such as war and forced migrations
- overcrowded and/or unsanitary living conditions
- poor agricultural practises
- poverty
- inadequate medical facilities

Social problems
- cultural and social practices that impose food taboos
- migration from traditional rural settings to urban slums

Ignorance
- poor infant- and child-rearing practices, e.g. inappropriate use of bottle milk
- misconception about the use of certain food
- improper food distribution among the family members

Fig. 1 **Characteristic features of marasmic kwashiorkur.**

decreased rate of glucose absorption
  – diarrhoea (secondary to malabsorption, altered intestinal motility and or bacterial overgrowth)
  – fat accumulation in the liver.

7. Changes in the central and peripheral nervous systems. Brain growth, nerve myelination, neurotransmitter production, and velocity of nervous conduction are all impaired.

This combination of changes can in time result in death. However, death can occur much more rapidly when the PEM is complicated by another illness, e.g. a respiratory infection. The mortality in severe PEM is around 40% and is highest in those children under 6 months who are markedly underweight.

ASSESSMENT OF NUTRITIONAL STATUS

In order to confirm the diagnosis of PEM and to plan treatment it is necessary to make an assessment of the child's nutrition. This should start with a dietary history. It is important to focus on early feeding practice, particularly:

- whether the child was breast fed and for how long
- when the child was weaned and what food the child has been offered.

This information has to be supplemented with details of how well the diet has been tolerated and whether there have been intercurrent illnesses.

ANTHROPOMETRC MEASUREMENTS

In children with evidence of PEM it is standard practice to grade the severity of their malnutrition. This is done by comparing the percentage difference in height or weight (or other body measurement) in comparison to a standard. A number of systems exist and all have shortcomings. However, they do permit individuals to be assessed in a simple but objective fashion. For example, the Gomez classification characterizes children according to weight in relation to the weight of a 'normal' child of the same age. In this classification, the 50th centile of the Boston standard is used as a reference standard. The pitfalls of this particular method (e.g. misclassifying oedematous children into less severe grades) are obvious but it does have strengths as a public health and epidemiological tool. In this system children are graded as summarized in Table 1.

Table 1 **Gomez classification system**

Weight for age (% of reference)	Wt. of subject / Wt. of normal child of same age × 100
90–110	Normal
75–89	Grade I – mild malnutrition
60–74	Grade II – mod. malnutrition
less than 60	Grade III – severe malnutrition

CLINICAL ASSESSMENT

At an individual level, clinical examination is important to ensure that an accurate diagnosis is reached not only in relation to nutritional status, but also in relation to the presence of other problems.

Some of the characteristic features of PEM are shown in Figure 2.

TREATMENT OF PEM

Uncomplicated cases should be treated outside hospital in order to reduce the risk of cross-infection. Hospital admission is required for those with severe PEM (as defined by the clinical picture or anthropomorphic measurements), total anorexia requiring nasogastric feeding, and cases with complications (e.g. intercurrent infection).

Treatment strategies can be divided into three stages:

- resolving life-threatening conditions
- homeostatic restoration of nutritional status
- nutritional rehabilitation.

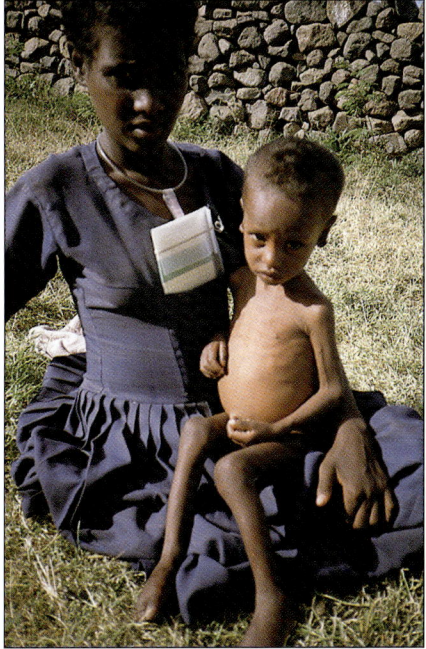

Fig. 2 **Gross wasting and ascites typical of PEM.**

Resolving life-threatening conditions
The following may require specific therapy:

- Fluid and electrolyte disturbances: these occur mainly when diarrhoea is a complicating factor. Cautious oral rehydration (or nasogastric for those refusing oral intake) is the method of choice.
- Infections: in severe PEM, clinical signs of infection may be absent.
- Cardiac failure (onset may be after rehydration).
- Severe anaemia.
- Hypothermia and hypoglycaemia.

Homeostatic restoration of nutritional status
In order to restore the nutritional status, a caloric intake of 180–200/kg/24 hours and a protein intake of 3–4 gm/kg/24 hours should be provided for the child. Gradual increment of the calorie and protein intake to attain the goal over 5–7 days should be planned to avoid intolerance, especially in severe cases. Weight will be the same or decrease in the first week, and increase by seven to fifteen days. Subjective improvements, such as an increase in appetite and interest in the environment, can be seen in the first week of management.

Nutritional rehabilitation
Introduce traditional foods with 120–150 kcal/kg and 3–4 gm of protein/kg/day.

PREVENTION

Given the huge range of factors involved in the aetiology of PEM, preventive measures are the responsibility of a large number of individuals and organisations. Attempts, at every level, to ensure that PEM is avoided are to be welcomed as they prevent not only the short-term effects of the condition, but also the long-term ramifications on child growth and well being as an adult.

The malnourished child

- Parasite infections may accompany PEM and, if untreated, impair recovery.
- Associated vitamin deficiencies may need treatment.
- Remember to check for the presence of problems such as TB which can be exacerbated by malnutrition.

GASTROINTESTINAL INFECTION

BACKGROUND

Acute diarrhoea, vomiting and abdominal pain are common symptoms in all young children around the world. However, children are at particular risk in disadvantaged countries, where acute gastroenteritis causes an estimated 10 million child deaths per year. This is because:

- where unclean water supplies and poor sanitation exist gut organisms are easily spread
- poor general health increases the vulnerability of individual children
- inadequate medical facilities may hinder treatment of complications, such as dehydration, which then becomes life threatening.

Therefore, this chapter will concentrate on those aspects of gastrointestinal infection that are of particular relevance to Developing Countries.

ACUTE GASTROENTERITIS

In about 70% of cases acute gastroenteritis are caused by viral pathogens, particularly rotavirus. In these cases the main symptoms are vomiting, watery diarrhoea and cramping abdominal pain. The remaining cases are caused by a variety of other pathogens, including *Salmonella typhi*, *Shigella* species, and *Vibrio cholera*. These bacterial pathogens often cause a more severe systemic upset, although each tends to have a fairly characteristic pattern of associated symptoms (e.g. cholera: profuse, watery diarrhoea; dysentery: blood in the stools). The most important complication common to all these conditions is dehydration (assessment of dehydration is covered on p. 66).

Treatment

The mainstay of treatment is oral rehydration using World Health Organisation (WHO) oral rehydration solution (ORS). This is made by mixing sachets, containing a mixture of electrolytes and sugar, with a set quantity of clean water. The sodium content is most important as active transport of this ion leads to associated uptake of water.

Where there is no significant dehydration (< 5%) the child can be treated with ORS at home. If there is moderate dehydation present (5-9%) the child should be given 75ml/kg of ORS over 4 hours, and then reassessed. In those unable to drink, a nasogastric tube should be used, and

where vomiting is a problem, very small, frequent amounts of ORS should be given. If severely dehydrated (≥ 10%) the child should receive intravenous rehydration with, for example, Ringer lactate solution. Similarly, intravenous fluid is required for children who have evidence of shock or who are unconscious.

The child should be reassessed at 4 hours. In those children who have adequate hydration, milk and solid feeds (in normal maintenance volumes and undiluted) can be reintroduced. In addition, oral rehydration fluid (10 ml/kg) must be given each time the child passes a loose stool. If the hydration state remains inadequate, a further 4 hours of the initial rehydration regime (described above) should commence before further reassessment.

Additional points

- If the child is hypernatraemic, rehydration must occur more slowly, over 12 hours, to reduce risk of seizures caused by rapid fluid shifts.
- Do NOT stop breast feeding during rehydration.
- NEVER give anti-diarrhoeal or anti-emetic agents to children, as these can make the child sleepy and cause severe side effects.
- Admission to hospital is required if the following are present:
  – severe dehydration
  – persistent vomiting

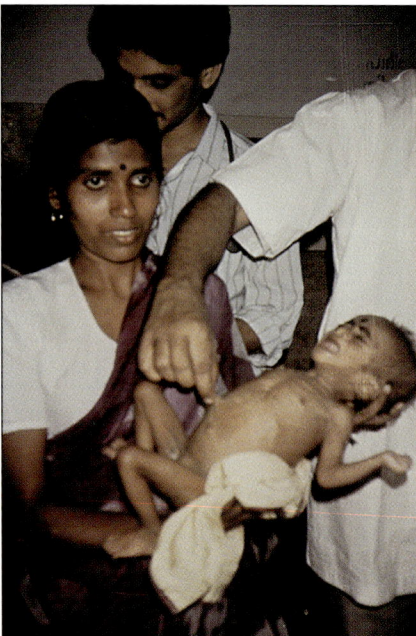

Fig. 1 **The reduced skin elasticity in this child indicates severe dehydration and the need for intravenous fluid.**

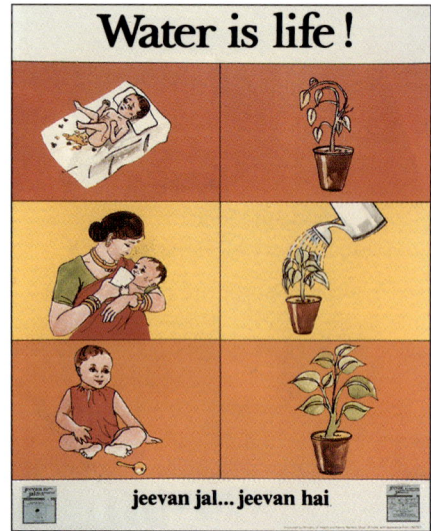

Fig. 2 **Education about the dangers of fluid loss, as in this poster from India, can help prevent severe cases dehydration.**

  – irritability or drowsiness
  – age ≤6 months.
- Antibiotics are not usually needed, and may do harm, unless treating a proven pathogen (e.g. salmonella or campylobacter).

CHRONIC GASTROINTESTINAL INFECTION

Giardiasis

This is an infection of the lumen of the small intestine with the flagellate protozoa *Giardia lamblia*. It occurs in all parts of the world, with the highest levels of endemicity occurring in areas with poor levels of sanitation, and particularly in disadvantaged countries. Infection follows ingestion of viable cysts of the parasite from contaminated food or water. Giardiasis is more frequently symptomatic in children than in adults. Symptoms begin with an acute onset after an incubation period of about 8 days. Typically these include diarrhoea, weight loss and cramping abdominal pain. There may be spontaneous resolution at this point but other affected individuals go on to suffer protracted diarrhoea with malabsorption. The diagnosis is made by demonstration of *G. lamblia* trophozoites or cysts from fecal or duodenal samples. (When the parasite cannot be found by any of these methods but giardiasis is still suspected on clinical grounds, treatment may be indicated.) Treatment is with metronidazole or tinidazole. Prevention requires good sanitation and clean water supplies.

Amoebiasis

This is an infection caused by the amoeba *Entamoeba histolytica*. It has a worldwide distribution but is more prevalent in tropical areas. Infection is established by ingestion of parasite cysts, which are resistant to gastric acidity and digestive enzymes. Excystation occurs in the small intestine to form trophozoites that colonize the lumen of the large intestine. Motile trophozoites passed with diarrhoea or dysenteric stools can survive only briefly outside the body, are destroyed by gastric secretions and, therefore, play no role in transmission. Most infected individuals are asymptomatic cyst carriers. Invasive amoebiasis leading to clinical manifestation occurs in only a small percentage (2–8%) of amoebic infections. The incubation period for amoebic dysentery is usually 7–21 days and the onset of symptoms is usually gradual. These include severe abdominal cramps, fever (nearly 30% of patients), prostration, nausea, headache and tenesmus. The stool contains blood and mucus. The course is typically chronic or subacute. Complications include amoebic liver abscess and local perforation. Diagnosis is made by identifying cysts or trophozoites of *E. histolytica* in the stool. Treatment is with metronidazole or tinidazole. Prevention requires good sanitation and clean water supplies.

Ascariasis

This infection is caused by *Ascaris lumbricoides*, the most prevalent human form helminthiasis. In tropical countries, where moist shaded soils and inadequate sanitation afford perfect conditions, the transmission of ascariasis is continuous. There is no intermediate host. Eggs are excreted in faeces after their production by female adult worms in the distal small intestine. The eggs become capable of infection after maturation under favorable (warm, moist) soil. After ingestion by humans, the eggs hatch in the jejunum, penetrate the intestine wall, and migrate to the lungs via the venous circulation. They then break into the alveolar space, ascend to the trachea, are swallowed and develop to adults in the small intestine.

Most light infestations are asymptomatic, except for vague abdominal pain and passage of adult worms. In heavy exposure, pulmonary ascariasis may occur with characteristic features of cough, wheezing, pneumonitis and eosinophilia. Heavy infestation may rarely lead to bolus obstruction of the bowel (worm colic). Where nutrition is marginal, infestation may provoke overt signs of malnutrition.

Diagnosis is made by stool examination where the characteristic eggs can be seen on direct microscopic examination. Treatment is with agents such as piperazine or mebendazole. Prevention requires good sanitation, clean water supplies and careful washing of vegetables before serving.

Hook worm

This infection (ancylostomiasis) is caused by three species of hookworm: *Necator americanus*, *Ancylostoma duodenal* and rarely *Ancylostoma ceylanicum*. *A.duodenale* and *N. Americanus* are widely distributed in the tropics. The hallmark of hookworm disease is iron deficiency anaemia due to chronic blood loss. Factors which favour the spread of hookworm infection, and which must be dealt with by preventive programmes, include poor sanitary practices, shaded moist soil, a warm climate and a population that does not wear shoes.

Hookworm ova are passed in the faeces. Under optimal conditions of moisture and temperature, eggs hatch in 1 to 2 days, liberating the larvae. The larvae mature and are able to infect the human by penetrating the skin. The larvae gain access to the venous circulation and are carried to the lungs, where they break out in to the alveoli, migrate upward and are swallowed to reach the upper small intestine where they mature to adult worms. Infection may also be acquired by the oral route, when the larvae are present on vegetables grown in contaminated soil.

The clinical features of hook worm infection correspond to the life cycle of the organism and the intensity of infection:

- Dermatitis: penetration of the skin by the larvae can produce intense pruritus. This has been termed 'ground itch' and persists for up to two weeks.
- Pulmonary manifestations: result from the migrating larvae and are usually mild.
- Gastrointestinal manifestations: epigastric pain and loss of appetite.
- Anaemia: the hallmark of chronic hookworm disease is iron deficiency anemia, hypoalbuminaemia and oedema. It results from the chronic presence of the worms which are physically attached to the wall of the small intestine.

Diagnosis is made by finding ova on microscopy of the stool. Although supportive therapy may be needed (e.g. for anaemia), specific therapy is with mebendazole, pyrantel pamoate or albendazole.

Trichuris trichuria (the whip worm)

This is one of the most prevalent helminths in the world. It is transmitted by ingestion of eggs from faecal contaminated soil. Upon ingestion, the eggs hatch and the larvae penetrate the intestinal mucosa. After maturing into adult worms, they reattach to the caecum. Matured female worms produce eggs which are passed in faeces, where they must mature before being capable of infection. Most infestations are asymptomatic, although the parasitic effect of the worms may be important where nutrition is marginal. Those with symptomatic infections complain of vague abdominal pain and distention. Heavy infection produces blood loss, anaemia, bloody diarrhoea and rectal prolapse. Diagnosis is made by finding the characteristic barrel-shaped eggs on microcopy. Treatment is with mebendazole. Prevention once again relies on measures to break the life cycle.

Gastrointestinal infection

- Clean water and education are essential in preventing gastroenteritis.
- ORS is effective in the large majority cases.
- In cases of gastroenteritis anti-emetics and anti-diarrhoeal preparations are not helpful and can do harm.
- Parasitic infections can exacerbate malnutrition.
- Parasitic infections can have a wide range of presentations which reflect the parasites life cycle.

ACUTE FEVER I

INTRODUCTION

In general, any of the acute fevers can occur in any part of the world; however, a number of factors influence what is actually observed in any one country. These factors include:

- nature and effectiveness of immunisation programmes
- extent to which local health services are able to identify and deal with outbreaks of infection
- natural immunity
- presence of natural reservoirs and vectors.

A number of acute infections and other causes of fever have been dealt with in earlier sections. This section focuses on those infections which are a particular problem in tropical countries.

MALARIA

Malaria is a common cause of acute febrile illness in the tropics. The world-wide distribution is shown in Figure 1. Almost one-third of the world's population is exposed to the risk of infection. It is caused by an obligate intracellular protozoa of the genus *Plasmodium*. The four species that causes human malaria are: *P. falciparum*, *P. vivax*, *P. malariae* and *P. ovale*. *P. falciparum* and *P. vivax* are the most common species that infect humans.

Malaria is transmitted by the bite of an infected female *Anopheles* mosquito or through direct inoculation of infected red blood cells (i.e. congenital malaria), transfusion malaria and malaria from contaminated needles. The normal life cycle is shown in Figure 2.

In non-immune children, symptoms include drowsiness, refusal of food, headache, vomiting, myalgia, arthralgia and sudden onset high fever with or without prodromal chill. The classic febrile paroxysm is usually observed in those under five and is commonly sustained in children without immunity. Physical findings include pallor, hepatosplenomegaly and labial herpes.

A number of factors increase the risk of suffering 'severe malaria'. These include:

- delayed initiation of treatment for acute malarial attack
- children – especially those aged six months to six years
- travelers from areas of little or no malaria to high malarial areas
- infection with *P. falciparum* malaria.

A patient is regarded as having severe malaria if there are asexual forms of *P. falciparum* on a blood film and the patient has any of the following:

- a change of behaviour, confusion or drowsiness
- altered state of consciousness or coma
- convulsions
- hypoglycaemia
- acidosis
- difficulty in breathing or pulmonary oedema
- acute renal failure.
- severe anaemia (Hct <20%)
- circulatory collapse
- haemoglobinuria
- jaundice
- bleeding tendency
- prostration.

These symptoms result from interference with the capillary circulation, destruction of erythrocytes and/or toxaemia

Diagnosis

Diagnosis is by demonstration of parasites in peripheral blood:

- thick film to detect low parasitaemia
- thin film for identification of species and parasitic count (Fig. 3).

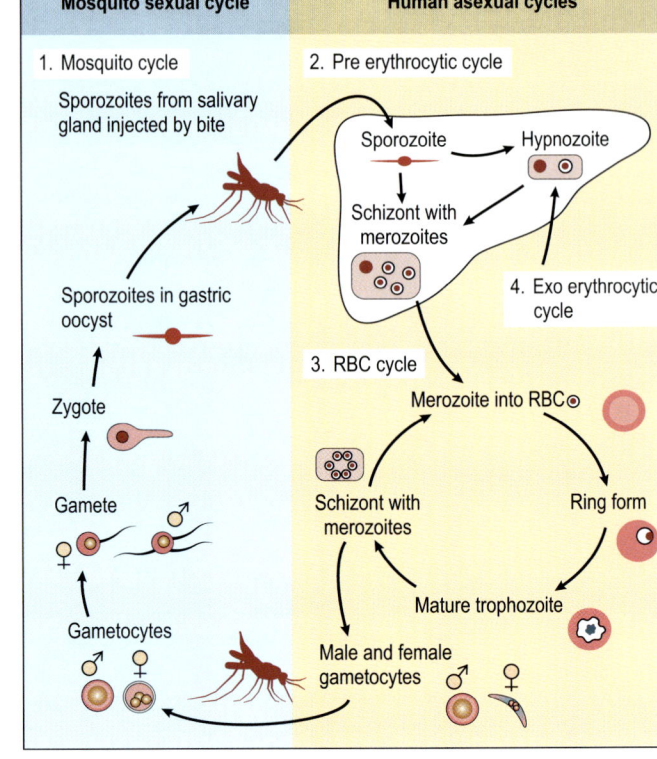

Fig. 2 **Lifecycle of the malaria parasite.** From Spicer WJ. Clinical Bacteriology, Mycology and Parasitology: An Illustrated Colour Text. Edinburgh: Churchill Livingstone; 2000.

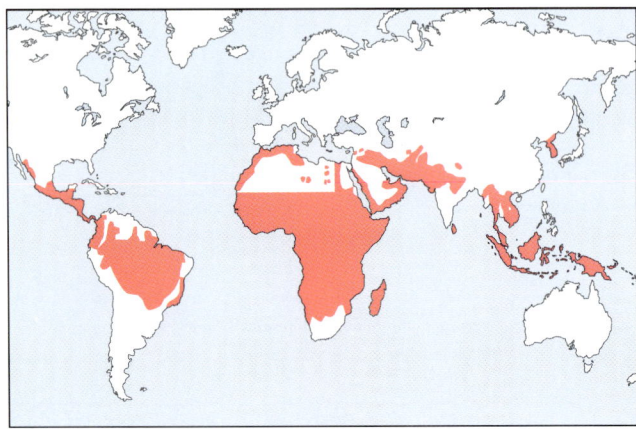

Fig. 1 **Map showing the worldwide distribution of malaria.**

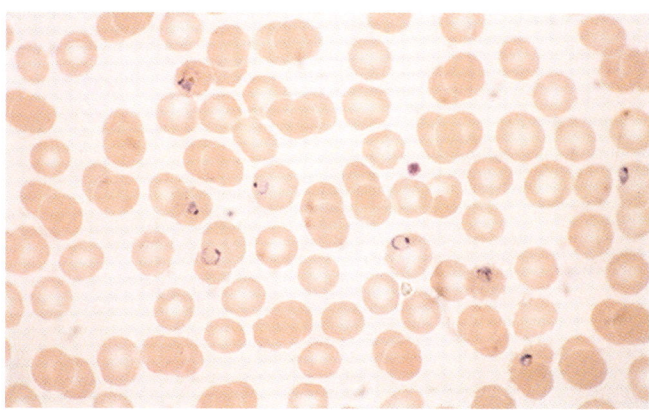

Fig. 3 **Blood film showing malarial parasites (***P. Falciparum* **'signet rings').** From Spicer WJ. Clinical Bacteriology, Mycology and Parasitology: An Illustrated Colour Text. Edinburgh: Churchill Livingstone; 2000.

Treatment

Acute malarial attack

- *P. vivax*, *P. ovale* and *P. malaria* infections and chloroquine-sensitive *P. falciparum* malaria can effectively be treated by chloroquine sulfate.
- Chloroquine-resistant *P. falciparum* malaria is effectively treated by pyrimethamine/sulfadoxime or quinine sulfate, orally.

Severe malaria

This is treated with quinine dehydrochloride by infusion. Oral therapy can be started (quinine or pyrimethamine/sulfadoxime).

Prevention

- Prevention of mosquito bites.
- Suppression of malaria parasite by chemoprophylaxis.
- Reduction or eradication of the *Anopheles* mosquito.

Living conditions may make it difficult to control exposure to mosquitos (Fig. 4).

RELAPSING FEVER (RECURRENT FEVER)

Relapsing fever is an acute febrile illness causes by spirochetes of the genus *Borrelia*, and is transmitted to man by lice or tick. There are two forms:

1. **Epidemic (louse-borne) relapsing fever** is caused by *B. recurrentis* and is transmitted from man to man by the human body louse (*Pediculus humanus*). It is a disease of poverty and commonly found at times of famine and war. Lice are not infective until 6 days after taking a blood meal, and man only becomes infected by crushing lice on the skin and not by bite.
2. **Endemic (tick-borne) relapsing fever** is caused by *B. duttoni* and is transmitted by the soft tick (genus *Ornithodorous*). Rodents are the principal reservoir. Human infection occurs when contaminated saliva or excrement is released by the tick during feeding.

The episodic nature of relapsing fever is explained by the ability of *Borrelia* organisms to continually undergo antigenic variation.

Presentation occurs after an incubation period of 2 days to 2 weeks (longer with louse-born disease), with a sudden onset of high fever, headache, photophobia, nausea, myalgia and arthralgia. CNS manifestations (lethargy, stupor, convulsion, focal neurological deficit and cranial nerve paralysis) may be the principal features of late relapse in tick-borne disease. Diagnosis is made by demonstrating the spirochetes in the blood during a febrile period.

Treatment for louse-borne disease is with erythromycin and penicillin. This invariably produces a severe reaction and hence is best done with the child in hospital. Delousing is essential in control of epidemics of louse-borne relapsing fever. In children younger than 12 years erythromycin can be used, and for older children and young adults, tetracycline is recommended.

TYPHUS

Typhus is caused by a ricketsial organism and transmission to man is by arthropods, such as lice. It occurs worldwide, but is endemic in the tropics and increases in frequency during times of war and famine. The onset is with high fever, prostration, myalgia, headache, a haemorrhagic rash and mental disturbance. The organs chiefly affected are the heart, lungs, brain and kidneys. The diagnosis must be considered in anyone with a fever of unknown origin who has been exposed to the vector. Laboratory diagnosis is serological and not always available. Treatment is with chloramphenicol.

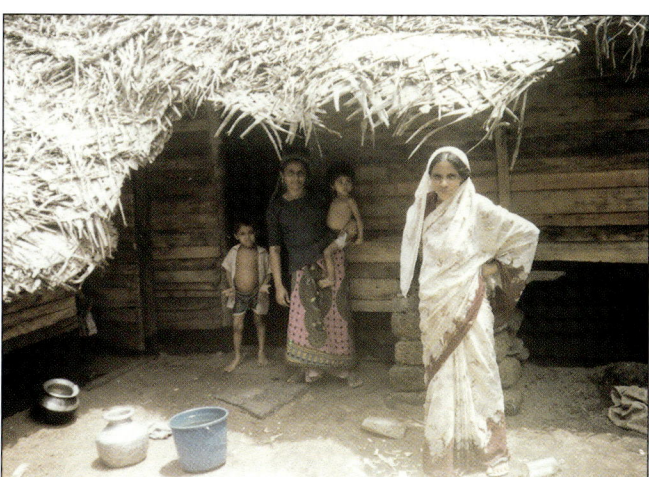

Fig. 4 **Example of the type of living conditions in which it is difficult to control exposure to mosquitoes.**

Acute fever I

- Malaria is a condition of global significance.
- During prophylaxis and in treatment against malaria it is important to be aware of resistance pattern in the area of acquisition.
- Typhus is particularly prone to appear in epidemics during periods of social disruption, e.g. during wartime when soldiers and those caught up in the conflict, such as refugees, can be affected.

ACUTE FEVER II

TYPHOID FEVER (ENTERIC FEVER)

Typhoid fever is an acute febrile illness which is spread by the faeco-oral route. It is common in Developing Countries where sanitation is inadequate. Peak incidence is in preschool children. It is caused by the Gram-negative *Salmonella typhi* and *Salmonella paratyphi* (paratyphoid fever).

The incubation period lasts a few days followed by the first phase of the illness in which abdominal symptoms dominate. Abdominal pain and diarrhoea are common at this point but constipation can occur. A septicaemic phase then occurs during which fever rises (characteristically in a step ladder fashion), usually reaching 40°C. At this stage the typical rash may be seen (erythematous papular lesions of 2 mm diameter – rose spots) Other features include headache, cough, malaise, lethargy, delirium, abdominal tenderness and meningismus. Examination may reveal hepatomegaly, splenomegaly and relative bradycardia for the degree of fever present.

Investigation

Although leucopaenia is common in the second week of disease, a definitive diagnosis is made by culture of the organism from blood or stools. Serology (Widal test) can also be helpful when a clear rise in antibody titre is seen.

Treatment

Treatment is with appropriate antibiotics. An immunization is available which will ameliorate if not prevent the disease.

CHOLERA

Although cholera is often considered, along with typhoid and paratyphoid, in the differential diagnosis of epidemic diarrhoea its presentation is quite different. The features of cholera result from its ability to induce severe diarrhoea typically containing a high concentration of potassium. Hence, hypoglycaemia and convulsions occur as a secondary consequence of the diarrhoea and dehydration; cardiac arrhythmias because of hypokalaemia. The systemic features typical of typhoid are not seen and fever, even in children, is often mild. It is important to note that not all cases are severe and, hence, severity of diarrhoea alone does not permit the diagnosis to be made with certainty.

TETANUS

The clinical picture of tetanus results from a potent neurotoxin, produced by

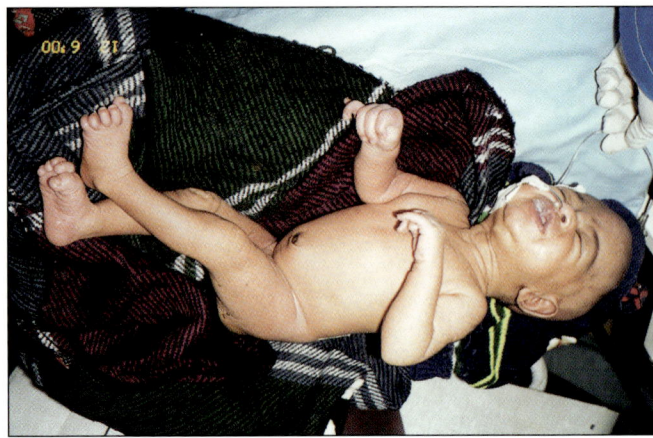

Fig. 1 **Infant suffering neonatal tetanus as a result of umbilical contamination.**

the causative organism *Clostridium tetani*. This neurotoxin prevents inhibition of spinal cord reflexes, causing increased muscle tone and rigidity, with super-imposed spasms occurring spontaneously or in response to stimulation. Early symptoms include lock jaw and, later, a grimacing faces known as 'risus sardonicus'. Mortality is high. It is a particular problem in Developing Countries because immunisation may be incomplete and spores are often plentiful in the soil. Entry into the body can occur through bites, wounds, burns or compound fractures. It can occur in neonates following contamination of the umbilicus (Fig. 1). Use of unsterilised instruments or the application of unhygienic 'dressings' (e.g. animal dung) are the usual mechanisms. Treatment is with penicillin, human tetanus immune globulin, cleansing of the wound, sedatives, muscle relaxants and careful nursing in a quiet and dark environment. Prevention is by immunisation and is highly effective.

PERTUSSIS (WHOOPING COUGH)

This bacterial infection is widespread around the world and is discussed in other parts of the book (pp. 56–59). In Developed Countries the infection is really only life threatening in non-immunised children in the first few weeks of life. In Developing Countries the combination of poor nutrition and low rates of immunisation can lead to large-scale severe outbreaks in children of all ages. However, most of those infected are under 6 years of age. The agent is highly infectious and spreads rapidly in overcrowded conditions exacerbates TB and predisposes those affected to malnutrition. Treatment is merely supportive.

Immunisation is effective but provides protection for only 3 to 5 years.

DIPHTHERIA

This condition occurs worldwide but particularly effects young children living in poor or overcrowded conditions. During the early phase of the illness the child may be toxic, but upper airway obstruction is the greatest potential source of danger. This results from a combination of inflammatory swelling and epithelial slough. At a later stage the toxin produced by the organism can lead to myocarditis and damage to a variety of peripheral nerves.

Treatment is with penicillin, antitoxin and supportive care, especially of the airway. Prevention is by immunisation with diptheria toxoid. This protects the individual from the effects of the toxin but does not prevent infection.

VIRAL HAEMORRHAGIC FEVERS

This term refers to a number of viral infections that are characterized by severe acute multi-system disease. Prominent features often include: high fever, headache, generalized myalgia, rash, diarrhoea, vomiting, confusion, fits, coma, renal failure, shock and haemorrhage from the nose, mouth and gastrointestinal tract. They are transmitted by insect vectors from mammalian reservoirs such as rodents or monkeys. Individual agents are associated with particular parts of the world, for example, yellow fever (Africa, Central America) (Fig. 2), dengue (South-East Asia), lassa fever (West Africa) and ebola virus (Central Africa). Treatment is supportive, with good nursing care and fluid resuscitation. Mortality rates are high in severe

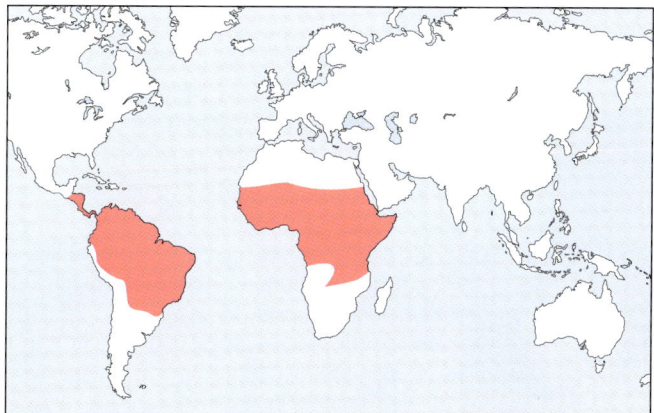

Fig. 2 **Map showing the distribution of yellow fever.**

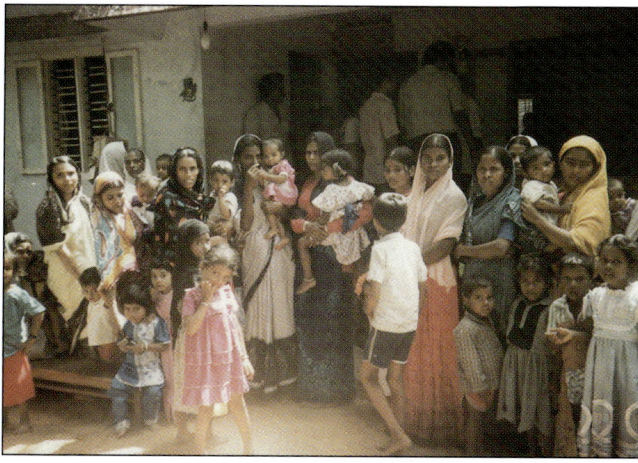

Fig. 4 **Good public health education is important in underpinning immunisation programmes.** These mothers clearly recognise the importance of attending the immunisation clinic.

cases. Immunisation is available for yellow fever and dengue.

POLIOMYELITIS

This viral infection is a major cause of disability in many countries (Fig. 3). It is an entero virus spread most commonly by the faecal–oral route. As a result, it is currently seen most commonly in those countries where sanitation is poor and immunisation rates are low. Infection may simply take the form of a severe non-specific viral infection with fever, myalgia headache and vomiting being prominent. In a proportion of cases the predisposition of the virus to attack nerves leads to anterior horn cell damage and paralysis (sensory impairment is not a feature). Death may occur during the acute phase. In those patients that suffer paralysis, some recovery may occur over a period of months. In many others, paralysis is permanent. Prevention can be achieved with immunisation, most commonly using an oral live attenuated virus.

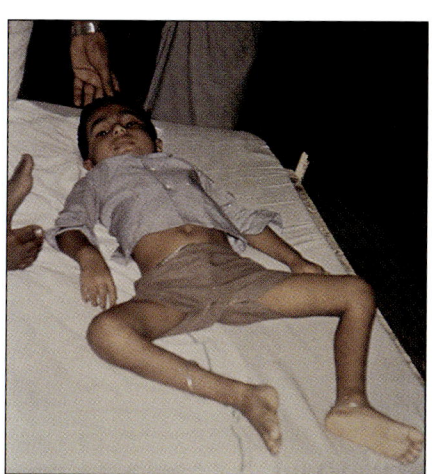

Fig. 3 **Child paralysed as a result of polio infection.**

MEASLES

This is a viral infection found throughout the world. It is associated with high fever and a characteristis rash (this is preceded by white spots on the buccal mucosa – Koplik's spots). The organism has a predilection for the respiratory tract so that pneumonia and a variety of upper respiratory complications are common. However, encephalitis and myocarditis are also well recognised. The severity of the infection reflects a variety of factors, but in particular:

- whether the child has been immunised
- the child's overall health
- the child's natural immunity.

It is in Developing Countries where the greatest numbers of vulnerable children are exposed to this condition and high rates of morbidity and mortality are common outcomes. Prevention is by immunisation.

IMMUNISATION

Immunisation programmes continue to be of major importance in the control of infectious disease (Fig. 4). However, it is important to understand that the nature and purpose of immunisations vary. For example, protection against tetanus and diphtheria is given in the form of a toxoid. A toxoid is a 'de-natured' form of the toxin which allows the individual to produce an effective anti toxin if they become infected. Infection itself is not prevented.

Immunisations designed to protect against bacterial infections often contain specific bacterial antigens to which the individual becomes primed. In some cases the protection provided (e.g. *Haemophilus influenzae*) is excellent and in others (e.g. *Bordetella pertussis*) less complete.

In general, vaccines developed to protect against viral infections are based on weakened (attenuated) strains of live viruses. They produce effective protection against acquiring the relevant organism (although the duration of protection varies). However, because they are live, they should not be given:

- to pregnant women
- individuals with immunosuppression.

Acute fever II

- Basic sanitation, reasonable living conditions and good nutrition are of major importance in reducing the incidence of acute infectious disease.
- Immunisation programmes can, where uptake is high, eradicate certain infections, e.g. smallpox.
- Education in relation to the above two points is essential to success.

CHRONIC INFECTION I

INTRODUCTION

Children within both Developed and Developing Countries are all capable of being affected by the same types of infection. However, a number of factors govern both the type of infections actually seen in a particular population and the usual clinical course. These factors include:

- Public health infrastructure: where this is well developed some diseases (e.g. those derived from infected water courses, such as schistosomiasis) can be eradicated.
- The general health of the population: individual well being can affect both whether a particular infection is acquired and its subsequent course.
- Genetic predisposition: some racial groups appear to be particularly susceptible to certain conditions (e.g. tuberculosis).
- Social structure/cultural differences: e.g. communal living can make it difficult to control the spread of infectious diseases.
- Access to medical treatment: where treatment is delayed or not given, conditions can progress far more extensively.
- Geography: some infections are dependent on intermediate vectors that are affected by climate.

Given these factors and the range of potential pathogens capable of causing chronic infection, there is no 'common presentation'. Described below are the clinical syndromes associated with some of the more important pathogens that operate in this role.

TUBERCULOSIS

This is a chronic bacterial infection caused by three species of *Mycobacteria: M. tuberculosis* is the most common. Tuberculosis has affected a third of the world population (2 billion people) with more than 80% of the burden being in Developing Countries. Droplet infection is the principal mode of transmission, while ingestion of bovine organisms may account for some cases in poor countries.

The first infection is known as primary infection and usually involves the lung or gut and the adjacent lymph nodes. In most cases, the child's immune response results in healing. In 5–15% of the infected children the condition progresses with either local extension or haematogenous spread to involve more

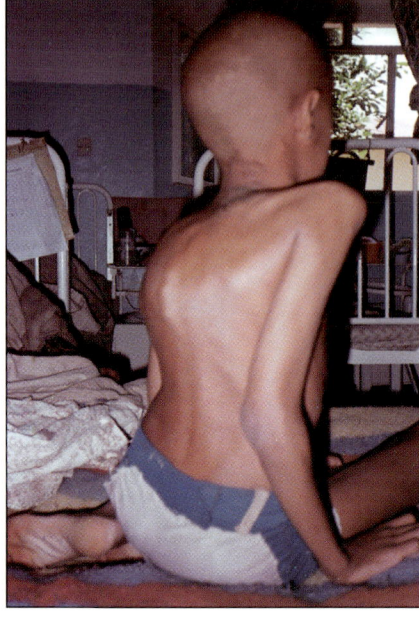

Fig. 1 **Spinal deformity caused by tuberculosis infecting and damaging the vertebrae.**

distant sites, such as lungs, lymph nodes, meninges and bones/spinal column (Fig. 1). The risk of progression is highest in younger children.

Post-primary disease in the lungs and/or other organs can occur either by endogenous reactivation of dormant bacilli in a healed primary lesion or by exogenous re-infection. Co-existing HIV infection increases the lifetime risk of progression of TB by up to 50%.

CLINICAL PRESENTATION AND DIAGNOSIS

Because the organism has the potential to affect any organ system in the body, a wide variety of clinical presentations are recognised. Although pulmonary infection is the most common, cough and haemoptysis are unusual. More common features at presentation include:

- intermittent fever
- failure to thrive
- painless swelling (any site including spine or limb where deformity may also be present)
- painless haematuria and/or pyuria
- unexplained neurological syndromes or behavioural changes.

Any of these presentations may be accompanied by erythema nodosum (Fig. 8, p. 95) or phlyctenular conjunctivitis, which are helpful in identifying the underlying diagnosis. Further confirmation can be obtained by carrying out a Mantoux test. This involves the intradermal injection of 0.1ml of 1 in 10 000 purified protein derivative (i.e. TB antigen); affected individuals mount a brisk immune response. The organism can sometimes also be identified in sputum, pus, CSF, or urine, depending on the site of infection.

In general the diagnosis of tuberculosis is made when at least two of the following are present:

- strongly suggestive symptom complex
- strong contact history with a case of open pulmonary TB
- positive Mantoux test
- compatible radiological findings

OR

- *Mycobacterium tuberculosis* seen on smear or grown
- Cyto-histological evidence of TB on needle aspiration or biopsy.

MANAGEMENT

Management is based on combination drug therapy. Nutritional supplementation will be necessary in the malnourished child. Additional measures may be required in certain cases (e.g. steroids to reduce a mediastinal lymph node

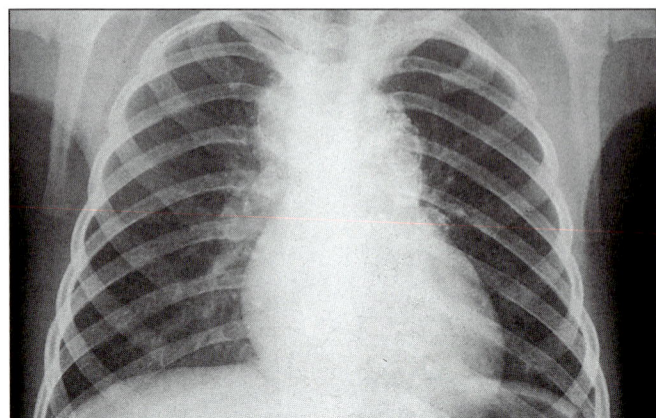

Fig. 2 **Chest X-ray showing a mass of paratracheal glands caused by TB.**

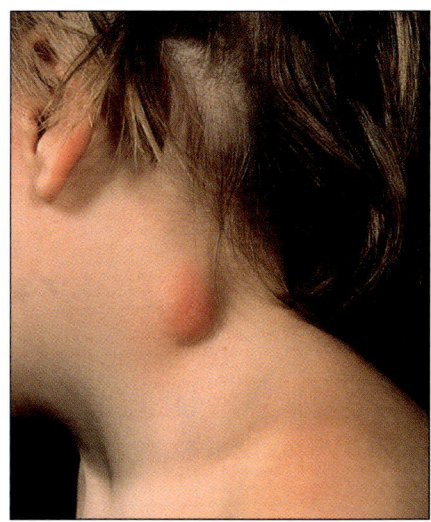

Fig. 3 Child with a 'cold abscess' as a result of TB infecting a neck gland.

mass [Fig. 2]; surgery to drain an abscess [Fig. 3]).

General measures of prevention are discussed separately (see pp. 122–3); however, pasteurization of milk and the use of mass BCG vaccination can have major impacts on the disease. The latter is contraindicated in symptomatic HIV infection/AIDS.

HIV

A WHO estimate suggests that there are 10 million children infected with HIV. Paediatric AIDS accounts for about 2% of all AIDS cases in the USA and Europe and 15–20% of all AIDS cases in Africa. It is thought the impact of these cases will increase infant and child mortality rates in Africa by 30%.

Most affected children (90%) are infected by vertical transmission (i.e. by an infected mother). Transplacental, intrapartum and postpartum routes of passage of the virus are all described. Breast feeding further increases the risk of transmitting the virus to the infant: the virus has been isolated from the breast milk of more than 73% of HIV positive mothers. The rate of vertical transmission varies in different geographic locations on the same continent, and the rate is twice as high in Africa as in Europe. This difference is still unexplained.

Clinical presentation
Vertically acquired HIV has a more rapid progression to symptomatic disease than HIV infection acquired at a later age. Initial manifestations are often non-specific, with presentations such as fever and failure to thrive, although multiple organ systems are often involved. Children display an increased incidence of bacterial

infections (not typical of adult disease) and, also unlike adults, opportunistic infections in children usually result from primary infection rather than reactivation of latent infection. Other clinical presentations in children include:

- HIV encephalopathy
- lymphocytic interstitial pneumonia (unique to children and affects 30–50% of vertically infected children)
- chronic parotitis
- hyper gamma-globulinaemia
- diarrhoea.

Table 1 **WHO clinical case definition of AIDS in children (modified – 1989)**

Major criteria	Minor criteria
Weight loss/ FTT	Generalized lymphadenopathy
Chronic diarrhoea	Oropharyngeal candidiasis
Prolonged fever	Repeated common infections
Recurrent pneumonia	Generalized pruritic dermatitis
	Confirmed maternal HIV infection
Diagnosis is made by the presence of 2 major and 2 minor criteria	

Diagnosis
Diagnosis of HIV in infants under 18 months is complicated by the persistence of maternal antibody. However, early diagnosis is important in order that anti-retroviral therapy and early prophylaxis against opportunistic infections can commence before the onset of clinical symptoms. Therefore, a diagnosis of HIV infection in infants born to an HIV positive mother is made if:

- there are AIDS defining illnesses according to WHO criteria (see Table 1) *or*
- there are suggestive clinical symptoms and laboratory evidence of immune dysfunction *or*
- HIV is cultured or the child's blood is positive for the p24 antigen (note that all virological and immunological tests may give false-negative results in the first 3-months of life in up to 50% of the cases).

The natural course of vertically acquired HIV infection is not yet fully described and the course of the disease is changing with the advent of diagnostic and therapeutic modalities. Prospective studies have suggested a bimodal clinical expression of vertical HIV infection in children:

1. early onset of rapidly progressing and fatal disease (25%–35%)
2. the remainder show a slower progression with survival into older childhood and early adolescence.

However, prospective studies in Africa show higher rates of morbidity and mortality in HIV-infected children. Possible reasons include:

- risk of infection from the environment
- poor nutrition
- poor access to standard medical care
- lack of specific therapy (e.g. antiretrovirals, immunoglobulin).

Management
The management of affected children should include access to a multidisciplinary team covering each of the following areas:

1. Supportive care:
   - counselling and psychosocial support; good nutrition (continued breast feeding in developing countries is recommended)
   - blood transfusions, haematinics/vitamins
   - chemoprophylaxis against *Pneumocystitis carinii* and toxoplasmosis
   - immunization:
     – asymptomatic – routine immunization
     – AIDS patients – all routine vaccines except BCG
     – post-exposure prophylaxis for measles and chickenpox.

2. Treatment of HIV-associated infections. TB infections are common and serious in symptomatic HIV patients. Active TB appears to enhance the rate of progression of the HIV infection.
3. Antiretroviral therapy.
4. Management of end-organ dysfunction, e.g. bone marrow failure, HIV encephalopathy.

There is good evidence that AZT given to the mother in labour and to the infant in the first few weeks after birth reduces the rate of vertical transmission.

Chronic infection I

- In relation to HIV education and prevention of infection offers the main hope of controlling the epidemic.
- Although effective treatment for TB is available, this is unlikely to control the world wide epidemic without an improvement in standards of general health and health care.

CHRONIC INFECTION II

LEPROSY

This disease is caused by the organism *Mycobacteria leprae* and mainly affects the nerves and the skin. Infection is acquired by inhalation or through abrasions in the skin. There is no animal reservoir. There are two types of infection:

1. Tuberculous characterized by strong cell-mediated immunity, localized disease with few bacteria and positive lepromin test. Clinically, individuals have a small number of hypopigmented skin lesions, which are dry, hairless and anaesthetic. Peripheral nerves such as the ulnar and median become thickened. Mutilation can result from the peripheral nerve damage.
2. Lepromatous characterized by low levels of cell-mediated immunity, large numbers of bacteria and negative lepromin test. Affected patients have a widespread macular rash with hypopigmentation on the face and extensor surfaces. The skin later becomes thickened nodular, dry and fissured.

Treatment is with dapsone or rifampicin. Prevention is by early detection and treatment to avoid spread.

TRACHOMA

This is a chlamydial conjunctivitis that is common in tropical countries. Simple therapy (e.g. erythromycin orally or tropical tetracyline or sulphanamide) is curative in the early stages. However, delayed treatment results in chronic infection and scarring of the eyelids, causing entropion. This can lead to blindness as a result of secondary corneal damage. Treatment of established entropion is surgical.

RABIES

Rabies is caused by a virus which is endemic in most parts of the world, especially in Africa. Animal reservoirs include jackals, civets, dogs and foxes. Transmission is by a bite from an infected animal. The incubation period is very variable, from 2 weeks to several years, but is usually 4 to 10 weeks. Clinical features include pain at the site of the bite, then hydrophobia (laryngeal and respiratory muscle spasm in response to attempts to drink water) leading to opisthotonus, convulsions and cardiorespiratory arrest. Spasms are precipitated by any mild stimulus. Death can occur during a spasm or by progression to flaccid paralysis and coma.

Treatment is by heavy sedation, analgesia, general supportive care and avoidance of stimuli that might produce spasms. However, the outcome of manifested rabies is poor. A rabies vaccine is available. In non-immunised individuals exposed to potential infection, prevention is by scrubbing the bite wound with soap, applying anti-viral agents such as iodine or alcohol, and administration of antiserum.

TRYPANOSOMIASIS

This is caused by an elongated protozoa which is transmitted by the tsetse fly (Fig. 1). As a result, certain lifestyles are associated with high risk of exposure, e.g. farmers and fishermen. The initial lesion (chancre) occurs on the skin as result of the insect bite. Days later there is fever, a characteristic serpiginous rash and progression to later symptoms, many of which are the result of an associated meningo-encephalitis (e.g. loss of weight, personality change and the characteristic sleepiness).

Lymphadenopathy and hepatosplenomegaly are also regularly seen. Diagnosis can be made by identifying the organisms on a thick blood film. Treatment is with suramin. Preventive programmes have focused on eradicating the insect vector.

LEISHMANIASIS

This condition is caused by a protozoa which is spread by sand flies. Rodents and dogs can act as reservoirs of infection. The species of infecting organism varies around the world and this affects the pattern of symptoms seen. Clinical features may be confined to the skin (*L. tropica* found in Africa; *L. mexicana* found in South America), or spread from skin to the viscera causing the clinical picture of kala-azar, (*L. donavani* found in Africa, South America and Asia). Visceral symptoms may be very slow to evolve (i.e. over many years) and include fever, huge swelling of the spleen (Fig. 2), hepatomegaly,

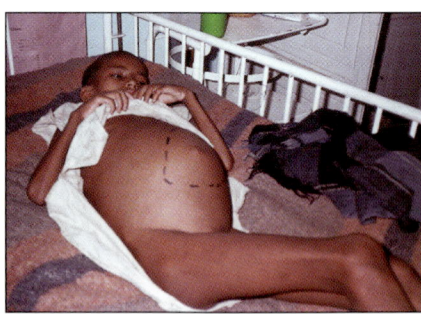

Fig. 2 **Massive splenomegaly caused by leishmaniasis.**

lymphadenopathy, cough and diarrhoea. Diagnosis is by serological means or isolation of the organism. Treatment is possible with antimony based agents; however, these can produce many side effects.

SCHISTOSOMIASIS (BILHARZIASIS)

This is a group of diseases caused by a trematode worm (fluke) and affects more than 200 million people worldwide (Fig. 3) — mainly children and young adults. There are three main species: *S. haematobium*, *S. mansoni* and *S. japonica*. Man is infected by contact with fresh water containing the cercariae (Fig. 4). They penetrate the skin, causing an itchy papular rash, and are carried in the blood stream to the liver. This stage may cause severe toxaemia and eosinophilia. The adult worm then reaches its final destination, causing a granulomatous reaction. *S. haematobium* goes to the genitourinal tract causing haematuria, dysuria and frequency, and later hydronephrosis; *S. mansoni* lodges in the gastrointestinal tract causing abdominal pain and rectal bleeding.

Diagnosis can be made by finding eggs in the urine or stool respectively (or via appropriate endoscopy). An immunological test is also available. Treatment is with a single dose of praziquantel. Control can be achieved by ensuring clean water supplies and destroying the intermediate host (a water snail).

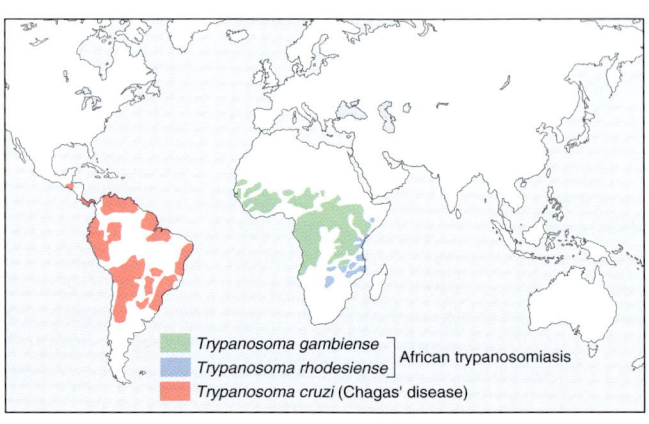

Fig. 1 **The worldwide distribution of trypanosomiasis.**

Trypanosoma gambiense / Trypanosoma rhodesiense — African trypanosomiasis
Trypanosoma cruzi (Chagas' disease)

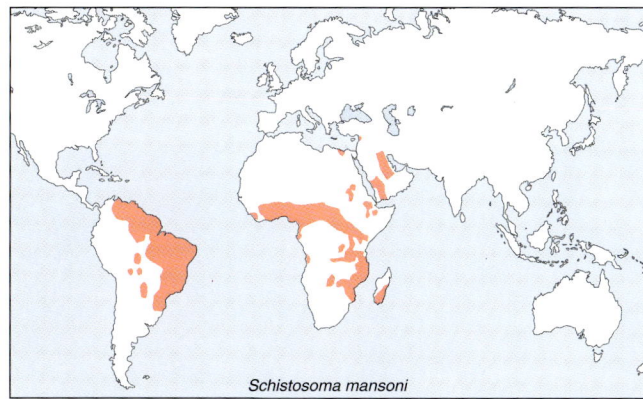

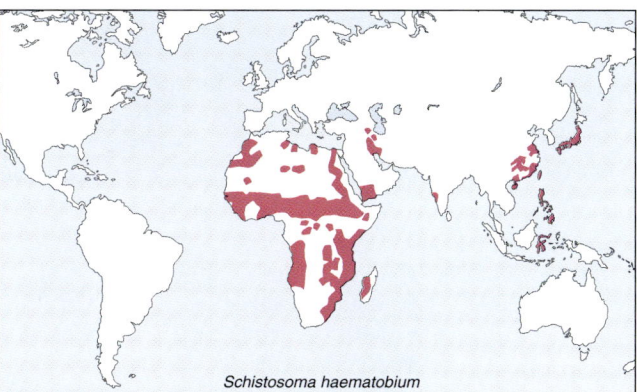

Schistosoma mansoni

Schistosoma haematobium

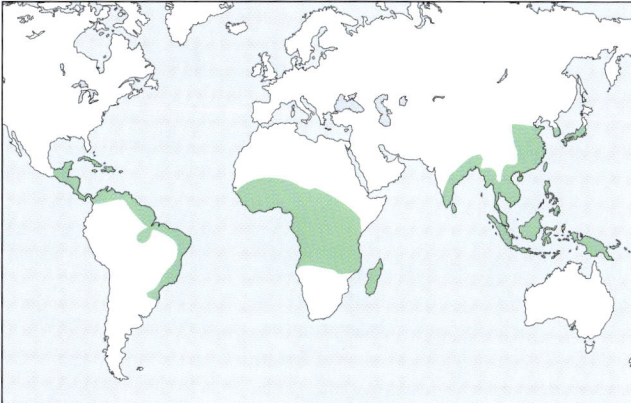

Fig. 5 **The worldwide distribution of filiariasis.**

Fig. 3 **The worldwide distribution of schistosomiasis.**

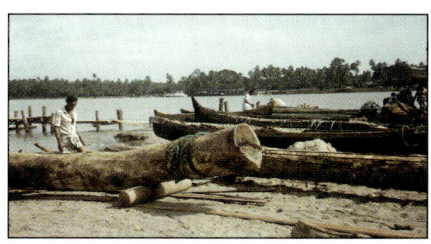

Fig. 4 **Certain occupations, such as these fishermen with their regular exposure to water, predispose to schistosomiasis.**

FILARIAL INFECTIONS

These organisms produce a range of conditions (Fig. 5). The causative agent is a worm with a complex life cycle, which is transmitted to the human blood stream by mosquito and other insect bites. Acute infection, depending on the precise nature of the infecting organism, causes fever, skin rashes, lymphangitis and myalgia. Later signs, such as eye damage and elephantiasis, are the result of chronic infection. Diagnosis is made by identifying the organisms on a thick blood film or in a skin nodule. Drug treatment is with diethylcarbazine. Prevention is achieved by controlling the appropriate insect vectors.

STREPTOCOCCAL INFECTIONS

Streptococcal infections are common in developing countries involving a variety of sites of which the pharynx and skin are the most important. Antibiotic treatment is not usually given and a variety of important, longterm, sequelae can result producing major morbidity involving, particularly, the kidneys (p. 76) and heart.

RHEUMATIC FEVER

Rheumatic fever is important since it is a major cause of acquired heart disease of children in disadvantaged countries. The condition results from an aberrant immune response to infection with Lancefield group A beta haemolytic streptococci. It is a disease of poverty. Inadequate treatment of streptococcal infections, overcrowding, bad housing and poor environmental conditions are known predisposing factors. It is most common between the ages of 5 and 15 years.

Clinical presentation and diagnosis

A history of streptococcal infection occurring 4–6 weeks before the onset of the illness may or may not be obtained. The clinical manifestations and some of diagnostic laboratory tests are defined as 'major and minor Jones criteria'.

Major manifestations include:

- Arthritis: this is migratory and affects several different joints (elbows, knees ankles and wrists). It need not be symmetrical.
- Carditis: this occurs in 40–80% of patients. Manifestations include tachycardia, valvular insufficiency, pericarditis, pericardial effusion and congestive heart failure.
- Erythema marginatum: occurs in 10–20% of cases. It starts as red maculae which fade in the center but remain red at the edges.
- Subcutaneous nodules: seen only in severe cases. They are small nodules, firm, non-tender and characteristically seen on extensor surfaces of the joints.
- Sydenham's chorea: characterized by emotional instability and involuntary movements. This is often the sole symptom. Spontaneous recovery is usual, though it may be followed by chronic cardiac disease.

Minor manifestations include:

- Polyarthralgia: pain in two or more joints without signs of inflammation. This is not counted in Jones criteria if arthritis is present.
- Fever: usually low-grade.
- Elevated acute phase reactants: ESR, C-reactive protein and leucocytosis.
- ECG changes: prolongation of PR interval.
- Evidence of recent streptococcal infection (raised ASO titre).

Two major or one major and two minor criteria justify the diagnosis of rheumatic fever.

Treatment

Treatment is largely symptomatic. However, anti inflammatory drugs are important in dealing with both the arthritis and cardiac involvement where steroids may be indicated. Subsequent healing/scarring can result in long-term heart disease requiring surgery. Children and adults who have had an attack of rheumatic fever are at increased risk of recurrence. This can be reduced by administration of regular penicillin.

Chronic infections II

- The majority of these conditions can be prevented by simple measures.
- Entropion secondary to Trachoma is a major cause of blindness in many developing countries.
- The longterm consequences of rheumatic fever on the heart may take years to become apparent.

PREVENTATIVE AND SOCIAL PAEDIATRICS IN DEVELOPING COUNTRIES

Within the Developed World there is debate about the value of measurements such as infant mortality (deaths of live births in the first year of life per 1000 live births). The differences, of 1 to 2 per thousand, between communities are often related to variation in the interpretation of the term 'live birth'. In Western European countries the infant mortality rate is about 5. These countries make no attempt to measure mortality under age 5, as deaths between ages 1 to 5 years are so few. This contrasts sharply with the situation in the Developing World. For example, in sub-Saharan African countries the rate of death under age 5 varies between 100 and 300 per 1000, and the figure is seen as a critical indicator of the well-being of children. These gross differences reflect the huge inequalities between countries in terms of economic wealth, debt, war and naturally occurring problems such as drought and crop failure.

This chapter will examine the background to these differences:

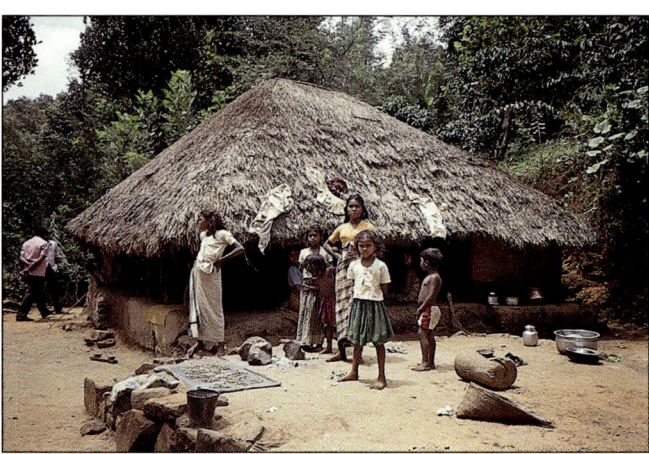

Fig. 1 **The nature of this Indian tribe house leads to children being regularly exposed to risk.**

- within the family
- in terms of the services available
- in relation to national priorities.

AT THE FAMILY LEVEL

Housing. The large majority of people in the Developing World are farmers living in rural areas. The houses are small, usually one-roomed, and made of easily available materials, perhaps mud and thatch. Animals may be brought inside at night and in cold weather. These cramped conditions increase the risk of spread of infection both between humans and from animals to human. Cooking tends to take place on an open fire, using wood or kerosene as fuel. As a result, accidents such as scalds and burns are common, and kerosene (as well as other fuels) is easily available for ingestion (see Fig. 1).

Occupation. It is usual for the entire family to help with work in the field. This puts a high degree of strain on the women of the household, who are usually responsible for fetching water (often over long distances) and other difficult tasks, while also being the chief carer of the family. Hard work over long hours and a sometimes irregular food supply, deficient in calories and essential vitamins, makes a woman more likely to have smaller babies and to have less milk, increasing the risk of ill-heath in her young children.

Organophosphates are commonly used in agriculture but storage is often inadequate, increasing the risk of ingestion (Table 1).

Family size. Where there is a high death rate among children, there is usually a corresponding high birth rate. Parents need children, and they are unlikely to reduce the number of their children until the death rate falls. However, children born too close together do not fare as well as children born after longer intervals, because of the increased demands on the mother. Evidence from around the world suggests that this cycle can be broken by improving public health measures and, as a consequence, reducing infant mortality. When parents are confident that their children will survive, the birth rate usually falls in less than a generation.

SERVICE PROVISION

It has been suggested that the following are the basic requirements for a healthy society:

- shelter
- clean water
- adequate sanitation
- adequate food
- medical help.

The first four have the greatest effect on reducing risk to health, i.e. more than providing medical care.

Water. In rural communities, water is usually obtained from a river or a spring. It may be contaminated by human and animal faeces, and also used for washing humans, animals and clothes. Water borne diseases, such as diarrhoea, are therefore spread easily. In some poor countries, each child averages 10 attacks before the age of 5 years, and diarrhoea kills 1 in 10 children. Simple rules such as defaecating well away from the water source, preferably in a latrine, and only washing downstream of the water source substantially reduces this risk. In some countries, less than 50% of the population have access to safe water, and the percentage is often far lower in rural areas.

Table 1 **Common poisonings/ingestions**

Hydrocarbons	Organophosphates

- Commonly used as fuels and included in other products
- Can be inhaled and absorbed through skin as well as swallowed
- Main risk of simple hydrocarbons is from aspiration and secondary hypoxia
- More complex products can be toxic to a variety of organs
- Management depends on the nature of the product – for simple hydrocarbons gastric emptying is not required but is indicated for aromatic compounds and those containing additives (because of potential systemic toxicity)
- Where inhalational pneumonia does occur effects may be very severe
- Because effects may be delayed always observe affected children for 24 hours
	- Commonly used insecticides
	- Can be absorbed from skin, respiratory tract and conjunctiva as well as gut
	- Acts as an anticholinesterase leading to over stimulation of relevant sites followed by blockade
	- Signs include:
	  – 'garlic breath'
	  – vomiting and diarrhoea
	  – confusion
	  – bradycardia
	  – excessive secretion of tears, saliva and from respiratory tract
	- Gastric emptying is not indicated — use measures to prevent further absorption
	- Always correct any secondary hypoxia before giving atropine (risk of arrhythmia)

Sanitation. Faeco-oral transmission is the pathway of spread of many diseases, but in many tropical countries, less than 50% of the population have adequate sanitation.

Access to health care. In rural populations, access to health care is limited, and there are few health professionals per head of population. Many people living in remote areas are unable to travel the distance required to get to a clinic. Even when clinics are not too far away, there may be inadequate provision of vaccines due to inadequate government funding (e.g. only 15% of routine vaccines are financed by the government in Ethiopia). Entire diseases can be wiped out with a simple vaccination programme. For example, in Brazil every child was vaccinated against polio on a single Saturday in 1980, and the previously high rate of paralysis fell to almost zero within weeks. People may fail to have their children vaccinated because of being too busy (in the fields dealing with the harvest), or because they have not been educated in the importance of vaccination.

Education. The rate of uptake of vaccinations and the general health of children improve dramatically when the female literacy rate increases. For example, in the state of Kerala, southern India, there is one of the highest population densities in the country, and it is not a wealthy state. However, there is almost 100% female literacy, almost all children are vaccinated, and the state has the lowest infant mortality rate in India. The female literacy rate in Ethiopia is 26% and vaccination rate is approximately 40% in the towns and less in rural areas. Educating parents to use oral rehydration solution (ORS), home made or otherwise, is one of the most effective ways of reducing child deaths from diarrhoea (Fig. 2).

Traditional beliefs. The influence of traditional beliefs and remedies is variable, with some being distinctly harmful. For instance, the practise of prelacteal feeding in new-born infants in India increases the risk of infection while reducing the calorie intake in this vulnerable group, and hampers the stimulation of breast milk in the mother. (Pre lacteal feeding is the practise of giving fluid, perhaps sugar water made from the local water supply, to a baby after birth before lactation is established.) Putting ash on eyes with conjunctivitis, a practise in Africa, causes further irritation to the eye, infection and possible scarring, while incising the face of a child with facial oedema can cause multiple abscesses.

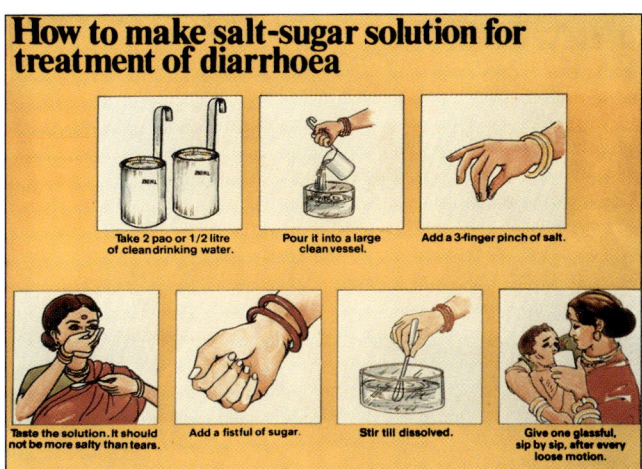

Fig. 2 **Health campaigns – such as the use of ORS – are of great importance in reducing infant mortality.**

Traditional procedures such as uvulectomy and blood letting cause injury, blood loss and risk of spread of HIV through use of undterile instuments.

NATIONAL PROBLEMS

Economics. Many Developing Countries are poor, with a low Gross Domestic Product. They are mostly agricultural, producing cash crops such as coffee, tea, sugar and grain. The big industrial nations hold most of the control on the international market, increasing the economic risk to less advantaged countries. National debts in these countries have built up over many decades, and are now a huge burden in terms of interest payments, hindering economic progress. There have been moves recently to cancel debt, but this is happening slowly and incompletely. The infant mortality rate can be directly correlated to the average income of the population: a baby born in a poor country has a 1 in 5 chance of dying before the age of one, while a baby born in a rich country has a 1 in 100 chance. In Uganda, a 2-year-old child has 5 to 10 times more illnesses per year compared to a child in England, and the illnesses are more varied and more serious.

War. Civil war is common in many Developing Countries, particularly those in Africa. Such wars are often driven by a lack of firm democratic structures and a desire to control the country's resources. Capital is diverted from health and education to the war effort, and young men are occupied with military activity instead of working to produce wealth and support their families. Clearly, many young lives (particularly men) are lost in war, leaving families without a father to support them. In turn, this further increases pressure on women. War causes disruption to existing services and, by diverting the national finances, prevents any further development of basic programmes, such as sanitation. To provide primary health care for the entire world would cost only 1/15 of world's military spending.

Drought and famine. Natural disasters are relatively common in tropical countries. Problems are compounded by factors such as:

- The population are often attracted to high-risk areas (e.g. the delta region of Bangladesh with its inherent high risk of flooding) because the resources these locations offer are seen as more important than the potential risks.
- Developing Countries have poorly developed social infrastructures. Natural disasters in Developed Countries are often planned for in advance and contingencies made, reducing the impact.

The impact of natural disasters can be huge. In the 1984 famine of Ethiopia, caused by several consecutive years of inadequate rainfall, 7 million people were affected and 1 million people died.

Preventative and social paediatrics in developing countries

- Improvements in basic amenities, such as provision of clean water and sanitation, are crucial to improving health of children in developing countries.
- Education reduces risk.
- Some measures, such as immunisation, can be very effective but are relatively inexpensive.
- Parasite infections may accompany PEM and, if untreated, impair recovery.

INDEX